Mangroves with Therapeutic Potential for Human Health

Global Distribution, Ethnopharmacology, Phytochemistry, and Biopharmaceutical Application

Mangroves with Therapeutic Potential for Human Health

Global Distribution, Ethnopharmacology, Phytochemistry, and Biopharmaceutical Application

Nabeelah Bibi Sadeer

Department of Health Sciences, Faculty of Medicine and Health Sciences, University of Mauritius, Mauritius

Mohamad Fawzi Mahomoodally

Department of Health Sciences, Faculty of Medicine and Health Sciences, University of Mauritius, Réduit, Mauritius

Centre of Excellence for Pharmaceutical Sciences, North-West University, Potchefstroom, South Africa

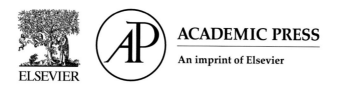

ACADEMIC PRESS

An imprint of Elsevier

ELSEVIER

Academic Press is an imprint of Elsevier
125 London Wall, London EC2Y 5AS, United Kingdom
525 B Street, Suite 1650, San Diego, CA 92101, United States
50 Hampshire Street, 5th Floor, Cambridge, MA 02139, United States
The Boulevard, Langford Lane, Kidlington, Oxford OX5 1GB, United Kingdom

Notices
Knowledge and best practice in this field are constantly changing. As new research and experience
broaden our understanding, changes in research methods, professional practices, or medical
treatment may become necessary.

Practitioners and researchers must always rely on their own experience and knowledge in evaluating
and using any information, methods, compounds, or experiments described herein. In using such
information or methods they should be mindful of their own safety and the safety of others, including
parties for whom they have a professional responsibility.

To the fullest extent of the law, neither the Publisher nor the authors, contributors, or editors, assume
any liability for any injury and/or damage to persons or property as a matter of products liability,
negligence or otherwise, or from any use or operation of any methods, products, instructions, or ideas
contained in the material herein.

ISBN: 978-0-323-99332-6

For Information on all Academic Press publications
visit our website at https://www.elsevier.com/books-and-journals

Publisher: Stacy Masucci
Acquisitions Editor: Andre G. Wolff
Editorial Project Manager: Tim Eslava
Production Project Manager: Sreejith Viswanathan
Cover Designer: Greg Harris

Typeset by MPS Limited, Chennai, India

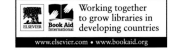

Working together
to grow libraries in
developing countries

www.elsevier.com • www.bookaid.org

Dedication

To my Mum and Dad,

who have shared all my joys and sorrows; my trials and achievements; who have indoctrinated in me the value of education since child and whose love, courage, and devotion have always been the strength of my striving,

this book is affectionately dedicated.

—Nabeelah Bibi Sadeer

To my Mum, Wife and Kids

—Mohamad Fawzi Mahomoodally

Contents

Preface

Mangroves are the roots of the sea. They are true ecotones that dominate coastlines in tropical and subtropical regions of the globe. Mangroves are popular halophytes that are vital for our future in so many ways, from being a protector against climate change to being a healer against many diseases. Though they are well-known for their ecological importance, they are rarely praised for their medicinal properties. On a few occasions, scientists have portrayed mangrove plants as intelligent plants possessing important pharmacological properties. Moreover, analysis of these plants has proved the possibility of isolating and identifying new and potential natural products having high specificity for various biopharmaceutical applications. However, research on mangroves is not enough and should not stop here, further studies are necessary.

Interestingly, numerous types of plants harbor a diverse array of microorganisms known as endophytes and mangroves are one of them. These endophytes living in the inner tissues of plants are acknowledged to produce the largest number of secondary metabolites having potential biological propensities than any other microorganisms. Thus, we propose that mangrove ecosystems should be regarded as a hot spot for natural product discovery and bioactivity survey.

To our surprise, we could not identify any contributions dealing with mangrove plants and human health on an adequate enough level that is deserved. We accepted this lack of detail as a challenge to sort out the needs of the scientific community and identify valuable topics that must be addressed to provide a narrow and well-defined picture of the pharmacological aspects of mangrove plants and their associated fungal endophytes. Therefore, with this book, we hope that this area of research becomes a reliable area for researchers interested in exploring the chemistry, analytical methodologies, and biotechnological and pharmacological activities of mangroves and their associated fungal endophytes. To facilitate reading and comprehension, we have carefully selected and added key figures, illustrations, and maps in each chapter and monograph, respectively. This authoritative, illustrative, and elegantly written book pairs the fascinating biodiversity of mangroves with their promising pharmacological propensities, as reported by experts from around the globe.

Of course, anything is possible when you have the right people there to support you. Similarly, this book would not have been a finished project without many others. We would like to express our sincere gratitude to all editorial and publishing staff members associated with Elsevier for their keen interest and support and for ensuring that the highest publications standards were maintained in making this project a success. Constructive comments and approach of the book from readers will be much appreciated. We also wish to acknowledge the support provided by our family members to complete this demanding task. And finally, we sincerely acknowledge the blessings from Almighty God, for helping us in the successful completion of this authored book.

Nabeelah Bibi Sadeer
Mohamad Fawzi Mahomoodally

A global overview on the biodiversity and biogeographical distribution of mangrove ecosystems and their connection with people

Introduction to mangrove plants: protectors of the marine environment and an asset for human health

1.1 Introduction

Coastlines of the tropics and subtropics are greatly known for their coral reefs or sandy beaches. Usually, nearby these coasts is found an ecosystem that is important for the health of the whole area of the coastlines but often overlooked. As waves carved into the coasts of the tropical and subtropical seashores, this unique ecosystem helped to diffuse the rage of the seas acting as a protective barrier. The protectors of these coasts are the mangrove forests. Mangroves are clusters of trees and shrubs that grow in tidal coasts. This tangle of groves which are salt tolerant, stabilize the coastline, curtail erosion from storm surges, currents, waves and tides. The intricate root system of mangroves is home to a multitude of organisms. Unfortunately, more than half of the world's mangrove forests have been damaged by flawed developmental activities. Yet, all is not lost. It is possible to reverse this damage and restore these vital biodiversity vaults. Small but significant efforts are sprouting up, regenerating the forests of the seashores which act as nurseries for many marine organisms. Conservation of these ecosystems is therefore of paramount importance. Actions to be taken to ensure sustainable management of the mangrove ecosystems have been listed at the end of Chapter 2.

Largely restricted to tropical and subtropical latitudes, mangroves are the only vascular flowering trees that can live in the confluence of land, freshwater, and ocean (Hogarth, 2015). This involves adapting to fluctuating environmental conditions such as changes in salinity, regular soil inundation, shifting sediments, and in-water low oxygen concentrations (Kathiresan and Bingham, 2001). As such, mangroves display a large set of morphological and ecophysiological adaptations to help them survive in these dynamic habitats. Among these adaptations are (1) the exclusion of salt by roots, (2) rapid canopy growth, (3) viviparous embryos, (4) tidally dispersed propagules, (5) exposed roots that breathe above ground, (6) highly vascularized wood, (7) efficient nutrient retention, and (8) salt-excreting leaves (Alongi, 2002; Duke, 2011).

Despite being considered a rare forest type because of their small global extent (less than 1% of tropical and subtropical forests worldwide), mangroves provide a wide range of ecosystem services and direct uses, including coastal protection, fuel (charcoal, firewood), food (fruit, leaves, associated vertebrates and invertebrates),

Mangroves with Therapeutic Potential for Human Health. DOI: https://doi.org/10.1016/B978-0-323-99332-6.00005-9

and construction material (Hogarth, 2015). Each ecosystem services are greatly discussed in Chapter 2. Mangrove plants are usually categorized into two subgroups, true mangrove and semimangrove plants. True mangrove plants are restricted to the typical intertidal mangrove habitats where seawater salinity is often 17.0−36.4. Usually, they are not found in the terrestrial marginal zones, which are subjected only to spring or storm high tides. Chapter 4 underscores that mangrove plants need the assistance of the endophytic community to be able to: (1) resist stress tolerance including climate change and (2) adapt themselves to their continuously changing environments. In general, true mangrove plants are distinguished from their terrestrial relatives at the generic level and the subfamily or family level. Semimangrove plants grow on the landward fringe of mangrove habitats or in the terrestrial marginal zones subjected to irregular high tides. True mangrove families include Avicenniaceae, Bombacaceae, Combretaceae, Maliaceae, Myrtaceae, Myrsinaceae, Pellicieraceae, Plumbaginaceae, Rhizophoraceae, Rubiaceae, and Sonneratiaceae, while semimangrove families comprise of Acanthaceae, Euphorbiaceae, Lythraceae, Palmae and Sterculiaceae (Wu et al., 2008).

Apart from the ecological importance mangroves provide to the marine environment, the various parts of the plants such as the leaves, roots, barks, or stems have been used in folk medicines to treat a panoply of maladies as reported by many ethnomedicinal studies. In general, mangroves are used medicinally to manage diabetes, hypertension, and gastrointestinal disorders such as constipation, diarrhea, dysentery, dyspepsia, hematuria, and stomach pain. Section III of this book comprises a set of monographs prepared carefully to discuss exhaustively on the traditional uses, pharmacological properties exhibited by different medicinally important mangroves and the different phytochemicals identified from these plants. Photos are also provided in each monograph to illustrate the morphological characteristics of each species. Chapter 3 covers the possible biopharmaceutical applications of mangroves as promising novel therapeutic agents and edible vaccines.

The focus of the current chapter explains how and when mangroves were discovered and their historical background is presented. The types and taxonomy of mangroves and their global distribution are also discussed. Moreover, the current pharmacological validation of mangroves is revised. This chapter also sets the stage to help understand how they adapt to their environment. The question to why mangrove plants manage to occur only in the tropics or subtropics and not in colder regions is addressed.

1.2 Discovery and historical background

The discovery of mangroves happened during the time of Alexander III of Macedon commonly known as Alexander the Great from 326−324 BC During Alexander's Indian expedition in 325 BC, Nearchus (admiral of Alexander the Great's army) was ordered to sail along the shores of Indus River to the Euphrates passing through the Persian Gulf. It was during the expedition that

Nearchus made the first discovery of the plant "Mangrove." Later in 305 BC, a Greek philosopher Theophrastus also reported and documented the existence of the mangrove vegetation in his book entitled as "Historia Plantarum" (Kathiresan and Bingham, 2001; Schneider, 2011). As a result, it is recognized that the most ancient written shreds of evidence on mangroves were documented by Nearchus and Theophrastus. Both described the plants as "held up by their roots like a polyp," and the leaves and flowers were *Rhizophora*. Consequently, in 323 BC, the ancient Greeks became aware of three mangrove areas namely the Red Sea, the Arabian Sea, and the Persian Gulf (Schneider, 2011).

Many tribes and indigenous people have relied heavily on mangroves as a source of raw materials and medicines. For instance, the tribal group of people living in the Orinoco Delta in Venezuela known as the Warao people has been dependent on mangrove forests for approximately 7000 years. The Warao people also known as the mangrove people used the roots of these plants to build houses and boats. Thousands of years later, mangroves attracted more people across the globe and till date has maintained its valuable importance for many people and also animals (Spalding et al., 2010). The array of benefits derived from mangroves includes wood and nonwood forest products; fisheries; recreation; ecotourism; bio-filtration; coastal protection; and carbon storage and sequestration. These benefits are the main focus of Chapter 3. Recently, a study conducted by Gardner in Madagascar showed that lemurs use mangroves as their natural habitats for sleeping and foraging (Gardner, 2016). For many years, mangroves have formed remarkable and highly prolific ecosystems along the coastlines of many countries around the world that are both environmentally and medicinally important (Spalding et al., 2010). Within the scope of knowledge, mangroves originate from the Indo-Malayan regions which grow most of the mangrove species around the world with Indonesia being the first country covering the most extensive mangrove area globally (Hamilton and Casey, 2016; Yong, 2018). The propagules and seeds produced by the plants have a unique feature which helped them to float in the water. Due to this characteristic, it was easy for the mangrove species to spread by water dispersal to Central and South America through India, East Africa about 23−66 million years ago (Yong, 2018).

1.3 Terms and definition

The term "mangrove" is of Guarani origin, the official language of Paraguay. In the early 1610s, the word was spelled as "mangrow" coming from Portuguese "mangue" or Spanish "mangle," but later in the 1690s the term "mangrow" turned into an English word as "mangrove" via folk etymology. Mangroves are associated with many terms, namely mangrove forest community or mangal and mangrove ecosystem. Other terms synonymous to mangrove forest are tidal forest, coastland woodlands, mangrove swamp, tidal swamp forest, and oceanic rainforests (Kathiresan and Bingham, 2001; Naidoo, 2016). For instance, the mangrove forest community or mangal is linked with microbes and fungi while animals associated with the plants form the mangrove ecosystem (MacNae, 1969). It is suggested that the word "mangrove" should be referred to specific mangrove species while the word "mangal" to the forest community instead.

Morphologically, a mangrove is a shrub or small tree that grows in coastal brackish or saline waters in muddy or rocky soils. Mangroves are halophytes as they are salt tolerant and are easily adapted to harsh coastal conditions due to their buttress root system or rhizophores and their aerial roots or pneumatophores (Kathiresan and Bingham, 2001). Different sources defined mangroves differently. For instance, Collins dictionary defined mangrove plants as a tree growing along the coastlines or on the bank of river in tropical countries (Collins, 2018) while Merriam-Webster (Merriam-Webster, 2021) defined the plant as 'any of a genus (*Rhizophora*, especially *Rhizophora mangle* of the family Rhizophoraceae) of tropical maritime trees or shrubs that send out many prop roots and form dense masses important in coastal land building and as foundations of unique ecosystems' or "any of numerous trees (of the genus *Avicennia*) with growth habits like those of the true mangroves" (Merriam-Webster, 2021). The Cambridge dictionary defined mangroves as tropical trees growing near water developing twisted roots growing partly above the ground (Collins, 2021). On the other hand, Spalding defined mangroves as "trees or large shrubs including ferns and palms growing in or adjacent to intertidal regions which can easily adapt themselves in their environment" (Spalding et al., 2010). However, these definitions sound paradoxical since many other plants can be mistaken for mangroves. For example, *Anemopsis california* (Nutt.) Hook. & Arn. (lizard tail) is an herb growing in wet or shallow waters (Dale, 1986), Atriplex (saltbush, genus of 250−300 species) is defined as a shrub growing in salty soils, and *Limonium* (sea lavender, genus of 120 species) is defined as a woody shrub growing along the coasts and in salt marshes (Welsh, 2003). These named plants are small in size and grow in saline conditions similarly to mangroves. Accordingly, it can be pointed out that mangroves do not have an appropriate and precise definition that demarcates the plants from other halophytes.

1.4 Botanical classification and types of mangroves

Global mangrove plants are distributed across the tropical and subtropical forests and are predominantly found in tropical regions. The majority of mangrove communities occur in tropical and subtropical areas where the water temperature is higher than 24°C in the warmest month and the annual rainfall exceeds 1250 mm. Asia and Australia have the greatest diversity and distribution of mangrove species in the world. For example, among 18 million hectares of mangrove forests, more than 40% are found along the Asian coasts. The largest mangrove formations are found in Bangladesh, Brazil, Indonesia, India, and Thailand (Lacerda, 2002; Valiela et al., 2001).

The mangrove plants of the world can be mainly divided into two main groups, the eastern group and the western group. The eastern group covers the region from west and central Pacific to the southern end of Africa. The western group covers the west coast of Africa and coastal regions of Caribbean, North and South America. In mangrove species, the eastern group is the majority, while the western group is the minority. Specifically, as far as the species are concerned, the number in the eastern group is five times than that of the western group (Ashton and Macintosh, 2002). According to the statistics, the eastern group is made up of 74 species (including twelve varieties) belonging to 18 genera and 14 families, however, the western group consists of only 10 species belonging to six genera and five families. In total, global mangrove plants have 84 species belonging to 24 genera and 16 families. Among them, 70 species are true mangroves pertaining to 16 genera and 11 families, and 14 species are semimangroves (or mangrove associates) belonging to eight genera and five families (Table 1.1) (Ashton and Macintosh, 2002). True mangrove families include Avicenniaceae, Bombacaceae, Combretaceae, Maliaceae, Myrtaceae, Myrsinaceae, Pellicieraceae, Plumbaginaceae, Rhizophoraceae, Rubiaceae, and Sonneratiaceae, while semimangrove families comprise Acanthaceae, Euphorbiaceae, Lythraceae, Palmae and Sterculiaceae.

Table 1.1 True mangrove and semimangrove species around the world.

Family	Species
True mangrove	
Avicenniaceae	*Avicennia africana* P. Beauv.
	A. alba Blume
	A. alba var. latifolia Moldenke
	A. balanophora Stapf & Moldenke
	A. bicolor Standl.
	A. germinans (L.) L.
	A. integra N.C. Duke
	A. lanata Ridl.
	A. marina (Forssk.) Vierh.
	A. marina var. acutissima Stapf & Moldenke
	A. marina var. anomala Moldenke
	A. marina var. australasoca (Walp.) J.Everett
	A. marina var. eucalyptifolia (Valeton) N.C.Duke
	A. marina var. intermedia (Griff.) Bakh.
	A. marina var. resinifera (G.Frost.) Bakh.
	A. marina var. typica Bakh.
	A. officinalis L
	A. rumphiana Hallier f.
	A. schaueriana Stapf & Leechm. ex Moldenke
	A. tomentosa Jacq.
Bombacaceae	*Camptostemon philippinensis* (S.Vidal) Becc.
	C. schultzii Mast.

(Continued)

Table 1.1 True mangrove and semimangrove species around the world. *Continued*

Family	Species
Combretaceae	*Conocarpus erectus* L.
	Laguncularia racemosa (L.) C.F.Gaertn.
	Lumnitzera littorea (Jack) Voigt
	L. littorea var. lutea
	L. racemose Willd.
	L. rosea (Gaudich.) C. Presl
Maliaceae	*Xylocarpus gangeticus* (Prain) C.E. Parkinson
	X. granatum J. Koenig
	X. mekongensis Pierre
	X. minor Ridl.
	X. moluccensis (Lam.) M.Roem.
	X. parvifolius Ridl.
Myrtaceae	*Osbornia octodonta* F.Muell.
Myrsinaceae	*Aegiceras corniculatum* (L.) Blanco
	A. floridum Roem. & Schult
Pellicieraceae	*Pelliciera rhizophora* Planch. & Triana
Plumbaginaceae	*Aegialitis annulate* Kurz
	A. rotundifolia Roxb.
Rhizophoraceae	*Bruguiera cylindrica* (L.) Blume
	B. exaristata Ding Hou
	B. gymnorhiza (L.) Lam.
	B. hainessii C.G.Rogers
	B. parviflora (Roxb.) Wight & Arn. Ex Griff.
	B. sexangula (Lour.) Poir.
	B. sexangula var. rhynchopetala W.C.Ko
	Ceriops decandra (Griff.) W.Theob.
	C. tagal (Perr.) C.B.Rob.
	C. tagal var. australasica C.T.White
	C. tagal var. typical
	Kandelia candel (L.) Druce
	Rhizophora apiculata Blume
	R. harrisonii Leechm.
	R. lamarckii Montrouz.
	R. mangle L.
	R. mucronata Lam.
	R. racemosa G.Mey.
	R. samoensis (Hochr.) Salvoza
	R. selala (Salvoza) Toml.
	R. stylosa Griff.

(Continued)

Table 1.1 True mangrove and semimangrove species around the world. *Continued*

Family	Species
Rubiaceae	*Scyphiphora hydrophylacea* C.F.Gaertn.
Sonneratiaceae	*Sonneratia alba* Sm.
	S. apetala Buch.-Ham.
	S. caseolaris (L.) Engl.
	S. griffithii Kurz
	S. x gulngai N.C. Duke & Jackes
	S. x hainanensis W.C. Ko, E.Y. Chen & W.Y. Chen
	S. ovata Backer
	S. paracaseolaris W.C. Ko, E.Y. Chen & W.Y. Chen
	Total number of true mangroves = 70
Semimangrove	
Acanthaceae	*Acanthus ebracteatus* Vahl
	A. ilicifolius Lour.
	A. volubilis Wall.
	A. xiamenensis R.T. Zhang
Euphorbiaceae	*Excoecaria agallocha* L.
	E. indica (Willd.) Mull.Arg.
Lythraceae	*Pemphis acidula* J.R. Forst. & G. Forst.
Palmae	*Mauritia flexuosa* L.f.
	Nypa fruticans Wurmb
	Phoenix paludosa Roxb.
	Oncosperma tigllarium (Jack) Ridl.
Sterculiaceae	*Heritiera littoralis* Aiton
	H. fomes Buch.-Ham.
	H. globosa Kosterm.
	Total number of semimangroves = 14

Twenty-eight mangrove species (including one variety), belonging to 15 genera and 12 families, are recorded in China. They contribute to about 38% of the total mangrove species in the eastern group and 33% in the world. *Sonneratia hainanensis* W.C. Ko, E.Y. Chen & W.Y. Chen, *Sonneratia paracaseolaris* W.C. Ko, E.Y. Chen & W.Y. Chen, *Bruguiera sexangula var. rhynchopetala* W.C. Ko, and *Acanthus xiamenensis* R.T. Zhang, are the four endemic mangrove species found in China. Though its terrestrial area does not exceed 34,000 km^2, Hainan island has the richest diversity of mangrove species in China. According to the statistics, 25 species are recorded in this tropical island (Lin and Fu, 2000).

Seven types of mangrove trees exist, among which three are most dominant namely the red, black, and white mangroves. The difference between the three

Table 1.2 Distinguishing characteristics between three dominant types of mangroves.[a]

Characteristics		Red	Black	White
	Leaves	Very shiny, very pointy green on both sides	Less shiny, pointy, gray in color in bottom surface	Shiny on both sides, round
	Roots	Rhizophores or arc-shaped prop roots, roots come out of the stem and grow downwards to end in the soil	Pneumatophores or pencil-like roots, roots grow against gravity from the soil surface	—
	Fruits	Cigar-shaped	Teardrop-shaped	Smallest in size
	Examples	*R. mucronata,* *R. mangle*	*B. germinans,* *B. gymnorhiza*	*L. racemosa*

[a]*Restoring Guyanas mangrove ecosystem, 2014. <http://www.mangrovesgy.org/home/index.php/2014-04-27-16-39-08/types-of-mangroves>.*

most common types of mangrove (red, black, and white mangroves) is distinctive from each other based on the morphology of their leaves, roots, and fruits (propagules). Table 1.2 describes the distinguishing characteristics between the three dominant mangrove types. However, most works of literatures have not specified which type of mangroves the studies were conducted which consequently results in only a few examples given in Table 1.2.

1.5 Biogeographical distribution

Mangrove forests are known as the world's most productive ecosystems, and they occur mainly in the tropical or subtropical regions (Saranraj and Sujitha, 2015). Mangroves are found in 123 countries across the globe (Spalding et al., 2010). Fig. 1.1 shows the distribution of mangroves across the globe. The total area covered by mangrove trees in the world was estimated to be 137,760 km^2 in 2000 (Giri et al., 2011) and currently mangroves covered about 152,000 km^2 (Yeo, 2014). Approximately 75% of mangroves are found in 15 countries, with only 6.9% of them protected (Thomas et al., 2017). The top 20 mangrove nations in the world with Indonesia covering the largest area followed by Brazil, Malaysia, and lastly Cameroon (Hamilton and Casey, 2016) are shown in Table 1.3. Overall, Asia consists of the largest amount of mangrove's forest (42%) in the world followed by Africa (21%), North/Central America (15%), and lastly by South America (11%).

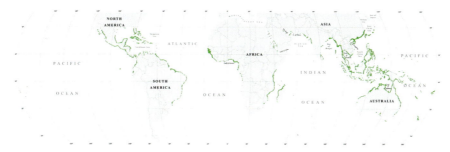

FIGURE 1.1

World map mangrove distribution (Wikimedia Commons, distributed under a CC-BY 2.0 license).

Table 1.3 Top 20 mangroves-holding nations in 2014 in km^2 and percentage of global total.

Rank	Country	km^2	% Global total
1	Indonesia	42,278	25.79
2	Brazil	17,287	10.55
3	Malaysia	7616	4.65
4	Venezuela	7516	4.59
5	Nigeria	6908	4.21
6	Papua New Guinea	6236	3.80
7	Colombia	6236	3.80
8	Mexico	6036	3.68
9	Thailand	3936	2.40
10	Gabon	3864	2.36
11	Myanmar	3783	2.31
12	Australia	3314	2.02
13	Panama	2673	1.63
14	Mozambique	2658	1.62
15	Cuba	2407	1.47
16	Bangladesh	2314	1.41
17	Philippines	2084	1.27
18	Ecuador	1906	1.16
19	United States	1554	0.95
20	Cameroon	1323	0.81

1.6 Why are mangroves tropical?

The key mangrove adaptations are the ability to survive in waterlogged and anoxic soil, and the ability to tolerate salt or brackish water. Many, but not all, mangroves show vivipary and have relatively large propagules. Why should this suite of characteristics be limited by latitude? Plants that tolerate salt, and plants that survive in waterlogged soils, are not unusual in temperate latitudes: in fact, salt marsh vegetation is as typical of temperate coastal environments as mangroves are of tropical ones. There are temperate trees that cope with waterlogging, or with high salt concentrations. It is only the combination of being a tree, tolerating salt, and coping with waterlogging that is restricted to the tropics. The geographical spread of mangroves is broadly delineated by the 20°C winter sea temperature isotherm. Apparent anomalies can largely be explained by the pattern of ocean currents: for example, on the west coast of South America, the limit to mangrove distribution is at 5°32′S, largely because to the south of this point, the cold Humboldt Current lowers the temperature below what is found at comparable latitudes in other oceans. Conversely, the extreme southern distribution of mangroves in Australia (38°45′S) and New Zealand (38°05′S) may be explained, at least in part, by the pattern of ocean currents (Hogarth, 2015).

In general terms, the ability of mangroves to cope with their environment declines with increasing latitude and decreasing temperature. In several cases, the extremes of range have been linked with variations in local temperature, specifically with the frequency and severity of frosts. In extreme cold, the contents of the water-conducting xylem vessels may freeze. Air bubbles form, and on thawing these may expand, causing an embolism—a blockage of the vessel. While plants can repair the damage by displacing the embolism, or develop new conduction routes to bypass it, an embolism clearly impairs hydraulic conductivity and a plant's ability to acquire and transport water. The risk of embolism formation can be mitigated by the development of narrower xylem vessels, which has been shown in some mangrove species at higher latitudes. The problem is more significant in trees than in smaller plants, and particularly acute in those that already struggle with water acquisition. Mangroves will be affected more than nonmangrove trees: and mangrove trees in more saline circumstance, and in arid environments are more likely to be affected than those in more congenial locations. Hence, the incidence of frost and the risk of embolism will curtail mangrove distribution in cold atmospheres (Morrisey et al., 2010; Stuart et al., 2007).

1.7 Critical analysis of the current pharmacological validation of mangroves

The importance of mangroves in the medical field for curing diseases cannot be undermined as the plants have much therapeutic potential. Mangroves were used in folklore medicines a long time ago, and different extracts from various parts of the plants (roots, leaves, fruits, bark, and resin) have shown exciting and significant inhibitory activities in many assays namely antidiabetic, antiinflammatory, anticancer, antiulcer, antitumor, antiviral, antioxidant, and antimicrobial among others. Since various parts of the plants were used for inhibitory assays and considering the fact that mangrove ecosystems are known to be threatened, it can be said that plant samples were being used sustainably. Although many mangrove species have been used traditionally by local inhabitants for an extended period following folk traditions in various countries as ailments, many among them have not been studied extensively yet, and thus their medicinal properties have not been reported. For example, in Mauritius, local people use the root decoction of *R. mucronata* Lam. against diabetes, but the plant has not been locally validated by researchers to confirm its pharmacological properties. Similarly, no scientific research has been carried out so far on *Ceriops tagal* and *Kandelia rheedii* to prove their efficacy against diseases that can be cured by folk medicine. Interestingly, although few studies have been conducted on the species *B. sexangula*, *R. stylosa*, and *Pelliciera rhizophorae*, these species are yet to be used in folk medicine (Table 1.4). Therefore

Table 1.4 Traditionally used and pharmacologically validated species of mangroves.

Species	Traditionally used	Pharmacologically validated
Acanthus ilicifolius	✓	✓
Aegiceras rotundifolia	✓	✓
A. corniculatum	✓	✓
Acrostichum aureum	✓	✓
Avicennia germinans	✓	✓
A. marina	✓	✓
A. officinalis	✓	✓
Bruguiera cylindrica	✓	✓
B. gymnorhiza	✓	✓
B. parviflora	✓	✓
B. sexangula	✓	✓
Ceriops decandra	✓	✓
C. roxburghiana	✓	✓
C. tagal	✓	✗
Excoecaria agallocha	✓	✓
Heritiera fomes	✓	✓
H. littoralis	✓	✓
Kandelia candel	✓	✓
K. rheedii	✓	✗
Lumnitzera racemosa	✓	✓
Nypa fruticans	✓	✓
Pelliciera rhizophorae	✗	✓
Rhizophora apiculata	✓	✓
R. mucronata	✓	✓
R. stylosa	✗	✓
R. conjugata	✓	✓
R. mangle	✓	✓
R. racemosa	✓	✓
Xylocarpus granatum	✓	✓
Total number of species	27	27

mangrove species require more attention from researchers to shed more light into the traditional and pharmacological uses of these unique plants as there is a dearth of knowledge on this particular area. Table 1.4 shows the number of species used in folk-lore medicines and those that are pharmacologically tested.

A series of monographs of different traditionally important mangrove plants are compiled and presented in Section III of this book. Each monograph gives a broader knowledge on the pharmacological activities of mangroves, and the different types of phytochemicals identified. Fig. 1.2 illustrates the types of extracts commonly used for validating the pharmacological activities of mangroves. Methanolic extracts (32.46%) were the most preferred extracts used in most studies followed by ethanolic (12.28%), ethyl acetate (10.53%), aqueous (7.89%), and chloroform (6.14%) (Sadeer et al., 2019).

On the other hand, Fig. 1.3 illustrates the types of plant parts most commonly used in studies. From the data shown, it can be said that the plant parts mostly studied are leaves (64%), roots (10%), stem bark (5%), and stem (5%) (Sadeer et al., 2019).

Fig. 1.4 illustrates the types of assays usually conducted on mangroves. It is evident that antioxidant (28.8%) and antimicrobial (24.0%) assays were the two most common in vitro studies performed. Interestingly, most in vivo studies were done for antidiabetic assays compared to in vitro. It is found that antipyretic, antiviral, thrombolytic activity, anticoagulant, antiparasitic, antiulcer, and antifilarial tests were less seldom conducted. However, it is important to highlight that many mangrove species are used as a remedy for the ulcer in folklore medicine. For instance, the leaf of *A. marina*, the leaf of *A. officinalis*, the bark of *B. cylindrica*,

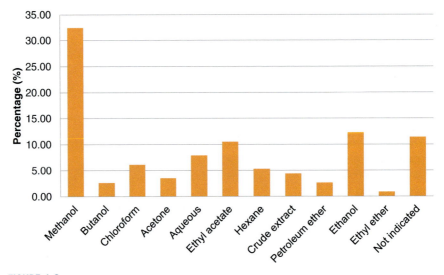

FIGURE 1.2

Types of mangrove extracts used in pharmacological assays.

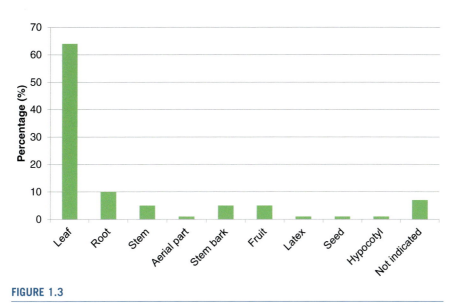

FIGURE 1.3

Types of plant parts of mangroves used in pharmacological assays.

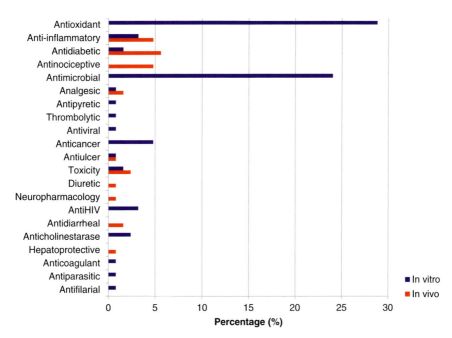

FIGURE 1.4

Types of assay conducted on mangroves.

bark, fruit, and leaf of *C. decandra*, whole plant of *C. roxburghiana*, and whole plant of *R. mucronata* are traditionally believed to cure ulcers. Nonetheless, the antiulcer potential of these named plants has not been extensively validated either in vivo or in vitro studies to confirm this belief in medical lore.

Species such as *B. gymnorhiza* (17%), *R. mucronata* (14%), *A. ilicifolius* (10%), and (9%) are widely used traditionally and possess an array of potential medicinal values compared to the other species. Briefly, *B. gymnorhiza* is used traditionally to treat diabetes, hypertension, diarrhea, fever, intestinal worms, amongst others. *A. ilicifolius* is used to treat asthma, diabetes, hepatitis, leprosy, rheumatism, snake bites, among others. In folklore medicine, *R. mucronata* is used against angina, dysentery, hepatitis, fever, toothache, malaria (Sadeer et al., 2019). Fig. 1.5 shows the most and least common mangroves used in folklore medicine.

A pie chart in Fig. 1.6 represents mangroves that have been pharmacologically validated. The five most reportedly investigated species are *R. mucronata* (19%), *A. officinalis* (11%), *A. marina* (9%), *B. gymnorhiza* (8%), and *R. apiculata* (7%). It is important to highlight that *B. gymnorhiza* is the most traditionally used

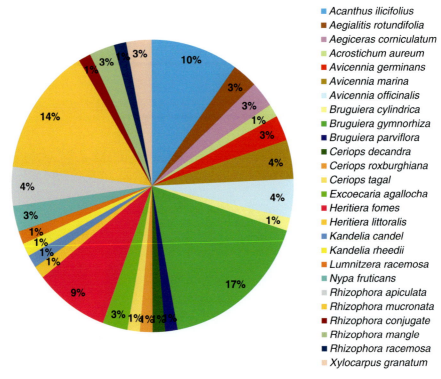

FIGURE 1.5

Most and least common mangroves used traditionally.

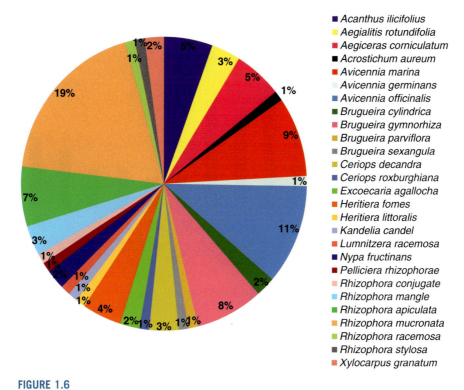

■ *Acanthus ilicifolius*
■ *Aegialitis rotundifolia*
■ *Aegiceras corniculatum*
■ *Acrostichum aureum*
■ *Avicennia marina*
■ *Avicennia germinans*
■ *Avicennia officinalis*
■ *Brugueira cylindrica*
■ *Brugueira gymnorhiza*
■ *Brugueira parviflora*
■ *Brugueira sexangula*
■ *Ceriops decandra*
■ *Ceriops roxburghiana*
■ *Excoecaria agallocha*
■ *Heritiera fomes*
■ *Heritiera littoralis*
■ *Kandelia candel*
■ *Lumnitzera racemosa*
■ *Nypa fructinans*
■ *Pelliciera rhizophorae*
■ *Rhizophora conjugate*
■ *Rhizophora mangle*
■ *Rhizophora apiculata*
■ *Rhizophora mucronata*
■ *Rhizophora racemosa*
■ *Rhizophora stylosa*
■ *Xylocarpus granatum*

FIGURE 1.6

Mangrove plants that have been pharmacologically validated till date.

species (Fig. 1.5), but it is found in the fourth place to be pharmacologically validated. This warrants an in-depth study on that particular species considering its importance in folklore medicine.

There is an undeviating link between pharmacological activities and phytochemicals. In this era in which most researchers are screening thousands of plants for the discovery of novel compounds, it is thus of high importance to scrutinize mangrove species with that very aim to isolate new phytochemicals which can be potential candidates for the development of pharmaceutical drugs. Histogram in Fig. 1.7 illustrates the 16 most common types of phytochemicals isolated from mangrove species. Generally, the seven most common chemical constituents present are terpenoids (16.25%), tannins (12.5%), steroids (10.0%), alkaloids (9.38%), flavonoids (8.75%), saponins (8.75%), and glycosides (8.13%) (Sadeer et al., 2019). Furthermore, mangroves also yielded other compounds namely fatty acid derivative, anthraquinone, amino acid, coumarin, quinine, ester, gum, phenol, terpene, quercetin, and anthranoid. However, these compounds are found at low levels and are present in only certain mangrove plants.

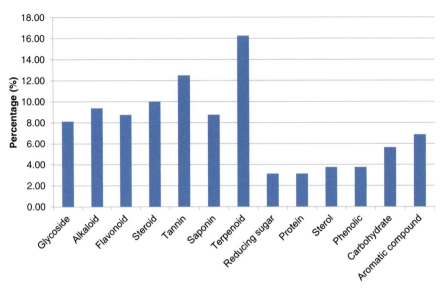

FIGURE 1.7

Classes of compounds isolated from mangroves.

1.8 Conclusion

This chapter introduces the mangrove plants to the readers, covering their discovery, historical background, the number and types of mangroves that exist, the biogeographical distribution of these plants across the globe, and ends with a critical analysis of the current pharmacological studies conducted so far on these traditionally important halophytes.

Collins, Merriam-Webster, and the Oxford English dictionaries defined mangroves simply as trees or shrubs with tangled roots growing along the coastlines of tropical countries while Spalding et al. (2010) generalized mangroves as trees or large shrubs growing in or adjacent to intertidal regions which can easily adapt themselves in their environment. Having said that, it can be concluded that there are still ambiguities in the definition of mangroves and thus require the attention of botanists to properly define the plant.

Also, mangrove taxonomy needs much attention. Several species are poorly identified. There are several natural hybrids, but their parental species are not clearly understood. Another problem in the taxonomy of mangroves is the confusion between the species of true mangroves and semimangroves (or mangrove associates). Often the same species is named differently at different sites. Molecular analyses may eventually help resolve the taxonomic problems.

It is acknowledged that there are 84 mangrove species. However, only 27 species are known to the folklore medicine and not all species have been tested for their pharmacological activities both in vivo and in vitro, which accounts for only about 31% of mangrove species that have been investigated till date. This rather low percentage can be linked to either a poor interest from the researchers' side on these particular plants or because these plants are considered as endangered species in some countries. Therefore, this might have created a gap between traditional medicines and the interest in developing drugs derived from mangroves. Consequently, to fill the gap between traditional medicines and pharmaceutics, more research is needed to provide a greater range of potential cures against a panel of diseases.

So far, we have seen that mangrove species has a long history in traditional medicine/ethnopharmacology and is still widely used because of a wide array of potential sources of natural compounds. Several classes of bioactive substances have been isolated and identified and investigations on different metabolic activities have been performed both in vitro and in vivo. While we present and discuss the evidence in this book chapter in connection with mangrove species and their beneficial medicinal properties, there are still doubts as to how far these bioactive compounds can be used as direct disease management agents. There is no conclusive report of human trials and up to what extent these beneficial medicinal properties are substantiated warrant further investigation. For proper ethnopharmacological use of mangroves, we believe there should be more direct scientific evidence substantiated with more clinical-based research with rationale impact assessed on human health.

Deeper scientific understanding of the mechanisms of those compounds, their molecular targets, and any drug interaction should further be investigated. Well-designed in vivo tests and randomized controlled clinical studies should be carried out to obtain statistically significant outcomes. There is also a dire need to ensure the efficacy and safety of mangrove preparations and not direct their use solely based on people's perceptions. Other pertinent questions that must be delved in are: How far can these mangroves be further exploited on a commercial scale by pharmaceutical companies? What are the optimized methods of extraction and characterization? What are the risk levels or adverse human effects? What types of pharmacological evaluations must be carried out to confirm activity of mangrove ingredients?

References

Alongi, D.M., 2002. Present state and future of the world's mangrove forests. Environmental Conservation 29, 331−349.

Ashton, E.C., Macintosh, D.J., 2002. Preliminary assessment of the plant diversity and community ecology of the Sematan mangrove forest, Sarawak, Malaysia. Forest Ecology and Management 166, 111−129.

Collins, 2018. Definition of 'mangrove'. <https://www.collinsdictionary.com/dictionary/english/mangrove> (accessed 06.04.21).

Collins, 2021. Portuguese translation of 'mangrove'. <https://www.collinsdictionary.com/dictionary/englishportuguese/mangrove> (accessed 06.04.21).

Dale, N., 1986. Flowering Plants: The Santa Monica Mountains, Coastal & Chaparral Regions of Southern California. Capra Pr, Bakersfield, CA.

Duke, N., 2011. Encyclopedia of Modern Coral Reefs: Structure, Form and Process. Springer, Dordrecht, the Netherlands.

Gardner, C.J., 2016. Use of mangroves by lemurs. International Journal of Primatology 37, 317–332.

Giri, C., Ochieng, E., Tieszen, L.L., Zhu, Z., Singh, A., Loveland, T., et al., 2011. Status and distribution of mangrove forests of the world using earth observation satellite data. Global Ecology and Biogeography 20, 154–159.

Hamilton, S.E., Casey, D., 2016. Creation of a high spatio-temporal resolution global database of continuous mangrove forest cover for the 21st century (CGMFC-21). Global Ecology and Biogeography 25, 729–738.

Hogarth, P.J., 2015. The Biology of Mangroves and Seagrasses, third ed Oxford University Press, Oxford.

Kathiresan, K., Bingham, B.L., 2001. Biology of mangroves and mangrove ecosystems. Advances in Marine Biology. Academic Press, Cambridge, MA, pp. 81–251.

Lacerda, L.D., 2002. Mangrove Ecosystems: Function and Management. Springer, Berlin.

Lin, P., Fu, Q., 2000. Environmental Ecology and Economic Utilization of Mangroves in China. Higher Education Press, Beijing, China.

MacNae, W., 1969. A general account of the fauna and flora of mangrove swamps and forests in the indo-west-pacific region. In: Russell, F.S., Yonge, M. (Eds.), Advances in Marine Biology. Elsevier, Amsterdam, the Netherlands.

Merriam-Webster, 2021. Definition of mangrove. <https://www.merriam-webster.com/dictionary/mangrove> (accessed 06.04.21).

Morrisey, D.J., Swales, A., Dittman, S., Morrison, M.A., Lovelock, C.E., Beard, C.M., 2010. The ecology and management of temperate mangroves. Oceanography and Marine Biology: An Annual Review 48, 43–160.

Naidoo, G., 2016. The mangroves of South Africa: an ecophysiological review. South African Journal of Botany 107, 101–113.

Sadeer, N.B., Mahomoodally, F., Mohamad, Gokhan, Z., Rajesh, J., Nadeem, N., et al., 2019. Ethnopharmacology, phytochemistry, and global distribution of mangroves—a comprehensive review. Marine Drugs 17, 231.

Saranraj, P., Sujitha, D., 2015. Mangrove medicinal plants: a review. American-Eurasian Journal of Toxicological Sciences 7, 146–156.

Schneider, P., 2011. The discovery of tropical mangroves in Graeco-Roman antiquity: science and wonder. Journal of the Hakluyt Society 3, 1–16.

Spalding, M., Kainuma, M., Collins, L., 2010. World atlas of mangroves. A Collaborative Project of ITTO, ISME, FAO, UNEP-WCMC. Earthscan, London.

Stuart, S.A., Choat, B., Martin, K.C., Holbrook, N.M., Ball, M.C., 2007. The role of freezing in setting the latitudinal limits of mangrove forests. New Phytologist 173, 576–583.

Thomas, N., Lucas, R., Bunting, P., Hardy, A., Rosenqvist, A., Simard, M., 2017. Distribution and drivers of global mangrove forest change, 1996–2010. PloS One 12, e0179302.

Valiela, I., Bowen, J.L., York, J.K., 2001. Mangrove forests: one of the world's threatened major tropical environments: at least 35% of the area of mangrove forests has been lost in the past two decades, losses that exceed those for tropical rain forests and coral reefs, two other well-known threatened environments. Bioscience 51, 807–815.

Welsh, S.L., 2003. Flora of North America. <http://www.efloras.org/florataxon.aspx?flora_id=1&taxon_id=103110> (accessed 06.04.21).

Wu, J., Xiao, Q., Xu, J., Li, M.-Y., Pan, J.-Y., Yang, M.-H., 2008. Natural products from true mangrove flora: source, chemistry and bioactivities. Natural Product Reports 25, 955−981.

Yeo, S., 2014. Save mangroves for people, planet and the economy, says UN. <https://www.climatechangenews.com/2014/09/30/save-mangroves-for-people-planet-and-the-economy-says-un/> (accessed 06.04.21).

Yong, J., 2018. Origin of mangroves and mangrove diversity. <http://mangroveactionproject.org/origin-of-mangroves-mangrove-diversity/#more-2692> (accessed 06.04.21).

Mangroves and people

2.1 Introduction

Mangroves have long been associated with human populations, as coastal communities rely on various ecosystem services that mangroves provide. Till date, human uses of mangrove ecosystems are significant. The most primordial uses derived from ecosystem services are: the provision of woods, the support of fisheries and the protection of coastlines from hurricanes and erosion. As a consequent of the dependence of humans on these important ecosystems, degradation and destruction of mangroves is prevalent (Friess et al., 2021). More than 90% of the world's mangroves are located in developing countries, where rates of destruction are increasing rapidly and on large scales. Since 1990, despite increasingly positive attitudes toward mangroves and their inclusion in protected areas and conservation policies, mangrove cover has continued to decline due to expanding human activities (agriculture, aquaculture, coastal development), even in the presence of laws prohibiting their removal (López-Angarita et al., 2016). Between 1980 and 2005, approximately 20% of the total coverage area were lost. Despite reliable statistics prior 1980 are not available, losses of mangroves were also noted as substantial. Most losses have been linked to the conversion of mangrove lands to artificial beaches, agriculture, aquaculture, urban and industrial space. Additionally, mangrove areas have been degraded through overextraction of timber, overfishing, pollution, and solid waste disposal (Spalding et al., 2010).

Timber and fisheries benefit from mangroves are probably as old as the history of human settlement in mangrove areas. However, as societies become more structured, so larger-scale and industrial uses of mangroves spread (Spalding et al., 2010). Coastal flood risks are increasing rapidly. It is estimated that if mangroves were lost, more than 15 million people would be flooded annually across the world. Some of the nations that receive the greatest economic benefits include the USA, China, India and Mexico. While Vietnam, India and Bangladesh receive the greatest benefits in terms of people protected (Menéndez et al., 2020). Hence, destruction of coasts by storms, failing aquaculture, decline in offshore fishing, coastal erosion has demonstrated how important mangroves are. Mangroves are important ecosystems that provide a wide range of goods and services to human communities living in coastal areas. The array of ecosystem services derived from mangroves includes wood and nonwood forest products, fisheries, recreation, ecotourism, bio-filtration, coastal protection, and carbon storage and sequestration

Mangroves with Therapeutic Potential for Human Health. DOI: https://doi.org/10.1016/B978-0-323-99332-6.00014-X

(Spalding et al., 2010). Large areas of mangroves are now under sustainable management and others have restored or replanted. Protected areas are helping to ensure that many mangroves are being maintained not as diminished and degraded patches but as vibrant ecosystems that are integrally connected with adjacent ecosystems, and with people. This chapter will elaborate on the various ecosystem services, impact of human interventions on mangroves, and the management of mangrove ecosystems.

2.2 Ecosystem services

Despite being considered a rare forest type because of their small global extent (less than 1% of tropical and subtropical forests worldwide), mangroves provide a wide range of ecosystem services and direct uses including coastal protection, fuel (charcoal, firewood), food (fruit, leaves, associated vertebrates and invertebrates), and construction material. Fig. 2.1 illustrates the various ecosystem services. Human uses of mangrove resources have been categorized into traditional, commercial and destructive uses (Field, 1995). The majority of people living in mangrove areas are fishermen, deriving their livelihood from fishing and related activities. Harvesting and processing of mangrove wood is a full-time occupation

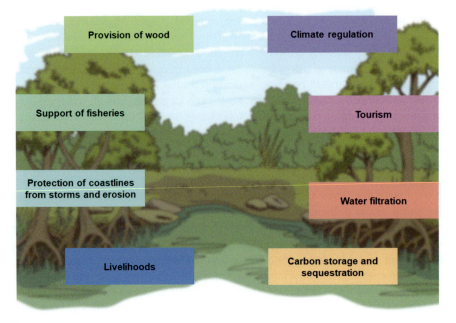

FIGURE 2.1

Ecosystem services derived from mangroves.

for the minority living near mangrove areas. In many countries, local communities rely on mangrove forest products to meet their subsistence needs for fuel and construction (Baba et al., 2013).

The impact of mangrove resource use by local villages can be sustainable as it forms an integral part of the ecology and functioning of the ecosystem (Spalding et al., 2010). However, with population growth and increasing demand, most mangrove forests are showing various levels of degradation due to overharvesting of forest products. In recent decades, large-scale commercial and destructive uses have led to the loss of mangrove forests.

2.2.1 Wood products

One of the most common uses of mangroves is as a source of wood for construction and fuel. Mangrove species from the Rhizophoraceae family are preferred for fuelwood and charcoal production because they burn with high calorific value. Coastal communities in many tropical countries continue to rely heavily on mangrove wood for domestic consumption, and commercial markets for mangrove fuelwood and charcoal are well established. Mangrove wood is strong, durable, and rot-resistant and is thus well suited for construction purposes. The extraction of poles is mostly for the construction of houses and fishing stakes. Mangrove poles are in great demand as piles for building and road construction. Mangrove timber is also used for the construction of houses and boats. In addition to wood for fuel and construction, mangrove wood has been an industrial source of pulp for manufacturing rayon, cellophane and paper (Baba et al., 2013).

2.2.1.1 Charcoal production

In Matang, Malaysia, the manufacture of charcoal from *Rhizophora* wood remains the most important industry. *Rhizophora apiculata* Blume and *Rhizophora mucronata* Lam. are the two species used for commercial charcoal production. Wood of *R. apiculata* and *R. mucronata* has densities of 890 and 900 kg/m^3, and calorific values of 18.5 and 18.0 MJ/kg, respectively (Baharudin and Hoi, 1987). The physical properties and calorific values of the wood of both species are therefore comparable. It has been reported that the calorific value of 5 tons of *R. mucronata* wood equals to 2−3 tons of coal (ACTI, 1980). In Vietnam, trees of *R. apiculata* and *Bruguiera parviflora* (Roxb.) Wight & Arn. ex Griff. are the main species converted into charcoal. Mangrove charcoal in Vietnam has a great variety of uses including domestic cooking, pig roasting and tea drying. The chemical and metal industries as well as the street food vendors are also major users of charcoal. The type of charcoal kiln presently used is the Siamese beehive kiln, which was first introduced to Matang in 1930 by charcoal manufacturers from southern Thailand as shown in Fig. 2.2 (Baba et al., 2013). Charcoal factories in Matang are usually constructed close to rivers or canals where transport boats can dock. On arrival of boats, mangrove billets are unloaded and stacked outside the factory ready to burn as shown in Fig. 2.3 (Baba et al., 2013).

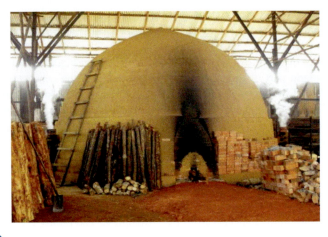

FIGURE 2.2

A typical beehive kiln in Matang, Malaysia. The kiln, a dome-shaped structure resembling an igloo, is made of bricks, sand and clay.

Reproduced with permission from Baba, S., Chan, H.T., Aksornkoae, S., 2013. Useful products from mangrove and other coastal plants. In: International Society for Mangrove Ecosystems (ISME). Okinawa, Japan.

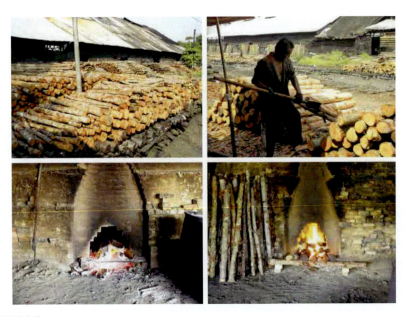

FIGURE 2.3

Mangrove billets outside the charcoal factory (*top left*), debarking billets (*top right*), firing schedule Stage I (*bottom right*) and firing schedule Stage II (*bottom left*).

Reproduced with permission from Baba, S., Chan, H.T., Aksornkoae, S., 2013. Useful products from mangrove and other coastal plants. In: International Society for Mangrove Ecosystems (ISME). Okinawa, Japan.

The present market value of high-grade charcoal is about USD 200 per ton. Some 30% of the charcoal produced from Matang is exported to Japan. Two local incorporated Japanese companies are involved in purchasing, grading and packing the charcoal for export to Japan. Charcoal from Matang has set an international benchmark for quality and attracts premium prices (Neilson, 2011). Fig. 2.4 illustrates how charcoal are packed.

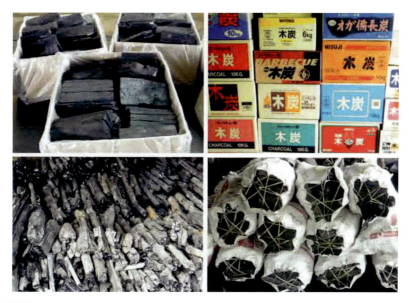

FIGURE 2.4

High-grade charcoal from Matang is packed for export (*top row*). Medium to lower grade charcoal (*bottom row*) is packed for the local market.

Reproduced with permission from Baba, S., Chan, H.T., Aksornkoae, S., 2013. Useful products from mangrove and other coastal plants. In: International Society for Mangrove Ecosystems (ISME). Okinawa, Japan.

2.2.1.2 Fish smoking purposes

In Cameroon, smoking is a popular method of fish preservation. Felling of *Rhizophora racemosa* G. Mey. trees is an important economic activity, with most of the wood harvested used for fish smoking (Ajonina and Usongo, 2001). Other mangroves species such as *Avicennia germinans* (L.) L., *Laguncularia racemosa* (L.) C.F. Gaertn. and *Conocarpus erectus* L. are also used (Atheull et al., 2009) (Fig. 2.5).

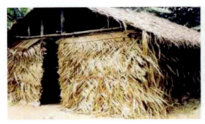 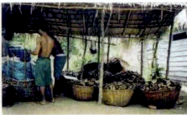

FIGURE 2.5

A *Nypa* thatched hut (*left*) and smoked fish for sale (*right*) in Cameroon.

Reproduced with permission from Baba, S., Chan, H.T., Aksornkoae, S., 2013. Useful products from mangrove and other coastal plants. In: International Society for Mangrove Ecosystems (ISME). Okinawa, Japan.

2.2.1.3 Poles

The felling of *Rhizophora* trees for poles is done using an ax, starting from the riverbank and progressively working inland. With the rapid development in housing and road building, mangrove poles are in great demand for piling purposes. Poles are also used as stakes for fish traps and as decorative panels of seafood restaurants in the coastal areas (Baba et al., 2013) (Fig. 2.6).

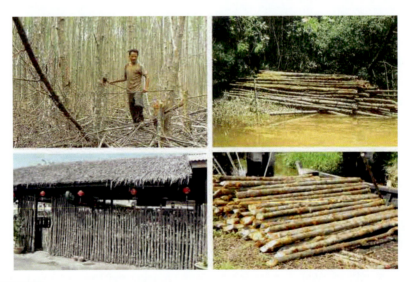

FIGURE 2.6

Stick thinning of mangrove poles (*top left*), poles are stacked at the riverbank (*top right*), poles are graded at the jetty (*bottom right*), and poles are used as decorative panel (*bottom left*).

Reproduced with permission from Baba, S., Chan, H.T., Aksornkoae, S., 2013. Useful products from mangrove and other coastal plants. In: International Society for Mangrove Ecosystems (ISME). Okinawa, Japan.

2.2.1.4 Construction materials

In Kenya, Madagascar and Zanzibar, the fishing communities are renowned for their boat building skills. Simple dug-out canoes, with or without stabilizers, are carved from large trunks of *Avicennia marina* (Forssk.) Vierh. (Dahdouh-Guebas et al., 2000; Rasolofo, 1997; Weiss, 1973). The ribs and keels of larger vessels such as the traditional dhows are built from *Sonneratia alba* Sm., *Heritiera littoralis* Aiton or *A. marina*. Mangrove species such as *R. mucronata, Bruguiera gymnorhiza* (L.) Lam., *Ceriops tagal* (Perr.) C.B. Rob., *Lumnitzera racemosa* Willd, *Xylocarpus moluccensis* (Lam.) M. Roem. and *S. alba* are used for masts, paddles and oars (Fig. 2.7).

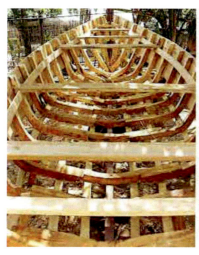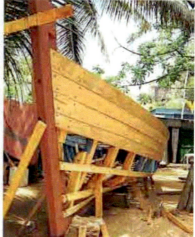

FIGURE 2.7

Dhows of different shapes being built in the Lamu Archipelago, Kenya.

Reproduced with permission from Baba, S., Chan, H.T., Aksornkoae, S., 2013. Useful products from mangrove and other coastal plants. In: International Society for Mangrove Ecosystems (ISME). Okinawa, Japan.

In Kenya, the most significant use of mangroves wood takes the form of poles for house construction (Dahdouh-Guebas et al., 2000). Poles of *R. mucronata, C. tagal* (Perr.) C.B. Rob. and *B. gymnorhiza* are often used. Each of these species occupies a particular place within the framework of a house. The long and strong poles of *B. gymnorhiza* are used for the rooftops. *R. mucronata* poles are used for the walls, especially the thicker supportive poles and corner pillars. The thinner poles of *C. tagal* are used to create an interweaving network for the walls. They are also used to construct structures such like shrines, cooking sheds and animal sheds (Fig. 2.8) (Baba et al., 2013).

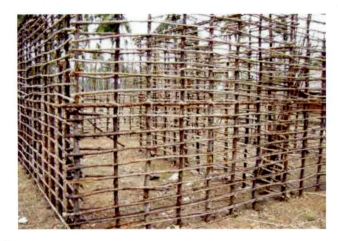

FIGURE 2.8

Poles used for construction of houses in Kenya.

Reproduced with permission from Baba, S., Chan, H.T., Aksornkoae, S., 2013. Useful products from mangrove and other coastal plants. In: International Society for Mangrove Ecosystems (ISME). Okinawa, Japan.

2.2.1.5 Wood handicrafts and decorations

Sculptures are made from the wood of *Xylocarpus*. Its wood is favored because of its attractive color and appearance, and its fine texture contributes to the smoothness of the finished product. The cream-colored sapwood can be easily distinguished from the reddish-brown heartwood. The wood of *X. moluccensis* (Lam.) M. Roem. is preferred over that of *Xylocarpus granatum* J. Koenig. It has been reported that the wood of these two species is also used to produce carvings in Tonga, one of the Pacific Islands (Baba et al., 2013). Besides sculptures, the Mah Meri people also make masks from the wood of *Alstonia spatulata* Blume, which is light, soft, and easy to carve (Fig. 2.9) (Baba et al., 2013).

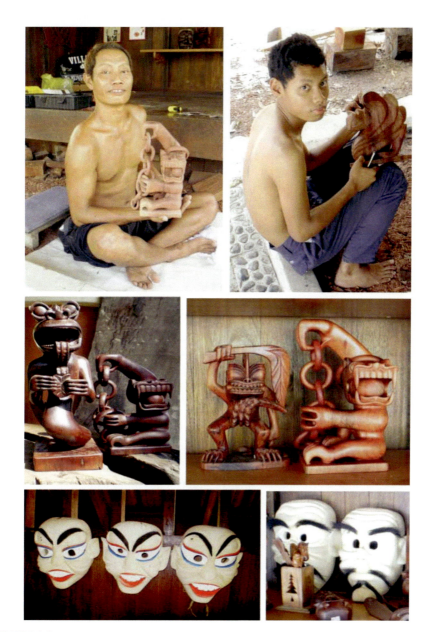

FIGURE 2.9

Mah Meri father and son displaying their wood sculptures (*top row*), beautiful mystical sculptures carved from *Xylocarpus* wood (*middle row*), and colorful masks carved from *Alstonia* wood (*bottom row*).

Reproduced with permission from Baba, S., Chan, H.T., Aksornkoae, S., 2013. Useful products from mangrove and other coastal plants. In: International Society for Mangrove Ecosystems (ISME). Okinawa, Japan.

Mangrove stumps found at the seashore can be used as driftwoods for aquaria and ponds. Besides tree stumps, roots and pneumatophores of *Xylocarpus* and *Heritiera*, when processed, resemble fossil bones of animals. They can serve as decorative wood for indoor use (Fig. 2.10) (Baba et al., 2013).

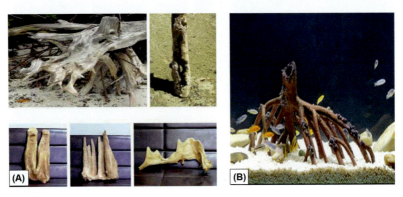

FIGURE 2.10

(A) Mangrove tree stumps that can be used as driftwood for aquaria and ponds (A: *top row*), peg-like pneumatophores of *Heritiera fomes* (A: *bottom left*) and *Xylocarpus moluccensis* (A: *bottom center*), and sinuous plank buttress of *Xylocarpus granatum* (A: *bottom right*). (B) Mangrove root in an aquarium.

Reproduced with permission from Baba, S., Chan, H.T., Aksornkoae, S., 2013. Useful products from mangrove and other coastal plants. In: International Society for Mangrove Ecosystems (ISME). Okinawa, Japan.

2.2.1.6 Fishing stakes and shrimp traps

Mangroves are critical habitats for fish and crustaceans and provide a number of ecosystem services to people. In Malaysia, fishing using gape nets is a popular traditional fishing method in mangrove rivers and estuaries. The net structures consist of a net, which is secured to a framework of 40−50 *nibong* poles. The framework of poles also acts as a working platform to facilitate operations (Fig. 2.11). Catch comprises mainly of shrimps. In Ambaro Bay, Madagascar, the traditional *valakira* is the best-known small-scale shrimp fisheries (Razafindrainibe, 2010).

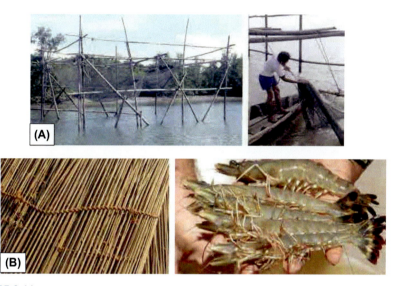

FIGURE 2.11

(A) A *ngian* showing the bag net and framework of mangrove stakes (*left*) and lifting the bag net during harvesting (*right*). (B) A *valakira* panel (*left*) and *Penaeus* shrimp harvested from the traps (*right*) in Madagascar.

Reproduced with permission from Baba, S., Chan, H.T., Aksornkoae, S., 2013. Useful products from mangrove and other coastal plants. In: International Society for Mangrove Ecosystems (ISME). Okinawa, Japan.

2.2.1.7 Pulp and paper

Excoecaria agallocha L. trees harvested for pulp and paper were crooked, and the wood was hard but of relatively low density. The white sap from the wood caused skin irritation and eye discomfort. The harvested woods darkened when exposed and had to be submerged in rivers before towing to the mill. Following the declaration of the Sundarbans as a world heritage site, the Forest Department imposed a ban on the felling of *E. agallocha* trees and the mill was forced to shut down in 2001 due to inadequate wood supply (Alam, 2006).

2.2.1.8 Wood vinegar

In recent years, charcoal operators have started to produce wood vinegar as a by-product of charcoal making. The by-product collected as raw distillate is pyroligneous acid. Before distillation, wood vinegar is almost black in color, resembling coffee (Chan et al., 2012a,b). After distillation, it becomes a golden-brown liquid, resembling tea. Wood vinegar has been traditionally used as sterilizer, deodorizer, fertilizer, and antimicrobial and growth-promoting agent (Loo, 2008). It has a wide range of industrial, agricultural, medicinal and home applications. In Thailand, wood vinegar is used to treat skin infections and dandruff (Rakmai, 2009) (Fig. 2.12).

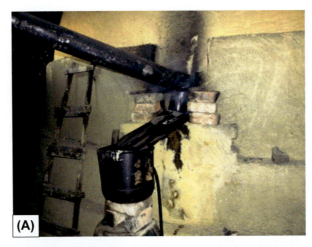

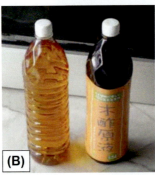
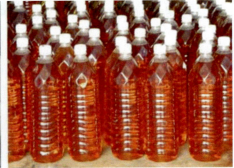

FIGURE 2.12

(A) On condensation, wood vinegar flows back into a drum. (B) Wood vinegar is almost black before distillation and golden-brown after distillation (*left*), and bottles of distilled wood vinegar produced by a factory in Matang (*right*).

Reproduced with permission from Baba, S., Chan, H.T., Aksornkoae, S., 2013. Useful products from mangrove and other coastal plants. In: International Society for Mangrove Ecosystems (ISME). Okinawa, Japan.

2.2.2 Nonwood products

Mangroves are also an important resource for a wide range of nonwood forest products. The mangrove palm *Nypa fruticans* Wurmb is commonly used for the production of thatch, beverage, sugar, alcohol and vinegar in Southeast Asia. Production of mangrove honey is an important economic activity in countries such as Bangladesh, Vietnam, Cuba and Guyana. Mangrove foliage is used as fodder for camels and cattle, notably in Pakistan, the Middle East and India. Harvesting of mangrove bark for tannin as dye remains a viable economic activity in countries of the Asia-Pacific region (Baba et al., 2013). Mangrove species with medicinal properties are also harvested as herbal remedies by coastal communities in some countries (Sadeer et al., 2019).

2.2.2.1 Thatches

In Malaysia, the weaving of thatches from leaves of *N. fruticans* continues to be an important traditional cottage industry among the coastal Malay villagers. There is still a strong demand for thatches as roofing and walling materials for poultry and pig farms, and charcoal kilns (Fig. 2.13) (Baba et al., 2013).

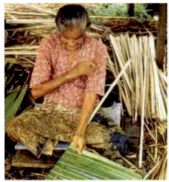
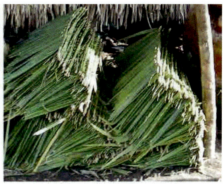
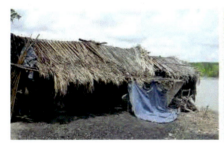
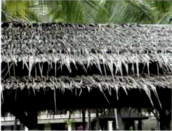

FIGURE 2.13

Weaving *Nypa* thatches is done by the womenfolk (*top left*), woven thatches are placed in the sun to dry (*top right*), and thatches for housing charcoal kilns (*bottom left*) and for ornamental use (*bottom right*).

Reproduced with permission from Baba, S., Chan, H.T., Aksornkoae, S., 2013. Useful products from mangrove and other coastal plants. In: International Society for Mangrove Ecosystems (ISME). Okinawa, Japan.

2.2.2.2 Cigarette wrappers

The manufacture of cigarette wrappers (*daun rokok*) from young leaves of *N. fruticans* (nipa) remained a flourishing industry in Malaysia, Indonesia. It requires special skills and many hours of patient work. A leaf is taken and one of the blades is stripped from the mid-rib with a swift tearing motion as shown in Fig. 2.14 (Baba et al., 2013).

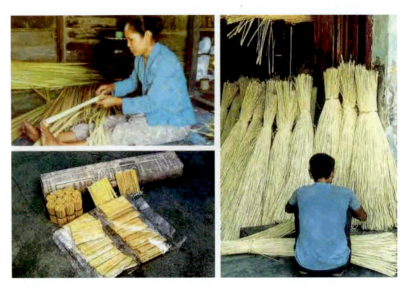

FIGURE 2.14

In Malaysia, stripping the cuticle from young leaves of *Nypa* is done by the womenfolk (*top left*), grading of bleached leaf blades (*right*), and cigarette wrappers are sold in small bundles and packets (*bottom left*).

Reproduced with permission from Baba, S., Chan, H.T., Aksornkoae, S., 2013. Useful products from mangrove and other coastal plants. In: International Society for Mangrove Ecosystems (ISME). Okinawa, Japan.

2.2.2.3 Sugar and beverages

It has been estimated that one hectare of *Nypa* forest yields 2,400−3,000 L of sap or 1,000 kg of sugar per month. Sap is generally collected from the fruit stalk after the almost full-grown fruiting head has been cut (Bamroongrugsa et al., 2004). Preparation of the stalk is essential to stimulate sap flow. It involves beating the stalk 40−50 times daily for 3 days. After an interval of 10 days, the beating process is repeated once or twice. Tapping begins by cutting off a thin slice of the stalk tip. When oozing commences, the sap is collected in bamboo tubes. It is estimated that a stalk can produce about 0.7 L of sap daily. A skilled worker is able to tap as many as 100 stalks per day (Fig. 2.15) (Baba et al., 2013).

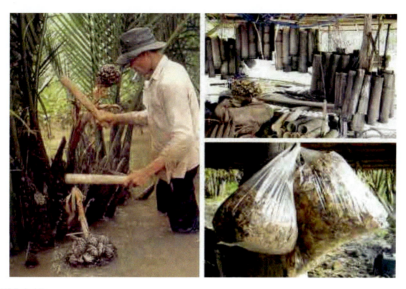

FIGURE 2.15

In southern Thailand, *Nypa* sap is tapped by beating the fruit stalk with a pair of wooden mallets (*left*), bamboo tubes are used as containers for the sap (*top right*), and shavings of *Rhizophora* wood are used as additive (*bottom right*).

Reproduced with permission from Baba, S., Chan, H.T., Aksornkoae, S., 2013. Useful products from mangrove and other coastal plants. In: International Society for Mangrove Ecosystems (ISME). Okinawa, Japan.

When freshly tapped, the sap is sweet. After several hours, it becomes alcoholic. In the production of *Nypa* sugar, the sap is immediately transported in plastic containers to the depot for processing (Thu Ha, 2004). At the depot, the sap is sieved and boiled under medium heat in large woks placed over earthen stoves for 1−2 h with continuous stirring till a thick golden-brown viscous sirup is formed as shown in Fig. 2.16. The sugar is allowed to cool with stirring continuing for another 25−30 min before it is sold in tin containers. From 100 L of sap, the yield of sugar is 20 kg (Bamroongrugsa et al., 2004). Containing 4%−17% of sucrose, *Nypa* sugar is used primarily as a confection for cakes and desserts, and as an elegant sweetener for coffee and tea (Thu Ha, 2004).

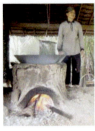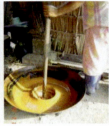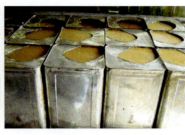

FIGURE 2.16

In southern Thailand, freshly collected sap is boiled in a wok under medium heat (*left*) with continuous stirring (*middle*) and on cooling, the sugar is sold in tin containers (*right*).

Reproduced with permission from Baba, S., Chan, H.T., Aksornkoae, S., 2013. Useful products from mangrove and other coastal plants. In: International Society for Mangrove Ecosystems (ISME). Okinawa, Japan.

Fresh tapped sap of *N. fruticans* (*nira*) is a popular drink that is sold in the coastal areas of Southeast Asia. The fruit bunch is shaken and the stalk is bent over to allow the *nira* to ooze out when cut. Tapping involves slicing off the cut end to sap out-flow. The milky white and sweet *nira* has to be consumed the day it is tapped, for it ferments spontaneously. After a day or two, it becomes an alcoholic drink with 6%−12% alcohol content (Fig. 2.17) (Päivöke, 1996).

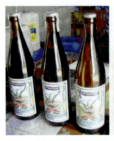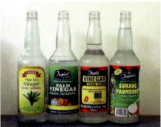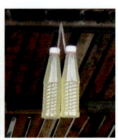

FIGURE 2.17

Bottled *Nypa* beverages sold as wine in southern Thailand (*left*), as vinegar in the Philippines (*middle*), and as fresh *nira* in Malaysia (*right*).

Reproduced with permission from Baba, S., Chan, H.T., Aksornkoae, S., 2013. Useful products from mangrove and other coastal plants. In: International Society for Mangrove Ecosystems (ISME). Okinawa, Japan.

In the southern and southwestern coast of Sri Lanka, local communities such as those at Kalametiya and Kahandamodara consume the fruit juice of *Sonneratia caseolaris* (L.) Engl. (*kirala*) (Jayatissa et al., 2006). Fruits are collected over a period of three months per year and each tree produces about 350 fruits annually (Batagoda, 2003). When freshly prepared, the drink is refreshing with a fruity flavor (Fig. 2.18). When kept for 24 h, the juice becomes unpalatable with a strong astringent taste due to fermentation and enzymatic browning. *Kirala* fruit juice is rich in dietary fiber, calcium and phosphorus (Jayatissa et al., 2006). Fruits have potent ability to scavenge free radicals and to inhibit lipid peroxidation (Bunyapraphatsara et al., 2002). Thus the fruit juice of *kirala* can be consumed as a natural health drink with cardiovascular protective properties. After adding sugar and preservatives, the fruit mixture can be used to prepare concentrated fruit cordial or ice cream with a shelf-life of more than six months. This procedure has now been patented in Sri Lanka.

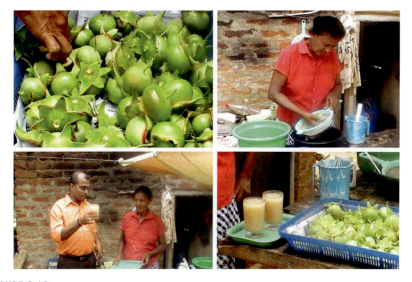

FIGURE 2.18

In Sri Lanka, mature fruits of *Sonneratia caseolaris* (*kirala*) are collected (*top left*), after removing the calyx, the fruits are hand squashed and sieved to obtain the fruit juice (*top right*), after adding some water and sugar, the drink is ready for serving (*bottom right*), and drinking the juice (*bottom left*).

Reproduced with permission from Baba, S., Chan, H.T., Aksornkoae, S., 2013. Useful products from mangrove and other coastal plants. In: International Society for Mangrove Ecosystems (ISME). Okinawa, Japan.

Aguardiente or "fiery water" is a generic term for alcoholic beverages that contain 29%−60% alcohol in Latin America. The use of pneumatophores of *Avicennia germinans* (L.) L. as colorant of alcoholic beverages is indeed very special as reflected in the brand name, *Aguardiente Especial*. Produced from sugar cane, *aguardiente* is the national liquor of Ecuador as it is most commonly consumed. A particular brand produced by *Frontera* in Manabi called *Aguardiente Especial* (48% alcohol content) has pneumatophores of *A. germinans* immersed inside each 0.75 L bottle (Baba et al., 2013) (Fig. 2.19).

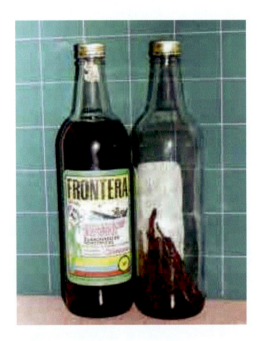

FIGURE 2.19

Aguardiente Especial, a liquor from Ecuador with pneumatophores of *Avicennia germinans*.

Reproduced with permission from Baba, S., Chan, H.T., Aksornkoae, S., 2013. Useful products from mangrove and other coastal plants. In: International Society for Mangrove Ecosystems (ISME). Okinawa, Japan.

2.2.2.4 Vinegar

In the Philippines, *Nypa* vinegar is commercially produced in Paombong, a town in Bulacan District. Cloudy white in color, the vinegar has a peculiar aroma. Compared to coconut vinegar, *Nypa* vinegar is less sour and has the tendency to darken as it ages (Baba et al., 2013).

2.2.2.5 Sirup

In Indonesia, mature fruits of *S. caseolaris* (*pedada*) are harvested to make sirup (Fig. 2.20) (Priyono et al., 2010).

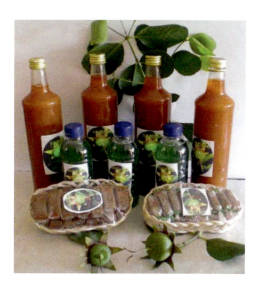

FIGURE 2.20

Brown *pedada* sirup bottled for the market in Indonesia.

Reproduced with permission from Baba, S., Chan, H.T., Aksornkoae, S., 2013. Useful products from mangrove and other coastal plants. In: International Society for Mangrove Ecosystems (ISME). Okinawa, Japan.

2.2.2.6 Edible plant parts
2.2.2.6.1 Nypa fruticans

Young seeds of *N. fruticans* are edible. The white and soft endosperm is eaten fresh as a refreshing dessert or snack. Known as *atap chi* in Malaysia, they are served as one of the ingredients in local ice confections (Fig. 2.21) (Baba et al., 2013).

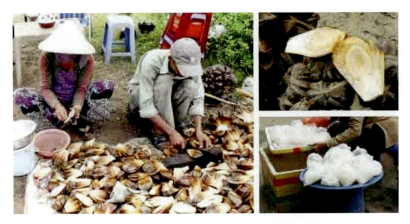

FIGURE 2.21

Young *Nypa* fruits are collected by the local people of Tra Vinh Province in Vietnam (*left*), spliced to obtain the white and soft endosperm (*top right*), and sold as a delicacy in the market (*bottom right*).

Reproduced with permission from Baba, S., Chan, H.T., Aksornkoae, S., 2013. Useful products from mangrove and other coastal plants. In: International Society for Mangrove Ecosystems (ISME). Okinawa, Japan.

2.2.2.6.2 Rhizophora apiculata

In Malaysia, the Bajau womenfolk at Kampung Penimbawan, Tuaran, Sabah, produce a condiment from flower buds of *R. apiculata*. Mature buds collected are removed of their calyx and pounded in a mortar, and mixed with shrimp paste (belacan), salt, chili, and tamarind or lime juice. The hot and spicy paste is eaten together with main dishes (Fig. 2.22) (Baba et al., 2013).

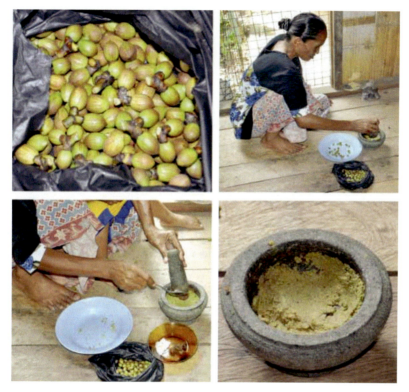

FIGURE 2.22

In Sabah, Malaysia, mature buds of *Rhizophora apiculata* are collected (*top left*) and crushed in a mortar (*top right*) with shrimp paste (belacan), salt, chili and tamarind or lime juice added for taste (*bottom left*), and the hot and spicy condiment is ready for consumption (*bottom right*).

Reproduced with permission from Baba, S., Chan, H.T., Aksornkoae, S., 2013. Useful products from mangrove and other coastal plants. In: International Society for Mangrove Ecosystems (ISME). Okinawa, Japan.

2.2.2.6.3 Bruguiera

Propagules of *B. gymnorhiza* are eaten cooked, after scraping or grating, washing, and drying (to remove tannins) and sometimes mixed with coconut in Melanesia and Nauru (Clarke and Thaman, 1993; Thaman, 1992). They are sold as a vegetable in the market of Honiara in Solomon Islands.

In the Maldives, propagules of *Bruguiera cylindrica* (L.) Blume, *B. gymnorhiza* and *Bruguiera sexangula* (Lour.) Poir. are consumed after removing the skin and boiling them several times, first with ash to remove their bitterness and then with salt for taste. Fruits of *S. caseolaris* are sold in the market. Taste like cheese, they are eaten raw and relished by the local people including children (Baba et al., 2013).

2.2.2.6.4 Acrostichum aureum

In Kiralakale, Sri Lanka, the young fronds or fiddleheads of *Acrostichum aureum* L. (karan koku) are sold in the market and eaten as a vegetable (Batagoda, 2003). A clump produces six edible shoots over a period of six month per year which are sold at USD 40 per ton. The fern is also eaten in Indonesia, raw but more often, steamed or blanched (Baba et al., 2013).

2.2.2.7 Dye

Dyeing of cotton fabric using the bark of mangrove trees was an important traditional industry on the Ryukyus Islands of Okinawa, Ishigaki and Iriomote in the southernmost part of Japan. This natural dye technique, known as *kusaki-zome*, uses the bark of *Rhizophora stylosa* Griff. (*yaeyama hirugi*). The dye color of the outer bark is brownish and that of the inner bark is reddish. The bark of *B. gymnorhiza* and *Heritiera littoralis* Aiton is sometimes used, yielding brownish and reddish-purple dyes, respectively (Fig. 2.23) (Baba et al., 2013).

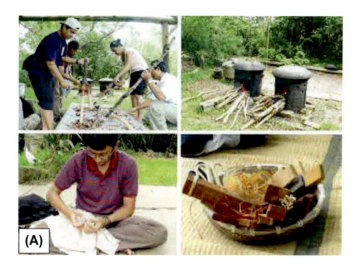

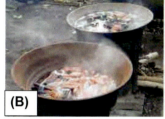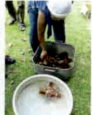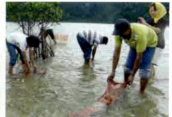

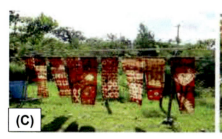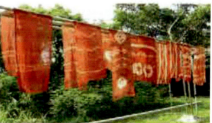

FIGURE 2.23

(A) Removing the *yaeyama hirugi* bark (*top left*), boiling the bark in pots of water to extract the dye (*top right*), knotting the cotton cloth for dyeing (*bottom left*), and creating color patterns using strings, elastic bands, sticks and blocks (*bottom right*). (B) Immersing the fabric into boiling dye solution (*left*), fixing the color of the dyed fabric in lye (*middle*), and untying and washing the dyed fabric in seawater to remove remaining dye (*right*). (C) Dyed fabrics drying in the sun.

Reproduced with permission from Baba, S., Chan, H.T., Aksornkoae, S., 2013. Useful products from mangrove and other coastal plants. In: International Society for Mangrove Ecosystems (ISME). Okinawa, Japan.

2.2.2.8 Fodder and forage

An important use of mangroves to the coastal populations in Gujarat is for fodder (GIDR, 2010). The foliage of *A. marina* is used as cattle feed. Propagules are also collected and fed to the calves (Fig. 2.24). Mangrove fodder is of high economic value to villagers as this has enabled them to make significant savings from having to buy fodder from the market. Livestock owners also noted an increase in milk production, which rendered them income gains from increased sale of milk.

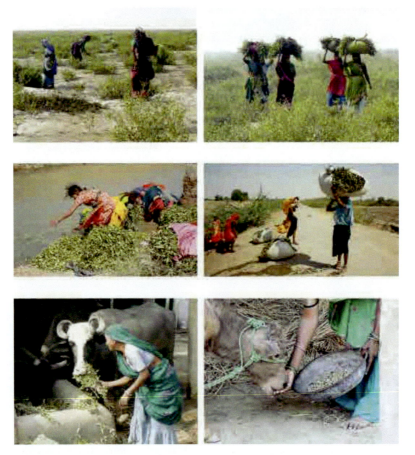

FIGURE 2.24

Women harvesting foliage from *Avicennia marina* bushes in Gujarat as fodder for cattle (*top row*), washing foliage in a stream before returning home (*middle row*), and feeding cattle with foliage and calves with propagules (*bottom row*).

Reproduced with permission from Baba, S., Chan, H.T., Aksornkoae, S., 2013. Useful products from mangrove and other coastal plants. In: International Society for Mangrove Ecosystems (ISME). Okinawa, Japan.

In the Red Sea and Gulf of Aden, mangroves of purely *A. marina* serve as livestock forage for camels (Baba et al., 2016). However, camel browsing has become a major problem causing degradation of the mangrove stands (Fig. 2.25).

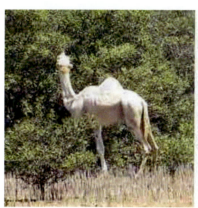 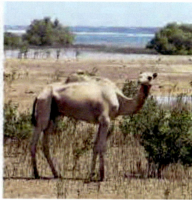

FIGURE 2.25

Camels browsing foliage of *Avicennia marina* in Egypt.

Reproduced with permission from Baba, S., Chan, H.T., Aksornkoae, S., 2013. Useful products from mangrove and other coastal plants. In: International Society for Mangrove Ecosystems (ISME). Okinawa, Japan.

2.2.2.9 Honey and wax

The Sundarbans in Bangladesh is one of the most fascinating places of the world where honey hunting maintains its historical traditions and importance. Occupying an area of about 10,000 km^2, the Sundarbans is home to the giant honey bee *Apis dorsata*. The main period of honey production is from April to June, and nectar is obtained mainly from *Aegiceras corniculatum* (L.) Blanco, *Ceriops decandra* (Griff.) W. Theob., *Sonneratia apetala* Buch.-Ham. and *X. moluccensis* (Lam.) M. Roem. The annual production of honey and wax has been estimated to be 50 and 200 tons, respectively (Baba et al., 2013).

In Florida, the main species for pollen and nectar production are *Avicennia germinans* (L.) L., *Conocarpus erectus* L. and *L. racemosa* (L.) C. F. Gaertn. (Bradbear, 2009). In Cuba, honey production remains an important and sustainable use of mangroves (Spalding et al., 2010). Some 40,000 hives are moved into the mangroves along the south coast during the four months of *Avicennia* flowering, producing 1700–2700 tons of honey per year (Fig. 2.26).

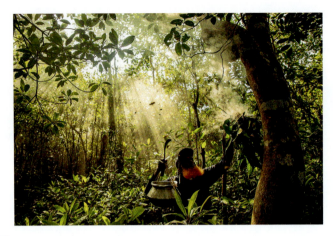

2.2.2.10 Handicrafts and ornaments

The Mah Meri women weave purses, pouches, mats and baskets from mengkuang leaves (Rahim, 2007). The Mah Meri people at Sungai Bumbun celebrate Hari Moyang (Ancestors' Day) a month after the Chinese New Year each year (Rahim, 2007). The morning begins with rituals and prayers in honor of their ancestors at the spirit hut. Music and dances then follow with the male dancers wearing their carved masks and the female dances wearing their elaborate woven nipa ornaments. After the dances, there is a pot-luck lunch for all present including guests and visitors, and all celebrations at the spirit hut end at noon. Hari Moyang is a major celebration for the Mah Meri people on Carey Island who take a 3-day mandatory holiday (Fig. 2.27).

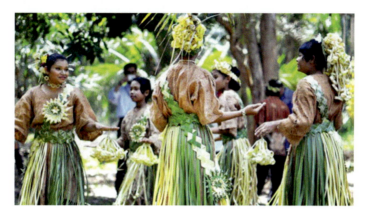

FIGURE 2.27

Mah Meri female dancers wearing their ornaments made from young and mature *nipa* leaves during the Ancestors' Day celebration.

Reproduced with permission from Baba, S., Chan, H.T., Aksornkoae, S., 2013. Useful products from mangrove and other coastal plants. In: International Society for Mangrove Ecosystems (ISME). Okinawa, Japan.

2.2.3 Support of fisheries

Mangroves are critical nursery habitats for fish and invertebrates, providing livelihoods for many coastal communities. Despite their importance, there is currently no estimate of the number of fishers engaged in mangrove-associated fisheries, nor of the fishing intensity associated with mangroves at a global scale (Ermgassen et al., 2021). Mangrove crabs are important fishery resources in all Brazilian coast, mainly in the north and northeast where many fishermen depend upon their catch. In addition to its social and economic importance, the mangrove crab is a "keystone" specie in ecosystem, they play an important role in the processes of nutrient cycling and energy transfer (Fish, 2021). A variety of mangrove crabs species exist for livelihood and commercial use. To cite a few, the red mangrove crab (*Neosarmatium meinerti* de Man), *Ucides cordatus, Cardisoma guanhumi, Episesarma chentongense, Callinectes bocourti*, amongst others. Swimming crabs, for example, include the large and fast-growing species of the genera *Callinectes, Charybdis* and *Scylla*, representing over half of the species listed in Table 2.1. Overall, the literature review yielded 27 exploited mangrove crab species in the Atlantic-East-Pacific and 40 in the Indo-West-Pacific. Fig. 2.28 illustrates some mangrove crabs. Salt marsh ecosystems also serve to maintain fisheries by boosting the production of economically and ecologically important fishery species, such as shrimps, oysters, clams, and fishes. Because of their complex and tightly packed plant structure, marshes provide habitat that is mostly inaccessible to large fishes, thus providing protection and shelter for the increased growth and survival of young fishes, shrimp, and shellfish. In Thailand, the net

Table 2.1 Mangrove crabs harvested for subsistence or commercial use in the AEP and IWP regions.

	AEP region			IWP region		
Americas[a]	**Caribbean**	**W. Africa**	**E. Africa**	**Asia**	**Oceania**	
Supra/intertidal (most active in air)						
Gecarcinidae	Gecarcinidae	Gecarcinidae	Gecarcinidae	Gecarcinidae		
Cardisoma guanhumi[WA]	*Cardisoma guanhumi*	*Cardisoma armatum*	*Cardisoma carnifex*	*Cardisoma carnifex*		
C. crassum[EP]	Ucididae	Grapsidae	Sesarmidae	Sesarmidae		
Grapsidae	*Ucides cordatus*	*Goniopsis pelii*	*Neosarmatium meinerti*	*Episesarma chentongense*		
Goniopsis cruentata[WA]		Sesarmidae		*E. mederi*		
Ucididae		*Sesarma angolense*		*E. palawanense*		
Ucides cordatus[WA]		Ocypodidae		*E. singaporense*		
U. occidentalis[EP]		*Uca tangeri*		*E. versicolor*		
Subtidal						
Portunidae	Menippidae	Menippidae	Matudidae	Calappidae	Portunidae	
Callinectes bocourti[WA]	*Menippe mercenaria*	*Menippe nodifrons*	*Ashtoret lunaris*	*Calappa lophos*	*Charybdis natator*	
C. danae[WA]	Portunidae	Panopeidae	Portunidae	*C. pustulosa*	*Portunus pelagicus*	
C. exasperatus[WA]	*Callinectes bocourti*	*Panopeus africanus*	*Charybdis feriata*	Matudidae	*Scylla serrataa*	
C. marginatus[WA]	*C. danae*	Portunidae	*C. natator*	*Ashtoret lunaris*		
C. sapidus[WA]	*C. exasperatus*	*Callinectes amnicola*	*Podophthalmus vigil*	*Matuta planipes*		

C. arcuatus [EP]	C. marginatus	C. marginatus	Portunus pelagicus	Menippidae	
C. bellicosus [EP]	C. rathbunae	C. pallidus	P.sanguinolentus	Myomenippe fornasinii	
C. toxotes [EP]	C. sapidus	Cronius ruber	Scylla serrata[a]	M. hardwickii	
		Portunus hastatus	Thalamita crenata	Oziidae	
		Sanquerus validus	Varunidae	Baptozius vinosus	
		Thalamita sp.	Varuna litterata	Epixanthus dentatus	
Total: 13 species	Total: 9 species (of which seven also occur in continental Americas)	Total: 13 species (one occurring in Americas/ Caribbean)	Total: 11 species (8 of them occurring in Asia also)	Total: 37 species (8 of them occurring in E-Africa also)	Total: 3 species (all fished in Asia also)

The list is not exclusive, particularly for species harvested for subsistence, which is often not reported in the scientific literature. *EP*, Eastern Pacific; *WA*, Western Atlantic.
[a]Also occurring in the lower intertidal, but most active in water.

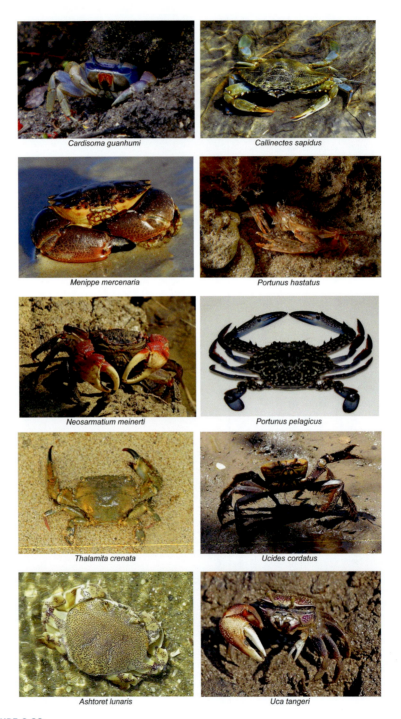

Cardisoma guanhumi

Callinectes sapidus

Menippe mercenaria

Portunus hastatus

Neosarmatium meinerti

Portunus pelagicus

Thalamita crenata

Ucides cordatus

Ashtoret lunaris

Uca tangeri

FIGURE 2.28

Representation of some mangrove crabs listed in Table 2.1 (Wikimedia Commons, distributed under a CC-BY 2.0 license).

present value of mangroves as breeding and nursery habitat in support of offshore artisanal fisheries ranged from $708 to $987/ha (Barbier et al., 2011).

2.2.4 Coastal protection

Since the 2004 Indian Ocean Tsunami, there has been considerable global interest in one particular service of mangroves: their role as natural barriers that protect the lives and properties of coastal communities from periodic storm events and flooding (Barbier et al., 2011). Eco-hydrological evidence indicates that this protection service is based on the ability of mangroves to attenuate waves and thus reduce storm surges.

2.2.5 Climate regulation

Mangroves play an important role in regulating climate by sequestering carbon within soils and to a lesser extent in forest biomass, as well as exchanging carbon dioxide with and emitting methane to the atmosphere. The ability of mangrove forests to develop, and thus capture and store carbon, is dependent on rate of sea level change relative to changes in accretion and subsidence. Mangroves are currently keeping up with the pace of sea level rise, but not all mangroves accrete, with geomorphological setting and water circulation being important drivers of net soil accumulation and net carbon sequestration (Alongi, 2016). Over the long-term, carbon is captured and stored belowground and, under the right conditions, as peat. Accumulation of carbon in soil depends on a number of factors including location of the forest in relation to the open coast, distance to adjacent aquatic habitats, tidal amplitude, forest position in the tidal zone, and primary productivity. A simple scaling up of the mean carbon burial rates to total mangrove area equates to a global sequestration rate of 13.5 GtC per year. However, if mangroves are disturbed, their high area-specific carbon stocks suggest the potential for significant greenhouse gas emissions. For example, deforesting mangroves on peat soils (Lovelock et al., 2011) results in CO_2 emissions (2900 $tC/km^2/year$) comparable to rates estimated from collapse of terrestrial peats (150−3200 $tC/km^2/year$). Mangroves thus contribute disproportionately as a carbon sink, having the highest per area rates of carbon capture and storage compared with all terrestrial and other marine ecosystems (Alongi, 2016).

2.2.6 Tourism

Mangrove recreation activities include hiking and boating—often centered around wildlife-watching—and fishing. While many visitors are participants in single-day or part-day trips, a few undertake extended stays for recreational fishing and overnight boating trips (Spalding and Parrett, 2019). Mangrove forest natural tourism based on an economic perspective is an alternative livelihood for coastal communities that can increase community income. Nature tourism activities can be carried out by the participation of surrounding community groups as a major component in driving the conservation of mangrove ecosystems. This will be able to encourage the economic growth of coastal communities and can increase public awareness of the importance of preserving the mangrove ecosystem (Kissinger et al., 2020). Fig. 2.29 gives an illustration of a number of tourists exploring the mangrove forests along the shore of Malanza river in Argentina.

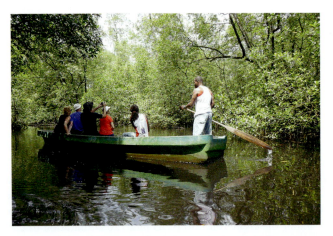

FIGURE 2.29

Tourists exploring mangrove forests in the Malanza river, Argentina (Wikimedia Commons, distributed under a CC-BY 2.0 license).

2.3 Human impacts

Mangroves are victims of dredging, filling, and diking, water pollution from oil spills and herbicides, and urban development. Dredging and filling activities have caused flooding of mangrove habitat. Standing water covers the aerial roots, making it impossible for oxygen to reach these specialized roots as well as the underground root systems. Eventually this leads to the deaths of mangrove trees. Oil spills cause damage to mangroves by coating roots, limiting the transport of oxygen to underground roots. Mangrove communities including invertebrates, fishes, and plants are also highly susceptible to damage from petroleum products (Museum, 2018). There have been at least 238 notable oil spills along mangrove shorelines worldwide. In total, at least 5.5 million tons of oil have been released into mangrove-lined, coastal waters, oiling possibly up to around 1.94 million ha of mangrove habitat, and killing at least 126,000 ha of mangrove vegetation since 1958 (Duke, 2016). On 25 July 2020, a 300 m long Japanese tanker that was sailing without cargo from China to Brazil, named MV Wakashio, ran aground on a barrier reef off the southeast coast of Mauritius (location Pointe d'Esny) (Fig. 2.30). Mauritius declared a "state of environmental emergency" on the same day and requested international help. The oil spill in Mauritius has affected sensitive ecosystems such as mangroves. The consequence for marine life could be disastrous as mangroves are the nursery of the marine environment. Mangrove communities are particularly susceptible to damage from large oil spills (Seveso et al., 2021).

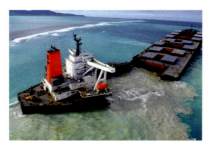 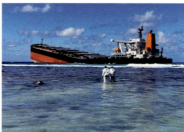

FIGURE 2.30

Wreck of MV Wakashio in Mauritius pictured on August 17, 2020 (*left*) and volunteers helping to remove oil spill from the sea (*right*) (Wikimedia Commons, distributed under a CC-BY 2.0 license).

2.4 Managing mangroves

It is gaining acceptance that conservation, economics, and social needs are not issues that can be dealt with separately (Barbier, 1987). To ensure sustainable management of ecosystems in a given area, the following goals need to be addressed:

- Ecological sustainability—maintaining genetic diversity, ecological resilience and biological productivity.
- Economic sustainability—satisfying the basic needs of local populations and reducing poverty; enhancing equity through ownership, management and participation in economic activities; and increasing useful goods and services.
- Social sustainability—maintaining cultural diversity; sustaining local institutions and traditions; ensuring social justice; and ensuring full participation through decision-making, employment, and training.

As mangroves have considerable socioeconomic values to human communities living in coastal areas, there is an urgent need for their sustainable management, conservation and rehabilitation (ITTO, 2012). These values need to be communicated to seek public and political support. In some countries, lessons have been learnt, and efforts are made to protect and use mangroves and adjacent ecosystems sustainably.

The sustainable utilization of mangrove ecosystems by traditional users shall be recognized and provided for to improve the welfare of the indigenous people. The decisions affecting the management of mangrove ecosystems shall be made only in the light of best existing knowledge and an understanding of the specific location. In the charter, decisions on the use of mangrove ecosystems include the following considerations:

- Utilize the mangrove resources so that their natural productivity is preserved
- Avoid degradation of the mangrove ecosystems
- Rehabilitate degraded mangrove areas
- Avoid overexploitation of the natural resources produced by the mangrove ecosystems
- Avoid negative impacts on neighboring ecosystems
- Recognize the social and economic welfare of indigenous mangrove dwellers
- Control and restrict nonsustainable uses so that long-term productivity and benefits of the mangrove ecosystems are not lost
- Introduce regulatory measures for the wise use of mangrove ecosystems.

2.5 Conclusion

We have discussed along the length of this chapter how important mangroves are to people. Mangroves around the world connect land and people with the sea, providing millions with food, clean water, raw materials and resilience against future climate change impacts including increasing storm intensity and sea level rise. Together with coral reefs, seagrass meadows and intertidal mudflats and marshes, these complex interconnected ecosystems are home to a spectacular range of visiting and resident species of birds, mammals, invertebrates and fishes, all of which helps to maintain the ecological functioning of mangroves. In turn, this rich mosaic of biodiversity supports people through fisheries, tourism, provision of wood and nonwood products (charcoal production, construction materials, fishing stakes, wood vinegar, thatches, cigarette wrappers, dye, handicrafts, herbal remedies, amongst others), coastal protection and cultural heritage.

It is emphasized that coastal developments that caused widespread mangrove destruction should have the legal requirement to replant mangroves and finance the costs, rather than leaving mangrove restoration solely to governments and local communities (Barbier et al., 2011). Detailed understanding of interactions between humans and their surrounding ecosystems is essential for designing sustainable use and management of these ecosystems. Mangroves are one of the most productive ecosystems worldwide, yet among the most threatened (Gnansounou et al., 2021). The contribution of mangrove to global forest carbon sequestration is small, but from a marine perspective, the mangrove contribution is impressive. Research is increasingly pointing to the role of mangroves as significant carbon storage systems, sequestering vast amounts of carbon. Understanding and quantifying the ecosystem services provided by mangroves to people will go a long way to helping secure their future and turn the tide on their devastation. Therefore the legislation, or its implementation should be revised to ensure that mangroves are protected, used, and restored properly for the benefits of future generations.

References

ACTI, 1980. Fuelwood Species for Humid Tropics, Firewood Crops: Shrub and Tree Species for Energy Production. Advisory Committee on Technology Innovation, National Research Council, National Academies, Washington, DC, pp. 32−69.

Ajonina, G.N., Usongo, L., 2001. Preliminary quantitative impact assessment of wood extraction on the mangroves of Douala-Edea forest reserve, Cameroon. Tropical Biodiversity 7, 137−149.

Alam, M., 2006. Khulna newsprint mill. Banglapedia. <http://www.banglapedia.org/http/docs/ht/k_0250.htm> (accessed 27.03.21).

Alongi, D., 2016. Climate regulation by capturing carbon in mangroves. In: Max Finlayson, C., Everard, M., Irvine, K., McInnes, R.J., Middleton, B.A., van Dam, A.A., Davidson, N.C. (Eds.), The Wetland Book. Springer, Germany, pp. 1−7.

Atheull, A.N., Din, N., Longonje, S.N., Koedam, N., Dahdouh-Guebas, F., 2009. Commercial activities and subsistence utilization of mangrove forests around the Wouri estuary and the Douala-Edea reserve (Cameroon). Journal of Ethnobiology and Ethnomedicine 5.

Baba, S., Chan, H.T., Aksornkoae, S., 2013. Useful products from mangrove and other coastal plants. In: International Society for Mangrove Ecosystems (ISME). Okinawa, Japan.

Baba, S., Chan, H., Oshiro, N., Maxwell, G., Inoue, T., Chan, E., 2016. Botany, uses, chemistry and bioactivities of mangrove plants IV: Avicennia marina. ISME/GLOMIS Electronic Journal 14.

Baharudin, Y., Hoi, W.K., 1987. The quality of charcoal from various types of wood. Fuel 66, 1305−1306.

Bamroongrugsa, N., Purintavarakul, C., Kato, S., Stargardt, J., 2004. Production of sugar-beating sap from nipa palm in Pak Phanang basin, southern Thailand. Bulletin of the Society of Sea Water Science 58, 304−312.

Barbier, E.B., 1987. The concept of sustainable economic development. Environmental Conservation 14, 101−110.

Barbier, E.B., Hacker, S.D., Kennedy, C., Koch, E.W., Stier, A.C., Silliman, B.R., 2011. The value of estuarine and coastal ecosystem services. Ecological Monographs 81, 169−193.

Batagoda, B.M.S., 2003. The economic valuation of alternative uses of mangrove forests in Sri Lanka. In: UNEP/Global programme of action for the protection of the Marine Environment from Land-based Activities, The Hague, Netherlands.

Bradbear, N., 2009. Bees and their Roles in Forest Livelihoods: A Guide to the Services Provided by Bees and the Sustainable Harvesting, Processing and Marketing of their Products. FAO, Bangkok, Thailand.

Bunyapraphatsara, N., Srisukh, V., Jutiviboonsuk, A., Sornlek, P., Thongbainoi, W., Chuakul, W., et al., 2002. Vegetables from the mangrove areas. Thai Journal of Phytopharmacy 9, 1−12.

Chan, E.W.C., Fong, C.H., Kang, K.X., Chong, H.H., 2012a. Potent antibacterial activity of wood vinegar from Matang Mangroves, Malaysia. ISME/GLOMIS Electronic Journal 10, 10−12.

Chan, E.W.C., Tan, Y.P., Chin, S.J., Gan, L.Y., 2012b. Antioxidant and anti-tyrosinase properties of wood vinegar from Matang Mangroves, Malaysia. ISME/GLOMIS Electronic Journal 10, 19−21.

Clarke, W.C., Thaman, R.R., 1993. Agroforestry in the Pacific Islands: Systems for sustainability. United Nations University Press, Tokyo, Japan.

Dahdouh-Guebas, F., Mathenge, C., Kairo, J.G., Koedam, N., 2000. Utilization of mangrove wood products around Mida creek (Kenya) amongst subsistence and commercial users. Economic Botany 54, 513−527.

Duke, N.C., 2016. Oil spill impacts on mangroves: recommendations for operational planning and action based on a global review. Marine Pollution Bulletin 109, 700−715.

Ermgassen, P.S.E.Z., Mukherjee, N., Worthington, T.A., Acosta, A., Rocha Araujo, A.R. D., Beitl, C.M., et al., 2021. Fishers who rely on mangroves: modelling and mapping the global intensity of mangrove-associated fisheries. Estuarine, Coastal and Shelf Science 248, 107159.

Field, C.D., 1995. Journey amongst mangroves. In: International Tropical Timber Organization and International Society for Mangrove Ecosystems. Okinawa, Japan.

Fish, T., 2021. Mangrove crab. <https://thisfish.info/fishery/species/mangrove-crab/> (accessed 27.03.21).

Friess, D.A., Chua, S.C., Jaafar, Z., Krauss, K.W., Yando, E.S., 2021. Mangroves and people: impacts and interactions. Estuarine, Coastal and Shelf Science 248, 107155.

GIDR, 2010. Socio-economic and ecological benefits of mangrove plantation: a study of community-based mangrove restoration activities in Gujarat. In: Knowledge Systems of Societies for Adaptation and Mitigation of Impacts of Climate Change, Springer, Germany, pp. 423−441.

Gnansounou, S.C., Toyi, M., Salako, K.V., Ahossou, D.O., Akpona, T.J.D., Gbedomon, R.C., et al., 2021. Local uses of mangroves and perceived impacts of their degradation in Grand-Popo municipality, a hotspot of mangroves in Benin, West Africa. Trees, Forests and People 4, 100080.

ITTO, 2012. Special edition summarizing the findings of the 2010 World Atlas of Mangroves. In: Tuck, C.H., Spalding, M., Baba, S., Kainuma, M., Sarre, A., Johnson, S. (Eds.), Tropical Forest Update. Yokohama, Japan, pp. 1−24.

Jayatissa, L.P., Hettiarachi, S., Dahdouh-Guebas, F., 2006. An attempt to recover economic losses from decadal changes in two lagoon systems of Sri Lanka through a newly patented mangrove product. Environment, Development and Sustainability 8, 585−595.

Kissinger, Alfi Syahrin, N., Muhayah, N.P.R., Violet, 2020. The potential of mangrove forest as natural tourism area based on the flora-fauna characteristics and social aspect case study: mangrove forest in Angsana Village. BIO Web Conf 20, 02004.

Loo, A.Y., 2008. Isolation and Characterization of Antioxidant Compounds from Pyroligneous Acid of *Rhizophora Apiculata*. Universiti Sains Malaysia, Penang, Malaysia.

López-Angarita, J., Roberts, C.M., Tilley, A., Hawkins, J.P., Cooke, R.G., 2016. Mangroves and people: lessons from a history of use and abuse in four Latin American countries. Forest Ecology and Management 368, 151–162.

Lovelock, C.E., Ruess, R.W., Feller, I.C., 2011. CO_2 efflux from cleared mangrove peat. PloS One 6, e21279.

Menéndez, P., Losada, I.J., Torres-Ortega, S., Narayan, S., Beck, M.W., 2020. The global flood protection benefits of mangroves. Scientific Report 10, 4404.

Museum, F., 2018. Impacts on mangroves. <https://www.floridamuseum.ufl.edu/southflorida/habitats/mangroves/impacts/> (accessed 27.03.21).

Neilson, T., 2011. King of charcoal: Japanese create new life for dying industry. Inwood Magazine 96, 32–33.

Päivöke, A.E.A., 1996. Plant Resources of South-East Asia No. 9: Plants Yielding Non-seed Carbohydrates. Backhuys Publisher, Leiden, Netherlands.

Priyono, A., Ilminingtyas, D., Mohson, S.Y.L., Hakim, T.L., 2010. Beragam produk olahan berbahan dasar mangrove. Kesemat, Semarang.

Rahim, R., 2007. Chita' Hae: Culture, crafts and customs of the Hma' Meri in Kampung Sungai Bumbun, Pulau Carey. Centre for Orang Asli Concerns (COAC), Selangor, Malaysia.

Rakmai, J., 2009. Chemical Determination, Antimicrobial and Antioxidant Activities of Thai Wood Vinegars. Prince of Songkla University, Thailand.

Rasolofo, M.V., 1997. Use of mangroves by traditional fishermen in Madagascar. Mangroves and Salt Marshes 1, 243–253.

Razafindrainibe, H., 2010. Baseline Study of the Shrimp Trawl Fishery in Madagascar and Strategies for By-Catch Management. FAO, Rome, Italy.

Sadeer, N.B., Mahomoodally, F.M., Zengin, G., Jeewon, R., Nazurally, N., Rengasamy Kannan, R.R., et al., 2019. Ethnopharmacology, phytochemistry, and global distribution of mangroves—a comprehensive review. Marine Drugs 17 (14), 231.

Seveso, D., Louis, Y.D., Montano, S., Galli, P., Saliu, F., 2021. The Mauritius oil spill: what's next? Pollutants 1, 18–28.

Spalding, M., Parrett, C.L., 2019. Global patterns in mangrove recreation and tourism. Marine Policy 110, 103540.

Spalding, M., Kainuma, M., Collins, L., 2010. World Atlas of Mangroves. Earthscan, London.

Thaman, R.R., 1992. Batiri Kei Baravi: the ethnobotany of Pacific island coastal plants. Atoll Research Bulletin 361, 1–62.

Thu Ha, L.T., 2004. Values of Nipa Palm (Nypa fruticans) and its Significance in Management Planning in Pak Phanang River Basin, Thailand. Prince of Songkla University, Thailand.

Weiss, E.A., 1973. Some indigenous trees and shrubs used by local fishermen on the east African coast. Economic Botany 27, 174–192.

Mangroves in medicines

Biopharmaceutical applications of mangrove plants: opening a new door to disease management and prevention

3.1 Introduction

Herbal remedies were the first medicines used by humans due to the many pharmacologically active secondary metabolites produced by plants. Until today, plants are an important source of numerous modern medicines. Bioinformatics and genomics can find application in drug discovery from plant-based products and biotechnological procedures can enhance and advance the studies of medicinal plants (Alamgir, 2018). Biotechnology could be described as a method for enhancing the formation and accumulation of desirable natural products, with possible product modification in medicinal plants. Increasing the production of pharmacologically attractive natural products represents on the main targets the genetic manipulation of medicinal plants. An increasing number of natural products are being biosynthesized (Julsing et al., 2007). An average approval of 10−15 products a year indicates that pharmaceutical biotechnology is a highly active sector. Amongst these, the number of genuinely new biopharmaceuticals is around 40%, indicating the high innovative character of research; some of these products are likely to be future blockbusters (Kayser and Warzecha, 2012). Examples are monoclonal antibody-based products such as Rituximab (Rituxan/MabThera) for the treatment of cancer with $8.58 billion sales in 2016 (Pierpont et al., 2018), insulin and insulin analogs ($16.7 billion/2011) (Davidson, 2014), and finally erythropoietin-based products ($0.95 billion/2020) (ReportLinker, 2021).

To date, biotechnology has produced more than 200 new therapies and vaccines, including products to treat cancer, diabetes, human immunodeficiency virus (HIV)/AIDS, and autoimmune disorders. There are more than 400 biotech drug products and vaccines currently in clinical trials, targeting more than 200 diseases, including various cancers, Alzheimer's disease, heart disease, diabetes, multiple sclerosis, AIDS, and arthritis. These few figures demonstrate the importance of biotechnological methods and techniques, which are increasingly dominating the process of drug research and development (Kayser and Warzecha, 2012).

Mangroves with Therapeutic Potential for Human Health. DOI: https://doi.org/10.1016/B978-0-323-99332-6.00011-4

The curative efficacy of medicinal plants is due to the bioactive metabolites (or pharmacologically active compounds) they possess, for example, alkaloids have an antispasmodic, antimalarial, analgesic, diuretic activities; phenols and flavonoids have an antioxidant, antiallergenic, antibacterial properties; terpenoids are known for their antiviral, anthelmintic, antibacterial, anticancer, antimalarial, antiinflammatory properties; glycosides are reported for antifungal and antibacterial properties; and saponins are reported to have antiinflammatory, antiviral activities. Biotechnology offers a valuable tool to produce these compounds of interest in a desired amount and an eco-friendly way. Plant tissue culture technology could be a potential alternative approach for bioproduction of phytoconstituents of therapeutic value. Different strategies can also be applied for the improvement of production of bioactive compounds of secondary metabolic origin. By employing biotechnological techniques (e.g., plant tissue culture or metabolite engineering), it is possible to regulate the biosynthetic pathway of a plant to enhance or decrease the synthesis of a particular compound (Alamgir, 2018).

In this chapter, we attempt at providing baseline information on the biotechnological applications on one of the marine resources in medicines to promote marine flora-based research. Therefore mangrove plants are opted as the focused research topic to elaborate on their biotechnological applications since they are well-known in traditional medicines, produce scads of interesting bioactive compounds and are increasingly being appraised for their medicinal values. Developing medicines or edible vaccines from mangroves are not impossible since several publications have already vouched the remarkable biological activities that various mangrove species exhibit (Sadeer et al., 2019a). In fact, scientists asserted that mangroves should be protected as they have the ability to produce vaccines that can be used to challenge chronic infections that existing synthesized drugs could not resist (Gayathri and Mahalingam, 2020). In this chapter, we also want to propose investigators to take modern biotechnological approaches including nanotechnology, vaccine biotechnology, enzyme engineering, and tissue culture, into account and apply them on mangrove plants with the aim to develop efficient and novel phytopharmaceuticals. Thus, this chapter forms a base of support and hastens urgent research on biomedical applications of mangroves.

3.2 Nanoparticles from mangroves

The advances in nanotechnology and its intersection with other fields, namely, biomedical science, cell and molecular biology, and medicine referred to as nanomedicine, have drawn significant interest from biomedical research due to its ability in diagnosing and treating pathological complications (Mauricio et al., 2018). Nanoparticles (NPs) are used as highly molecular specific theranostic agents in nanomedicine. With a size ranging from 1 to 100 nm, NPs possess large surface area-to-volume ratio allowing them to absorb high quantities of drugs (Borm et al., 2006) and to be easily distributed in the bloodstream (Stapleton and Nurkiewicz, 2014). Furthermore, NPs can act as nanocarriers for drug delivery. Nanocarriers are applied to preserve the therapeutic values of drugs by carrying the optimum quantity of herbal drugs to the required site of action bypassing the first pass metabolism and the acidic environment of the stomach (Mahomoodally et al., 2020). Some other examples of the applications of nanomaterials in medicine are fluorescent biological labels, gene delivery, bio detection of pathogens, tumor destruction via heating, and tissue engineering (Salata, 2004).

Since nanomaterials are the leading edge in the rapidly developing field of medicine, producing NPs on an industrial scale in an eco-friendly and cost-effective way is of prime interest (Das and Thatoi, 2020). Numerous literatures have suggested that plant-based NP synthesis or phyto nanotechnology could pave new ways to produce NPs in an environmental-friendly and low-cost way. Indeed, the involvement of biological resources, namely, microorganisms, enzymes, seaweeds, plant extracts or different plant parts (leaves, fruits, seeds, flowers, roots, barks, and fruit peels) in the synthesis of numerous NPs not only lead to cheaper but also to highly biocompatible and low toxicity NPs. Among the various sources used for the synthesis of metallic NPs, leaves are considered as the best due to their high stability and faster rate of synthesis (Das and Thatoi, 2020; Kumar and Rajeshkumar, 2018).

Despite considerable effort were directed toward the development of plant-based NP synthesis during the last decades, there has been only a few studies investigating on the use of mangrove plants for green synthesis of metallic NPs (Gouda et al., 2015) although on many occasions, mangroves have proved to be a potential source of bioactive compounds exhibiting high pharmacological activities (Chiavaroli et al., 2020; Sadeer et al., 2019a, b, 2020). In fact, biomolecules present in plant extracts, namely amino acids, proteins, vitamins, together with secondary metabolites including phenols, flavonoids, alkaloids, terpenoids, polysaccharides, can act as reducing agents to reduce metal ions into NPs in a single-step green synthesis. These phytocompounds may also act as important stabilizing and capping agents in the synthesis process. Several factors, namely, types of phytochemicals present in the extracts, pH and temperature of experimental conditions, concentration of extracts, ratio between extracts and metal salt may affect the size, shape and yield of NPs (Das and Thatoi, 2020). Fig. 3.1 illustrates the steps involved in NP synthesis using mangrove as the biological resource.

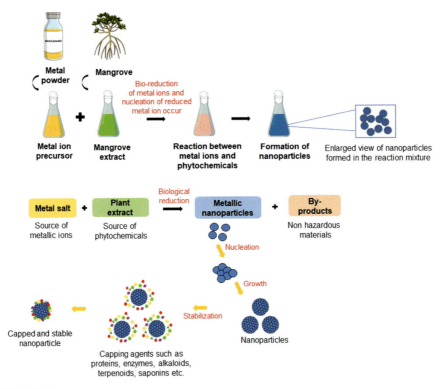

FIGURE 3.1

Steps involved in the synthesis of nanoparticles using mangrove extracts.

Mangrove plant-mediated synthesized NPs were reported to possess interesting biological activities including but not limited to antioxidant, antidiabetic, antiinflammatory, and larvicidal activity. Out of a total of 84 mangrove species that exist, existing literatures reported only a few of them in the biosynthesis of NPs which are applicable in the medical field, namely, *Acanthus ilicifolius* L., *Avicennia marina* (Forssk.) Vierh., *Ceriops tagal* (Perr.) C.B. Rob., *Rhizophora mucronata* Lam., among others. Table 3.1 summarizes the NPs synthesized using mangroves and the following sections elaborate in details on the type and size of NPs synthesized and their respective therapeutic applications.

Table 3.1 Therapeutic applications of mangrove plant-mediated synthesized nanoparticles.

Mangrove species	Part used	Types of NP	Size (nm)	Therapeutic applications	References
Acanthus ilicifolius L.	Leaf	AgNPs	50	• Antilarvicidal agent against mosquito borne diseases	Syed Ali et al. (2015)
Avicennia alba Blume	Leaf	AgNPs	60–110	• Antibacterial agent	Bakshi et al. (2015)
Avicennia marina (Forssk.) Vierh.	Leaf	AgNPs	71–110	• Antibacterial agent	Gnanadesigan et al. (2012)
	Seed	AgNPs	5–10	• Antibacterial agent	Naidu et al. (2019)
	Leaf	FeO-NPs	10–25	• Antibiofilm agent	Ramalingam et al. (2019)
	Leaf	AgNPs	60–95	• Antilarvicidal agent against mosquito borne diseases	Balakrishnan et al. (2016)
	Leaf	AgNPs	1–75	• NI	Abdi et al. (2018)
	Seed	AuNPs	2–40	• Antibacterial agent	Naidu et al. (2019)
	Leaf	CuNPs	48–29	• Antibacterial agent	Asghar and Asghar (2020)
	Leaf	AuNPs	4–13	• NI	Nabikhan et al. (2017)
	Leaf	AgNPs	NI	• Anticancer agent	Tian et al. (2020)
	Leaf	NiO-NPs	30–100	• NI	Karpagavinayagam et al. (2020)
	Leaf	AgNPs	25–30	• Therapeutic agent against lung cancer	Varunkumar et al. (2020)
	Flower	FeO-NPs	30–100	• NI	Karpagavinayagam et al. (2020)
Avicennia officinalis L.	Leaf	AgNPs	25–80	• Antiinflammatory agent • Antioxidant	Kumaran (2018)
	Leaf	AgNPs	50–1000	• Antiinflammatory agent • Antidiabetic agent	Das et al. (2019)

(Continued)

Table 3.1 Therapeutic applications of mangrove plant-mediated synthesized nanoparticles. *Continued*

Mangrove species	Part used	Types of NP	Size (nm)	Therapeutic applications	References
Excoecaria agallocha L.	Leaf	AgNPs	20	• Anticancer agent	Bhuvaneswari et al. (2017)
	Leaf	AgNPs	228	• Anticancer agent	Banerjee et al. (2017)
	Leaf	AgNPs	18–50	• Antilarvicidal agent against mosquito borne diseases	Kumar et al. (2016)
	Leaf	AgNPs	15–45	• Antioxidant	Satyavani et al. (2014)
Heritiera fomes Buch.-Ham.	Bark	ZnO-NPsAgNPs	40–5050–400	• Antiinflammatory agent • Antidiabetic agent	Thatoi et al. (2016)
	Leaf	AgNPs	15–40	• Therapeutic agent against dengue, zika, malaria	Alshehri et al. (2020)
Rhizophora mucronata Lam.	Leaf	AgNPs	4–26	• Antibacterial agent	Umashankari et al. (2012)
	Stem, root, leaf	AgNPs	1–80	• Antibacterial agent	Abdi et al. (2018)
	Leaf	AgNPs	12	• Efficient drug carrier	Singh et al. (2013)
	Leaf	Fe_2O_3-NPs	65	• NI	Nathan et al. (2018)
Sonneratia apetala Buch.-Ham.	Leaf	ZnO-NPsAgNPs	NI	• Antibacterial agent	Thatoi et al. (2016)
	Leaf	AgNPs	60–110	• Antibacterial agent	Bakshi et al. (2015)
Sonneratia caseolaris (L.) Engl.	Leaf	AgNPs	60–110	• Antibacterial agent	Bakshi et al. (2015)
Xylocarpus granatum J. Koenig	Bark	AgNPs	20–1000	• Antioxidant	Das et al. (2019)

3.2.1 *Avicennia marina* (Forssk.) Vierh

From the different organs (leaf, bark, root) of *A. marina*, Gnanadesigan et al. (2012) biosynthesized a higher yield of AgNPs from the leaf extract. Formation of silver NPs was observed by the appearance of a yellowish-brown color which could be the result of the excitation of surface plasmon vibration of the biosynthesized NPs (Jayaseelan et al., 2011). Fourier Transform Infrared (FTIR) results showed important peaks in various ranges (620, 1061, 1116, 1187, 1280, 1353, 1384, 1598, 1629, 2854 and 2927 cm^{-1}). Atomic Force Microscopy demonstrated that the size of the NPs ranged between 71 to 110 nm. Additionally, the x-ray diffraction pattern confirmed the synthesis of AgNPs since sharp bands of Bragg peaks were observed. It is anticipated that the sharp peaks could be the result of the stabilization of AgNPs by reducing agents present in the leaf extract of *A. marina* (Nabikhan et al., 2017). Antibacterial findings demonstrated that the synthesized NPs strongly inhibited the growth of Gram-negative bacterial strains. Since NPs play a key role in pharmaceutical applications, Gnanadesigan et al. (2012) concluded from their findings that the biosynthesized NPs derived with the help of this mangrove species could be used as future potential antibacterial agents.

Despite *A. marina* is used in traditional medicine to treat diseases such as skin diseases, rheumatism, ulcers, and smallpox, the biomedical property of the seeds remains poorly understood. Therefore the research group of Naidu investigated on the antibacterial activity of AgNPs derived from aqueous seed extract of *A. marina*. Transmission Electron Microscopy and UV analysis suggested that the size of the NPs is 5–10 nm. Since the spectrum from FTIR revealed the presence of eight absorption peaks at 3333, 3305, 2927, 2107, 1565, 1301, 1135, and 773 cm^{-1}, it is suggested that the amide, carboxylic, aliphatic amines, and amino acid groups in the plant extract could act as capping agents for the NPs. Bacterial strains, namely, *Escherichia coli, Klebsiella pneumonia*, and *Pseudomonas aeruginosa* were sensitive to the synthesized AgNPs which lead to the conclusion that the biosynthesized NPs can be used to fight against antibiotic-resistant bacteria (Naidu et al., 2019). For decades, silver ions were used as an antimicrobial source to resist a panoply of microorganisms including fungi, bacteria and viruses. To date, synthesizing silver NPs have gained momentum and they are widely used as bacterial agents in the pharmaceutical and biomedical field (Abdi et al., 2018).

Another type of NPs synthesized from the aqueous leaf extract of this gray mangrove (*A. marina*) was iron oxide NPs (FeO-NPs). The size of the NPs was determined using a Field Emission Scanning Electron Microscope. The magnified images showed that NPs formed were mostly spherical in shape of size ranging from 10 to 25 nm. There is currently a leading problem in the medical, food and marine industries concerning bacterial biofilms. These biofilms are difficult to deal with once the bacteria have adhered to a surface (Beolotto et al., 2016). Thus, the antibiofilm activity of FeO-NPs was determined. Results showed that the initial attachment and biofilm development of bacterial strains *E. coli, P. aeruginosa* and *Staphylococcus aureus* was inhibited by 200 μg/mL of FeO-NPs. Nearly 72% of quorum sensing of *P. aeruginosa* was recorded followed by 63% for *S. aureus* and 46% for *E. coli*. The study concluded that FeO-NPs could be used as a future antibiofilm agent against marine and medical pathogenic bacteria causing biofilm formation (Ramalingam et al., 2019). Other interesting NPs synthesized from *A. marina* include but not limited to gold NPs (Nabikhan et al., 2017), copper NPs (Asghar and Asghar, 2020), nickel oxide NPs (Karpagavinayagam et al., 2020) as shown in Table 3.1.

3.2.2 *Avicennia officinalis* L

In the medical lore, *Avicennia officinalis* is used to manage a manifold of diseases, namely, boil, ulcer, inflammation, snake bite, hepatitis, asthma, hemorrhage, bronchitis, stomach disorders as detailed in a review compiled by Sadeer et al. (2019a). It is considered as an excellent source of phytocompounds with important therapeutic potential which could provide great scope for the production of biocompatible NPs (Das and Thatoi, 2020). In a study, the biosynthesized silver NPs derived from aqueous leaf extract of this mangrove species could scavenge DPPH radicals at IC50 value of 0.14 mg/mL, depressed α-amylase activity and possessed antiinflammatory property. The phytochemicals involved in the synthesis of the NPs could result in unpreceded opportunities in producing NPs on an industrial scale for medicinal applications (Das and Thatoi, 2020).

3.2.3 *Ceriops tagal* (Perr.) C.B. Rob

Phytochemicals present in the stem extract of *C. tagal* act as bioreducers in the formation of copper NPs (Ramteke et al., 2018). Copper NPs have been reported by previous studies to possess antioxidant, antifungal, antibacterial and wound healing property (Rajeshkumar et al., 2019; Sriramulu et al., 2020; Zangeneh et al., 2019). Recently, Ramteke et al. (2018) biosynthesized a number of monometallic and alloy NPs from the aqueous leaf extract of *C. tagal*. Silver NPs successfully inhibited the growth of all tested microorganisms i.e., *K. pneumoniae, P. aeruginosa, S. aureus, E. coli, Enterococcus faecalis, Bacillus subtilis* while AuNPs were effective only against Gram-positive microorganisms. Also, both AgNPs and AuNPs exhibited effective toxicity against nosocomial pathogens. Another report synthesized AgNPs with average size of 30 nm. The NPs exhibited antimicrobial activity against a panoply of bacteria and the study has suggested to develop a bio-based approach to synthesis antimicrobial AgNPs (Dhas et al., 2013).

3.2.4 *Excoecaria agallocha* L

Excoecaria agallocha (*E. agallocha*) is also known as blind-your-eye mangrove since the latex that it produces is poisonous and can cause temporally blindness.

It is used in traditional medicine to manage rheumatism, epilepsy, leprosy, ulcers and paralysis (Sadeer et al., 2019a). Exploring the ability of its phytocompounds in synthesizing, stabilizing, reducing or capping NPs could reveal interesting outcomes. Indeed, synthesized AgNPs derived from the leaf extract exhibited substantially high cytotoxic effect against human breast carcinoma cell lines (MCF-7). The report suggested to develop the synthesized AgNPs as potential nano-drug formulation to control pathogenic diseases and used in breast cancer therapy (Bhuvaneswari et al., 2017). Developing NPs as part of cancer therapeutics is becoming a topic of intensive research in the field of nanomedicine. Compared to traditional anticancer drugs, NPs provide a targeted approach with less discouraging side effects (Chugh et al., 2018). The findings of Bhuvaneswari et al. (2017) are consistent with Banerjee et al. (2017) stating that AgNPs derived from *E. agallocha* could be a new medicinal approach to confront a wide spectrum of malignancy. Further examples are given in Table 3.1.

3.2.5 *Heritiera fomes* Buch.-Ham

The photo-mediated silver and zinc oxide (ZnO) NPs derived from the bark extract of this mangrove plant were investigated for their biomedical applications. The FTIR results suggested that oxime and other heterocyclic compounds could be the responsible compounds in reducing and stabilizing NPs in the solutions. The ZnO-NPs demonstrated higher antiinflammatory activity (79%) compared to AgNPs (69.1%). In addition, AgNPs exhibited significantly high antidiabetic property in terms of α-amylase inhibition activity (Thatoi et al., 2016). A study proposed *Heritiera fomes*-mediated AgNPs as potential standard care in a near future to manage dengue, zika and malaria since experimental data showed excellent toxicity against *Anopheles stephensi* with LC50 values ranging from 7.44 to 15.61 ppm and 8.39 to 17.66 ppm for *Aedes aegypti* (Alshehri et al., 2020).

3.2.6 *Rhizophora mucronata* Lam

Rhizophora mucronata is one of the most widely used mangrove plants in traditional medicine after *Bruguiera gymnorhiza* (L.) Lam (Sadeer et al., 2019a). The geometry of AgNPs biosynthesized from the leaf extract of *R. mucronata* revealed to be face-cubic at 4−26 nm in size. Resistance against fungal infection has emerged as a major health issue in the last decades, which needs great and immediate concern. The study reported that synthesized NPs were equally potent to synthetic antibiotics (Umashankari et al., 2012). Another study synthesized AgNPs from the stem, root and leaf extract of this mangrove species. The leaf extract yielded the highest production of NPs. The FTIR results revealed that aromatic loops, alcohol, phenol group, alkanes and alkyl halides were responsible in the biosynthesis of the NPs. Interestingly, results from antibacterial test suggested that AgNPs could be potential antibacterial agents against some bacterial strains (Abdi et al., 2018) and can be integrated in various medical applications (Singh et al., 2013). Nathan et al. (2018) managed to synthesis iron oxide NPs (Fe_2O_3-NPs) from the leaf extract through reduction of ferric chloride. The dynamic light scattering technique was used to determine the size of the NPs which was 65 nm. Several lines of evidence outlined that Fe_2O_3-NPs can form part of various biotechnological advancement, namely, magnetic resonance imaging, tissue repair, cell separation and detection, drug delivery due to their exceptional properties, namely, superparamagnetic, size and possibility of receiving a biocompatible coating (Arias et al., 2018).

3.2.7 *Sonneratia apetala* Buch.-Ham

Sonneratia apetala has been used in traditional medicine to treat gastrointestinal disorders (dysentery, diarrhea, constipation) and lack of appetite. Silver NPs synthesized from the leaf extract of the plant displayed potential inhibitory effect against *S. aureus*, *Shigella flexneri*, *E. coli*, *Vibrio cholerae*, *Staphylococcus epidermidis* and *B. subtilis* with inhibition zones ranging from 10 to 16 mm (Thatoi et al., 2016). Silver NPs synthesized by Nagababu and Rao (2017) possessed antibacterial property with potent antagonism toward *Proteus mirabilis* resulting in an inhibition zone of 27.3 mm. These NPs may be promising remedy against antibiotic drug-resistant diseases. Other studies are summarized in Table 3.1.

3.2.8 Other mangrove species

A study biosynthesized AgNPs from *Avicennia alba* Blume, *Sonneratia caseolaris* (L.) Engl. and *S. apetala* Buch.-Ham. at size of 60−110 nm. The NPs successfully inhibited the growth of six microorganisms (*E. coli*, *Agrobacterium tumefaciens*, *Streptococcus mutans*, *S. aureus*, *Tricophyton rubrum*, and *Aspergillus flavus*). However, the most significant activity was reported against *E. coli* resulting in an inhibition zone of 13.5 mm (Bakshi et al., 2015). Silver NPs were synthesized from aqueous leaf extract of *A. ilicifolius L.* mixed with $AgNO_3$ solution. The NPs characterized by Ali and coworkers confirmed the involvement of alcoholic and phenolic groups, namely, flavonoid and terpenoid with the metal ion to subsequently form the resulting silver NPs with an average size of 50 nm. Larvicidal activity of the synthesized NPs was tested against *Armigeres subalbatus* and *Armigeres aegypti*. Results showed that lethal concentration (LC) 50 values against the respective larvae were 0.532 and 0.754 mg/L, accordingly. Furthermore, the LC90 values were also determined as 2.13 and 5.98 mg/L against the same larvae (Ali et al., 2015). The aqueous bark extract of *Xylocarpus granatum* J. Koenig was a potential source of phytochemicals having the ability to synthesis AgNPs. The FTIR results reported that phenolic groups were responsible in stabilizing the biogenic AgNPs. The AgNPs derived from *X. granatum* was better α-amylase and α-glucosidase inhibitors compared to *A. officinalis* which lead to the conclusion that these NPs can be exploited in pharmaceutical applications (Das et al., 2019).

3.3 Plant edible vaccines: a revolution in vaccination

Plants have been as medicinal mediators for centuries. Recent trends in agro-biotechnology however, improved the therapeutic roles of plants to a significant level and introduced plant-based oral vaccine which can arouse an immune response in consumers. Although conventional vaccines against infectious diseases have been administrated for years the discovery of plant-based oral vaccines can potentially replace them completely in the future. The probable limitations in conventional vaccines are found to be overcome by plant-based oral vaccines. Humans and animals will no longer be dependent upon local or systemic administration of vaccines but they will just receive the vaccines as a routine food (Shakoor et al., 2019). An edible vaccine is when the antigen is expressed in the edible part of the plant. This reduces the cost of production of the vaccine because of ease of culturing (Gunasekaran and Gothandam, 2020).

Edible vaccines present numerous advantages. The specific proteins can be expressed into desired plants with very less cost and can be grown to the required locations so that, an edible vaccine can be available to the needy population globally, especially in the developing countries. Due to high cost, storage, refrigeration, transportation, and requirements of trained medical personnel, an injectable vaccine cannot be easily taken in developing countries. Apart from that, the plant-based vaccines are the most suitable for children as an oral delivery. Capsules can be made from dried leaf tissue powder. The edible vaccines do not have any risk of contamination and disease spread (Sohrab, 2020). Many medicinal plants possess significant antiviral properties owing to the presence of a large array of different bioactive molecules in them. Lin et al. (2014) summarized the antiviral activities from several natural products and herbal medicines against some notable viral pathogens including coronavirus, coxsackievirus, dengue virus, enterovirus 71, hepatitis B virus, hepatitis C virus, herpes simplex virus, HIV, influenza virus, measles virus, and respiratory syncytial virus and found that natural products and herbal ingredients possessed high antiviral activity.

Edible vaccines are mucosal-targeted vaccines that stimulate both the systematic and mucosal immune network, activating the first line of defense of human body through mucosa. The mucosal surfaces are found lining the digestive tract, respiratory tract and urinoreproductive tract. Mucosal immune system is the first line of defense and the most effective site of vaccination, nasal and oral vaccines being the most effective. When edible vaccines are eaten, they degrade majority of the plant cells in the intestine as a result of the action of digestive and bacterial enzymes. This degradation results in the release of antigens present in the plant product. The whole process occurs near the Peyer's patches where M cells recognize the released antigen and lead to the production of immunoglobulin (Ig) A antibodies in mucosal lymphoid tissues (Rudzik et al., 1975). These IgA antibodies get transported across the epithelial cells into the lumen where they interact with released antigens depicting immunogenic response. The whole process is elicited in Fig. 3.2.

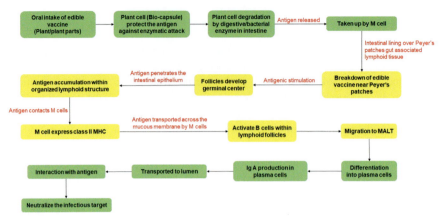

FIGURE 3.2

The steps that stimulates mucosal immunity in a very fine way which is elucidated by this diagram (Sahoo et al., 2020). *MALT*, Mucosa-associated lymphoid tissue.

Adapted from Sahoo, K., Dhal, N., Das, R., 2014. Production of amylase enzyme from mangrove fungal isolates. African Journal of Biotechnology 13, 4338–4346.

Certain foods, such as bananas, tomatoes, carrots, peanuts, corn and tobacco have a promising potential as edible vaccines as they can be eaten raw, not only because they are commonly available, but since genetic engineering efficiently developed these kinds of vegetable plants (Sahoo et al., 2020). Interestingly, several species of mangrove plants have edible parts that can be eaten raw. Details on the edible parts and how they are consumed are given in Chapter 2. The young seeds of *Nypa fruticans* Wurmb, the young fronds or fiddleheads of *Acrostichum aureum* L., fruits of *S. caseolaris* (L.) Engl. and mature flower buds of *Rhizophora apiculata* Blume are widely consumed raw, especially in Asia. However, since propagules of *Bruguiera cylindrica* (L.) Blume, *B. gymnorhiza* (L.) Lam. and *Bruguiera sexangula* (Lour.) Poir. are eaten cooked, frying or boiling can degrade certain antigenic proteins. Therefore, propagules of these mangroves cannot be considered for edible vaccines. Since mangroves are found in tropical and subtropical countries where facilities are usually underdeveloped and in turn contribute in poor health, edible vaccines develop from mangroves could be advantageous for these developing countries. However, will genetic engineering be able to efficiently develop mangrove fruits or other edible parts into successful edible vaccines, remain an unanswered research question that need to be urgently addressed. Fig. 3.3 illustrates the procedures involved in the development of edible vaccines from mangrove fruits.

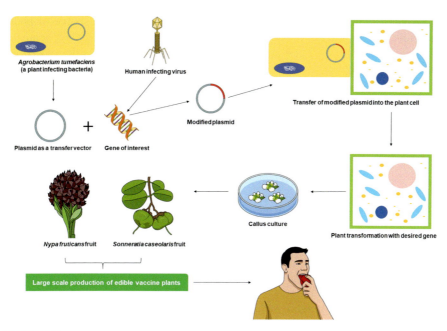

FIGURE 3.3

The procedure involved in the development of the edible vaccine from mangrove fruits. The development of an edible vaccine starts with the identification of desired genes or proteins which is biotechnologically modified with plant-bacteria or virus plasmid and introduced into it. Then the modified plasmid containing bacteria or virus is introduced to the desired plant cell and cultured in the lab with controlled environment. When plant successfully grew then moves for mass production in the crop field, from where these edible vaccines can be distributed to the whole world. After an edible vaccine has been consumed orally, it will trigger a response to B-cell and T-helper cell and induce an individual immune system as they are the main factors.

Adapted from Sahoo, K., Dhal, N., Das, R., 2014. Production of amylase enzyme from mangrove fungal isolates. African Journal of Biotechnology 13, 4338–4346.

3.4 Pharmacological applications of enzymes derived from mangroves

Enzymes are present in every living entity as all forms of life live by enzymes and also produce enzymes. Consequently, enzymes can be derived from three different sources, namely, plants, animals and microorganisms. Among these three sources, microorganisms are the main and most optimum source of pharmaceutically important enzymes owing to their diversified biochemistry (Volesky et al., 1984). They act as important biological catalysts that speed up chemical reactions without being consumed in the process and address elementary causes of numerous health issues. Enzymes that are pharmaceutically important form essential part of the pharmaceutical industries. These biological catalysts are defined as prodrugs that target specific reversible or irreversible reactions to treat a particular ailment. Some examples of enzymes that have pharmacological applications are proteinases, asparaginases, streptokinases, urokinases, deoxyribonuclease I, hyaluronidases, pegademases, and glucocerebrosidases (Das and Goyal, 2014).

The mangrove ecosystem hosts a variety of fauna and flora since the estuary acts as a connecting point between the marine water and river terrestrial water. Since the marine and coastal environment are rather complex in nature, there is a difference between the enzymes produced by the terrestrial and marine organisms (Volesky et al., 1984). Numerous enzymes of industrial importance have been derived from the microbial species hosted by the mangrove ecosystem as well as a myriad of different fungi. The different types of microorganisms (i.e., bacteria, fungi and yeasts) isolated from various mangrove species include *Acremonium* sp., *Alternaria* sp., *Fusarium* sp., *Aspergillus* sp., *Actinomycetes* sp., *Lactobacillus*, yeasts, *Trichoderma*, *Azotobactor*, among others. These microorganisms can be isolated from different tissues of the mangrove plants, namely, roots, propagules, petioles, rhizomes, fresh, dead or decaying leaves, stems and also from soils and water samples (Sengupta et al., 2020). Microorganisms from mangrove ecosystems contain useful enzymes, proteins, antibiotics and salt tolerant genes of much biotechnological significance (Thatoi et al., 2013). Microorganisms particularly fungal endophytes are exceptional extracellular enzyme producers. Fungal endophytes isolated from different mangrove plants and the promising biological activities they exhibit is the focus of Chapter 4.

Mangrove fungi, namely, *Pestalotiopsis microspora* and *Aspergillus oryzae* are important producers of α-amylase enzymes (Joel and Bhimba, 2012). α-Amylase is a starch degrading enzyme since it catalyzes the hydrolysis of $\alpha - 1,4$-glucosidic bonds in starch and associated α-glucans. Several studies have demonstrated that α-amylase inhibitors can be helpful in managing diabetes mellitus by reducing postprandial glucose levels (Agarwal, 2016; Janeček et al., 2014). *Cladosporium herbarum, Fusarium moniliforme, Cirrenalia basiminuta, Hyphomycetes* and *Halophytophthora vesicular* isolated from the leaves of *R. apiculata* Blume were reported to produce lignin cellulose enzymes (Raghukumar et al., 1994). Endophytic fungi *Acremonium,*

Cladosporium, Curvularia, and *Saccharomyces* isolated from *A. officinalis* L. produced a panoply of important enzymes including cellulase, tyrosinase, lipase, L-glutaminase, and L-asparaginase (Job et al., 2015). Tyrosinase is a multicopper enzyme responsible for the synthesis of melanin, a pigment responsible for the color of human skin, eyes and hair (Pillaiyar et al., 2017). A number of findings have suggested that tyrosinase inhibitors from mangrove resources can be a potential ingredient in cosmetic products and depigmenting agents (Chiavaroli et al., 2020; Sadeer et al., 2019b, 2020). Lipase enzyme is a biological catalyst that hydrolyze ester bonds of triglycerides. Lipase inhibitors interact directly with the enzyme to inhibit lipase action. Orlistat is the only approved drug for treating obesity in several countries and lipase is vital for lipid absorption. As a result, fat absorption or obesity can be controlled by lipase inhibition, especially pancreatic lipase which is responsible for hydrolyzing over 80% of total dietary fats (Bialecka-Florjanczyk et al., 2018). Since L-asparaginase acts as an antineoplastic agent, the enzyme is of vital significance in medicine and is reported to prevent protein synthesis in tumor cells (Usha et al., 2011).

Mangrove environment is also constituted of numerous bacteria mainly used in detergents, leather, and medicine. Marine bacteria have been exceptional sources of halotolerant enzymes since decades. Reports stated that several strains of bacteria that generate enzymes possessing antifungal properties are sheltered by mangrove plants. Enzymes were found to inhibit the growth of a number of fungi, namely, *Pythium ultimum, Phytophthora capsici, Aspergillus mali*, and *F. moniliforme* (Bibi et al., 2017; Mayanglambam et al., 2020). The abundance of *Bacillus* as an enzyme-producing genus has been confirmed by many researchers. Taking advantage of its abundance, *Bacillus* could be considered for biotechnological approaches, for instance in terms of mass enzyme production (Mayanglambam et al., 2020). The bacterial endophytes from the genera *Pantoea, Curtobacterium*, and *Enterobacter* identified from *Rhizophora mangle* L. and *Avicennia nitida* Jacq. have the potential to produce enzymes. For instance, 75% of the isolates exhibited protease activity and 62% demonstrated endoglucanase activity (Castro et al., 2014). Endoglucanase and exoglucanase activities were also detected in the bacterial strains isolated from mangrove sediments collected in Brazil (Soares et al., 2013).

As evidenced by a number of publications, a plethora of pharmacologically important enzymes can be derived from mangrove-associated fungi and bacteria. Therefore, there is a need to gather essential information on the microbial enzymes produced by the mangrove habitat and provide a better understanding on their applications. Table 3.2 aimed to provide more information on the fungal- and bacterial-derived enzymes.

Table 3.2 Enzymes recovered from mangrove-associated fungi and bacteria.

Enzymes	Mangrove-associated microbes	Source	Region/country	References
Fungi: α-amylase	Pestalotiopsis microspora VB5 and Aspergillus oryzae VB6	Leaves of Rhizophora mucronata, Avicennia officinalis, and Avicennia marina	Chidambaram area, India	Joel and Bhimba (2012)
α-amylase Lignocellulolytic enzyme	Penicillium citrinum JQ249898 Laetiporus sulphureus	Mangrove sediment Mangrove forests	Odisha, India Dar es Salaam, Tanzania	Sahoo et al. (2014) Mtui and Masalu (2008)
Amylase, protease, cellulase, pectinlyase, lipase	Aspergillus niger, A. ochraceous, A. flavus, A. luchuensis, A. terreus, Halocyphina villosa, Helicascus kanaloanus, Lignicola longirostris, Rhizopus nigricans, and A. sydowi	Mangrove forests	Tamil Nadu, India	Immaculatejeyasanta et al. (2011)
Laccase, peroxidase, caseinase, gelatinase, nitrate reductase, lipase, amylase, cellulase, laminarinase	Halocyphina villosa	Rhizophora mangle	NI	Rohrmann and Molitoris (1986)
Amylase, cellulase, lipase, chitinase, protease	Thraustrochytrids sp., Pichiasalicaria, Geotrichum sp., Pichiafermentans, Cryptococcus dimennae, Trichoderma asperellum, T. aaggerssivum, T. spirale, T. polysporum, Trichosporon sp., Aspergillus sp., Fusarium sp.	Decomposing leaves of Rhizophora mucronata and Avicennia marina	Vellar estuary, India	Kathiresan et al. (2011)
Lytic polysaccharide monooxygenases	Pestalotiopsis sp. NCi6	Rhizophora stylosa	Saint Vincent Bay, Southern province, New Caledonia	Patel et al. (2016)

Enzyme	Organism(s)	Source	Location	Reference
Pectolytic enzyme	Colletotrichum gloeosporioides and Coniella musaiaensis	Mangrove forests	West Bengal, India	Purkait and Purkayastha (1996)
Cellulase, tyrosinase, lipase, L-glutaminase, and L-asparaginase	Acremonium, Cladosporium, Curvularia, and Saccharomyces	Avicennia officinalis	Ernakulam district, India	Job et al. (2015)
Endoglucanase, cellobiohydrolase, and β-glucosidase	Hypoxlon oceanicum, Julella avicenniae, Lignincola laevis, Savoryella lignicola, and Trematosphaeria mangrovei	Mangrove forests	Hong Kong	Pointing et al. (1999)
Xylanase	Staganospora sp.	Mangroves decaying wood	Hong Kong	Luo et al. (2005)
Cellulase, amylase, lipase, protease	Acremonium sp., Alternaria Chlamydosporus, Alternaria sp., Fusarium sp., Aspergillus sp. 2, Aspergillus sp. 3, Pestalotiopsis sp.	Acrostichum aureum	Southwest coast of India	Maria et al. (2005)
Amylase	Penicillium fellutanum	Rhizosphere soil of Rhizophora annamalayana	India	Kathiresan and Manivannan (2006)
Laccase, xylanase, lipase	Rhizopus stoloniferm, Aspergillus flavusm, A. versicolor, Mucor sp., R. nigricans, and R. oryzae	Mangrove sediment	Tamil Nadu, India	Prakash (2013)
Bacteria:				
Protease	Pantoea, Curtobacterium, and Enterobacter	Rhizophora mangle and Avicennia nitida	Bertioga and Cananéia, Brazil	Castro et al. (2014)
Amylase, cellulase, lipase, protease, chitinase	Bacillus sp., Heterotrophic bacteria, Lactobacillus, Actinobacteria, Trichoderma, Azotobacter, Thraustrochytrids	Decomposing leaves of Rhizophora mucronata and Avicennia marina	Vellar estuary, India	Kathiresan et al. (2011)
Agarase	Gram-negative bacteria	Mangrove forests	Andamans, India	Shome and Shome (2001)

(Continued)

Table 3.2 Enzymes recovered from mangrove-associated fungi and bacteria. *Continued*

Enzymes	Mangrove-associated microbes	Source	Region/country	References
Cellulase	*Micrococcus* spp., *Bacillus* spp., *Pseudomonas* spp., *Xanthomonas* spp. and *Brucella* spp.	Mangrove forests	Odisha, India	Behera et al. (2016)
Cellulase	*Bacillus cereus* JDO404	Mangrove sediment	Thailand	Chantarasiri (2015)
Endoglucanase and exogluconase	Bacterial strains	Mangrove sediment	Brazil	Soares et al. (2013)
L-Asparaginase	*Bacillus cereus*	Rhizosphere soil of mangrove	Vellar estuary, India	Thenmozhi et al. (2011)
Cellulase	*Brucella* sp. and *Bacillus licheniformis*	Rhizosphere soil of mangrove	Mahanadi river delta, Odisha, India	Behera et al. (2016)
L-Asparaginase	*Bacillus* and *Pseudomonas* sp.	Rhizosphere soil of mangrove	Nizampatnam and Chollangi, A.P. India	Audipudi et al. (2013)
Pectinase	*Streptomyces* sp. GHBA10	Mangrove forests	Kerala, India	Das et al. (2014)
Fibrinolytic protease	*Bacillus circulans*	Mangrove sediment	Pitchavaram, India	Sadeesh et al. (2015)
Alkaline protease	*Bacillus circulans* BM15	Mangrove sediment	Cochin, India	Venugopal and Saramma (2008)
Amylase	*Bacillus megatorium*	Leaves of *Avicennia marina*	Tamil Nadu, India	Gurudeeban et al. (2011)
Carbonic anhydrase	*Bacillus altitudinis*	Mangrove forests	Gujarat, India	Bhagat et al. (2014)
Adenosine deaminase	*Lysinibacillus* sp.	Leaves of *Avicennia marina*	Tamil Nadu, India	Kathiresan et al. (2014)
Cholesterol oxidase	*Micrococcus* sp.	Rhizosphere soil of mangrove	Goa, India	Kanchana et al. (2011)
L-Asparaginase	*Pseudonocardia endophytica* VUK-10	Mangrove sediment	Andhra Pradesh, India	Kiranmayi et al. (2014)

3.5 Therapeutic applications of microbial pigments

As discussed in the previous section, microbes from mangrove ecosystems have the potential to produce key clinical enzymes that have a great boon for the pharmaceutical industry. Interestingly, apart from the production of enzymes, microbes residing in mangroves have the ability to produce another biogenic substance known as natural pigments. Natural pigments are nontoxic, biodegradable and noncarcinogenic secondary metabolites derived from the natural fauna and flora (Numan et al., 2018). Microbial pigments isolated from mangrove ecosystems thrive in extreme coastal conditions such as high salinity and temperature, which consequently help these pigmented microbes to produce manifold compounds possessing therapeutic benefits (Gopal and Chauhan, 2006). Microbial pigments have been proven to be efficient in controlling numerous pathological disorders and have outstanding biological activities, namely, antibiotic, anticancer, wound healing, and immunosuppressive compounds (Chidambaram et al., 2020).

Heterotrophic bacteria that produce pigments have been reported in mangrove environment, and the source of pigmentation is pivotal to obtain novel secondary metabolites. Pigments are known to safeguard bacterial cells from their environment against extreme temperatures, salinity, and lack of nutrient (Ghizelini et al., 2012). The pigments have biotechnological potential in the pharmaceutical, food, and cosmetics. For example, two novel red-pigmented *Vibrio* strains, MSSRF3T and MSSRF10, isolated from the rhizosphere region of mangrove-associated wild rice (*Porteresia coarctata* Tateoka) were found to exhibit antibacterial activity against phytopathogenic bacteria (Nair, 2007). Twenty antagonistic red-pink pigmented strains were isolated from two different mangrove species, *A. marina* and *R. mucronata*, belonging to the genus *Vibrio* (Nair, 2007). Saha et al. (2017) studied pigment-producing bacteria derived from the mangroves collected from the Sundarbans forests of Bangladesh. Thirty pigmented bacterial strains were isolated with most strains belonging to the genus *Bacillus*, including *B. subtilis, Bacillus firmus, Bacillus pumilus, Bacillus licheniformis, Bacillus pantothenicus, Bacillus lentus, Bacillus acidocaldarius*, and *Bacillus schlegelii*, to cite a few. However, a lack of information was noticed concerning the biological properties of the isolated bacterial pigments by different studies conducted.

In terms of fungal pigments, filamentous fungi are known to produce a vast range of pigments such as carotenoids **phytoene (1)**, α-**carotene (2)**, **lycopene (3)**, β-**carotene (4)**, γ-**carotene (5)**, **melanin (6)**, **flavins (7)**, **phenazine (8)**, **quinone (9)**, **monascin (10)**, **violacein (11)**, and **indigo (12)**. More than 200 fungal species have been recorded to produce carotenoids (Dufossé et al., 2014). Carotenoids are a family of naturally occurring organic pigmented compounds produced not only by bacteria and fungi but also algae and plants. They are highly effective antioxidants and is reported to manage a number of diseases like dementia, cardiovascular diseases, diabetes mellitus, and osteoporosis (Tan and

Norhaizan, 2019). Quinones, including anthracycline antibiotics: **doxorubicin (13)** and **daunorubicin (14)**, are among the most prospective group of natural and synthetic compounds which possess substantially high antitumor activity against several types of tumor cells (Grushevskaya and Krylova, 2018).

Pigments such as **anthraquinone (15)**, **naphthoquinone (16)**, **1,8-dihydroxy naphthalene melanin (17)**, **flavins (7)**, **chrysophanol (18)**, **cynodontin (19)**, **helminthosporin (20)**, **tritisporin (21)**, and **erythroglaucin (22)** were reported by genera, namely, *Eurotium, Fusarium, Curvularia* and *Drechslera* (Babitha, 2009). From known literatures, anthraquinone especially chrysophanol, is widely used in the pharmaceutical industries since it exhibits a variety of biological effects including anticancer, antibacterial, antiviral, neuroprotection, and regulating blood lipids among others (Xie et al., 2019). Despite mangrove-associated fungi produced promising metabolites, experimental data are insufficient yet to understand their therapeutic applications. Regardless of the lack of information, Table 3.3 tends to gather all existing information on both bacterial and fungal pigments isolated from mangrove plants and their respective therapeutic applications and Figs. 3.4—3.6 show the chemical structures of the isolated secondary metabolites/pigments.

Table 3.3 Mangrove bacterial and fungal pigments and their therapeutic applications.

Mangrove-associated microbes	Pigments	Therapeutic applications	References
Bacteria:			
Halobacillus trueperi MXM-16	Carotenoids	Antioxidants	Kharangate-Lad and Bhosle (2016)
Streptomyces sp.	Melanin	Antimicrobial agent	Yasmeen et al. (2017)
Streptomyces xiamenensis	Dark brown pigment	Antimicrobial agent	Das et al. (2014)
Micromonospora sp. K3–13	Blue diffusible pigment	Antimicrobial agent	Abidin et al. (2018)
Streptomyces sp. K2–03	Purple diffusible pigment	Antimicrobial agent	
Talaromyces	Anthraquinone	Neuroprotective agent	Nicoletti et al. (2018)
Streptomyces fradiae	Red pigment	Antioxidant, and hemolytic activity	Chakraborty et al. (2015)
Fungi:			
Penicillium	Brownish red pigment	Antioxidants	Chintapenta et al. (2014)
Eurotium rubrum	Anthraquinone	Antioxidants	Li et al. (2009)

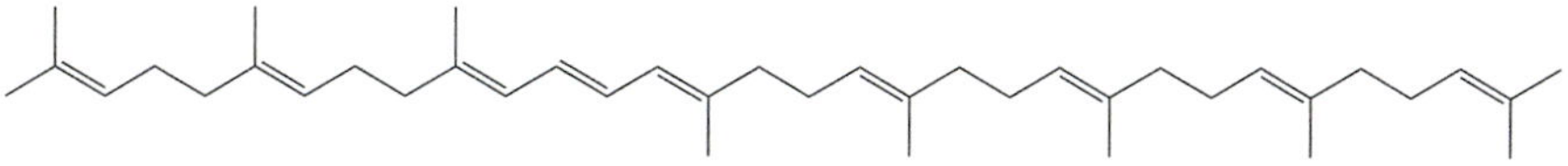

1

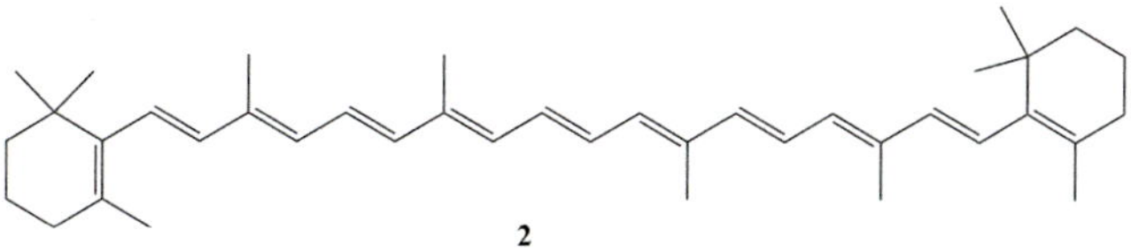

2

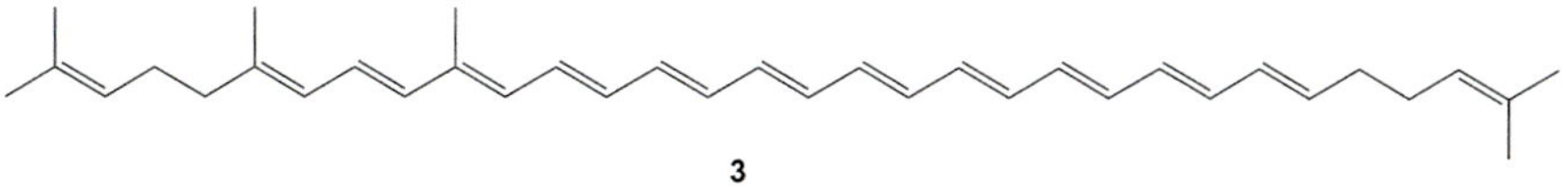

3

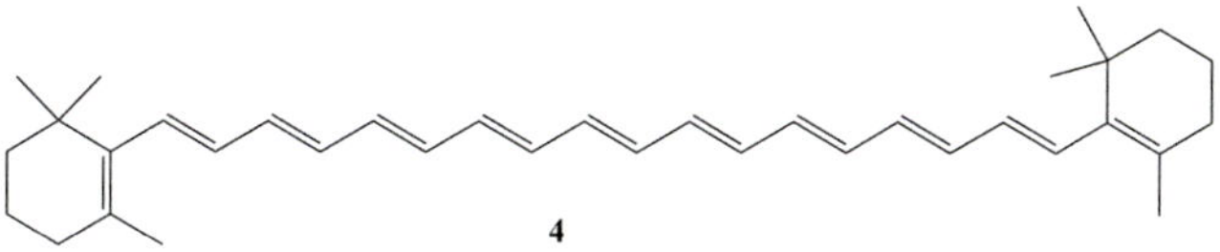

4

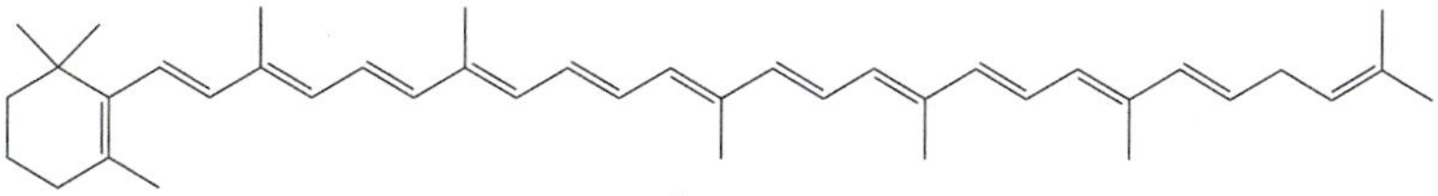

5

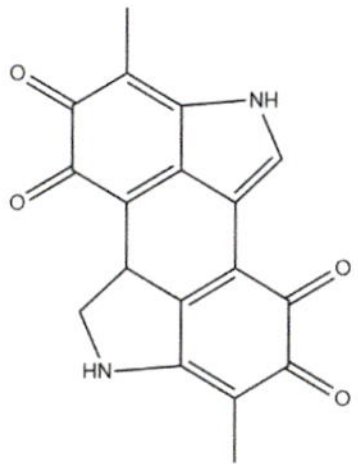

6

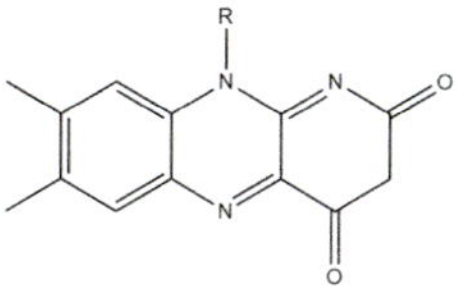

7

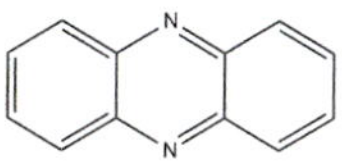

8

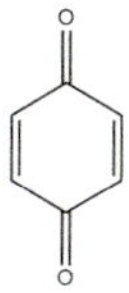

9

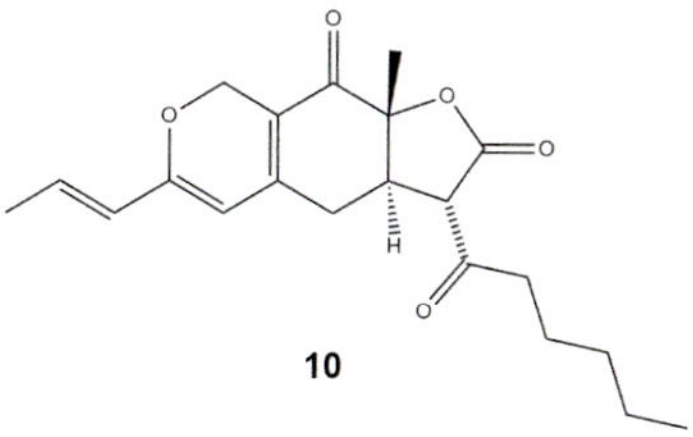

10

FIGURE 3.4

Chemical structures of secondary metabolites isolated from mangrove-associated microbes.

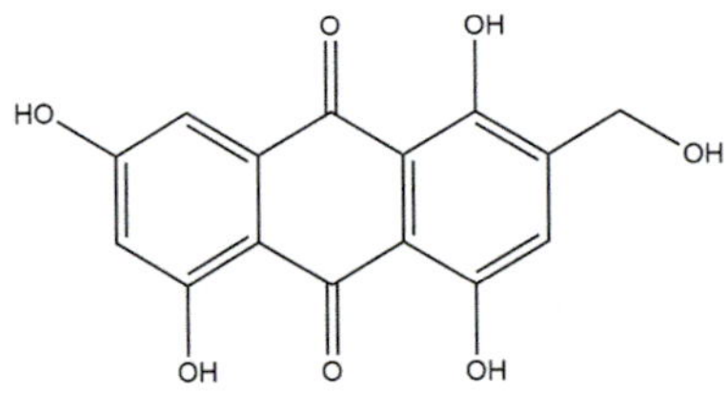

FIGURE 3.5

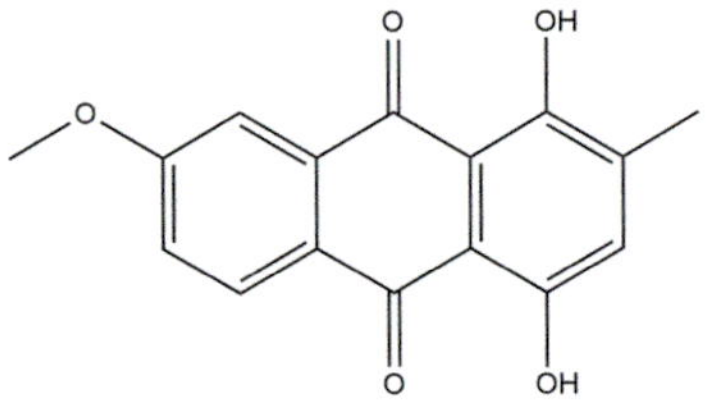

Chemical structures of secondary metabolites isolated from mangrove-associated microbes.

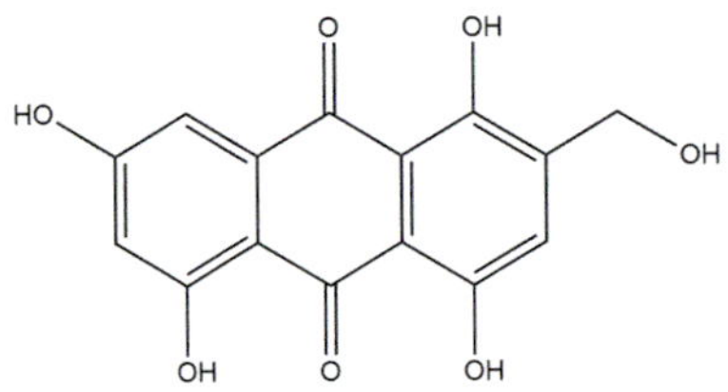

FIGURE 3.6

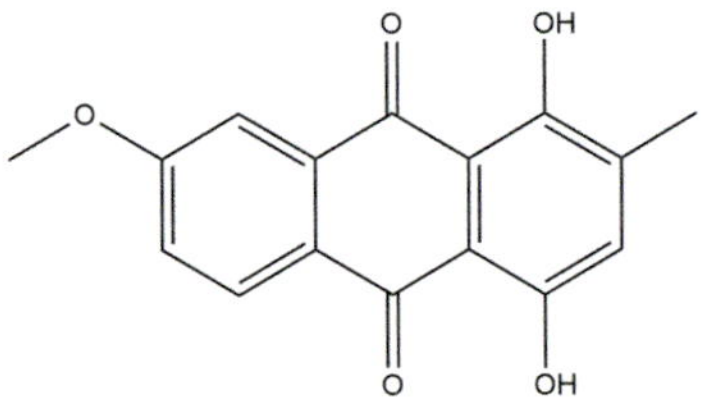

Chemical structures of secondary metabolites isolated from mangrove-associated microbes.

3.6 In vitro production of phytomedicinal secondary metabolites: a ray of hope of novel pharmaceutical drugs from mangroves?

Plant tissue culture is an important area of research in plant biotechnology which eventually lead to the production of a vast number of phytoactive compounds in laboratory conditions. A number of medicinal plants have been successfully introduced into tissue culture to produce biologically active compounds. Typically, these tissue cultures involve either callus cells growing on a semisolid media, or liquid suspension cultures. Both systems, involving the unorganized growth of plant cells, have the advantage of allowing straightforward, continual propagation of cultures and in the case of liquid suspension cells, cell production can be scaled up to high levels using bioreactors. In this respect, suspension cell cultures have the advantage of higher growth rates than callus cultures (Wink, 1999). Moreover, secondary metabolites can be more easily extracted from liquid suspension culture than organized growth systems. Hence, if adequate levels of secondary metabolites can be produced by such system, this would be advantageous for the commercial production of these compounds (Briskin, 2007). Table 3.4 shows some medicinal plant growth and the successful production of secondary metabolites in cell cultures.

Table 3.4 Production of secondary metabolites from some plants in cell cultures (Briskin, 2007).

Plants	Culture type	Secondary metabolites	Pharmacological property
Catharanthus roseus (L.) G.Don	Suspension culture	Vinblastine/ vincristine	Antitumor
Glycyrrhiza glabra L.	Callus culture	Triterpenes	Antiinflammatory
Hypericum perforatum L.	Suspension culture	Hypericins	Antidepressant
Papaver somniferum L.	Suspension culture	Opiates	Anesthetic
Podophyllum hexandrum Royle	Suspension culture	Podophyllotoxin	Antitumor

Unorganized cell systems, such as callus and suspension cells, may lack the biochemical control mechanisms that specify secondary metabolite production, and secondary metabolite production may be restored or elevated with the induction of organized cell growth in organ cultures. Moreover, herbal medicines often represent a complex mixture of secondary metabolites, and cell cultures may not produce the appropriate spectrum and relative levels of secondary metabolites necessary for an effective phytomedicinal preparation. Nevertheless, it has been possible to increase secondary metabolite production in some medicinal plant callus or suspension cultures. The achievement of elevated levels of secondary metabolite production in cell culture can require modification of the growth media components, including levels of plant hormones, the addition of fungal elicitors, or the addition of metabolic precursors for the secondary metabolite (Briskin, 2007; Wink, 1999).

At the time of writing, tissue culture technique is usually applied on mangrove plants but not in terms of metabolite production. For example, micropropagation has been used on B. cylindrica L. with the aim to strengthen large-scale plantation activities toward the conservation and restoration of mangrove forests (Vartak and Shindikar, 2008). Other mangrove species that have been successfully micropropagated are limited to Sesuvium portulacastrum (L.) L., E. agallocha L., A. officinalis L., and Acanthus illicifolius Lour (Al-Bahrany and Al-Khayri, 2003). Studies attempting to produce bioactive compounds from mangrove species using tissue culture are rather scarce, although mangroves produce scads of valuable secondary metabolites due to their extreme coastal conditions, they thrive in. A plethora of studies have showed that mangroves possessed a well-characterized set of phytochemicals. A recent comprehensive review entitled "Ethnopharmacology, Phytochemistry, and Global distribution of Mangroves-A Comprehensive Review" has already successfully gathered a large amount of information on the different compounds identified so far from various mangrove species (Sadeer et al., 2019a). Phytochemicals and pharmacological activities have an undeviating correlation. To cite a few instances, the compound tannin isolated from *B. sexangular* (Lour.) Poir. showed anticancer activity against lung cancer cells (Boopathy and Kathiresan, 2010; Kathiresan et al., 2006). The bark extracts containing the alkaloids; brugine and tropine, and its acetic ester acid was reported to exhibit antitumor activity. Secondary metabolites yielded by *R. mangle* L. also exhibited substantially high activity against carcinomas, melanomas, and lymphomas (Kathiresan et al., 2006). Phytocompounds such as flavonoids, reducing sugars, gums, saponins, and tannins identified from the roots of *B. gymnorhiza* (L.) Lam. are responsible for antinociceptive and antidiarrhea effects (Rahman et al., 1963). The wide spectrum of biogenic substances yielded by mangroves reflects their potential to be projected as unique and effective therapeutic drugs.

With respect to strategies to enhance secondary metabolite production, other useful approaches such as metabolite engineering can be applied. It involves the overexpression of an enzyme (or enzymes) at a key limiting step(s) in a pathway, decreasing the expression of enzymes in competitive pathway branches, increasing an entire pathway through expression of regulatory factors (excluding transcription factors), and the introduction of novel enzymes utilizing a pathway intermediate for the generation of a different secondary metabolite (Oksman-Caldentey and Inzé, 2004; Verpoorte and Memelink, 2002; Verpoorte et al., 2000). At present, a limited number of examples are available where these approaches have been utilized in cell cultures resulting in the enhanced production of secondary products. Moreover, to the best of our knowledge, the usage of metabolite engineering on mangrove plants have not been tried yet, despite studies demonstrated the potential of such application for producing phytomedicinal compounds from medicinal plant cells in culture. For instance, in cell cultures of *Coptis japonica* (Thunb.) Makino, isoquinoline alkaloid metabolism leads to the production of berberine, as well as to other alkaloid components (Wink, 1999). By overexpressing an enzyme located at a key branch point in this pathway (scoulerine 9-Omethyltransferase), Sato et al. (2001) enhanced berberine (and columbamine) production over that of an alternative metabolite, coptisine. Overexpression of this enzyme resulted in a ca. 20% increase in enzyme activity and an elevation of the amount of berberine and columbamine levels ranging from 79% to 91% of the total alkaloid level.

Based on previous evidences on production of compounds by tissue cultures and metabolite engineering and bearing in mind that mangrove is a storehouse of phytocompounds exhibiting essential pharmacological potentialities, we therefore encouraged investigators to conduct such experiments on various species of mangroves with the aim to produce vital biocompounds in large-scale and with the hope to develop efficient therapeutic drugs. Fig. 3.7 illustrates a scheme proposing how mangrove plant culture can be conducted for producing natural medicine.

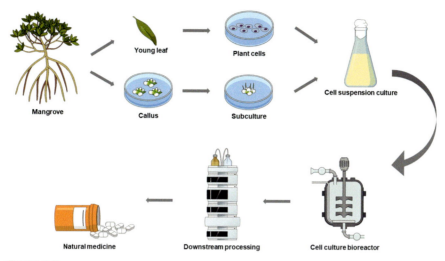

FIGURE 3.7

Proposed schematic depiction of mangrove plant cell suspension culture process for producing natural medicine. The callus produced, can be utilized directly to regenerate plantlets or to extract or manipulate some primary and secondary metabolites. The bioreactor is used to scale-up plant culture system allowing industrial production of secondary metabolites.

3.7 Conclusion

Biotechnology in general is a fast-moving area, and this development can be noticed in the field of pharmaceutical biotechnology. In the different sections of this chapter, we have focused on mangrove plants and have attempted to structure the latest biotechnological developments of these plants. The information collated and shared in this chapter open the door to multiple research questions. Here, the major questions are: How do mangrove plants and pharmaceutical biotechnology fit together, how mangrove as a promising "bio factory" can be used in an integrative drug discovery process, how mangroves can be developed into edible vaccines in the future, how enzymes produced by microorganisms hosted by the plants can be used in pharmacology. This chapter has indeed clearly showed how important it is to integrate mangroves in the biotechnology sector for the manufacturing of drugs or vaccines to continuously help people across the globe confront infectious and noninfectious diseases. Despite being an underexploited species, mangroves possess promising potential and require urgent research attention on a wide array of topics as discussed in detail along the length of this chapter.

Within an open scientific environment, the discovery and development of botanical therapeutics and medicinal plant biotechnology must be accepted, as its expansion is very unlikely to cease. During the compilation of this chapter, we noticed a lack of experimental data connecting biotechnology and mangroves on a comprehensive level that deserves the subject of today. We accepted this lack as a challenge to sort out the needs of the scientific community and to identify valuable topics that must be addressed to provide a narrow and well-defined picture on mangrove plants and pharmaceutical biotechnology. To fill this niche, we encouraged experts from the field of pharmaceutical biology, biotechnology, biochemistry, genetics, pharmacognosy, medicinal chemistry or any other related fields to fully engaged themselves in the investigation of biopharmaceutical applications of mangroves; as experiments can reveal key details on these plants. We therefore conclude that mangroves are worthy of further and continued exploration and development.

References

Abdi, V., Sourinejad, I., Yousefzadi, M., Ghasemi, Z., 2018. Mangrove-mediated synthesis of silver nanoparticles using native *Avicennia marina* plant extract from southern Iran. Chemical Engineering Communications 205, 1069−1076.

Abidin, Z.A.Z., Chowdhury, A.J.K., Malek, N.A., Zainuddin, Z., 2018. Diversity, antimicrobial capabilities, and biosynthetic potential of mangrove actinomycetes from coastal waters in Pahang, Malaysia. Journal of Coastal Research 174−179.

Agarwal, P., 2016. Alpha-amylase inhibition can treat diabetes mellitus. Research & Reviews: Journal of Medical and Health Sciences 5.

Al-Bahrany, A.M., Al-Khayri, J.M., 2003. Micropropagation of grey mangrove *Avicennia marina*. Plant Cell, Tissue and Organ Culture 72, 87−93.

Alamgir, A.N.M., 2018. Biotechnology, In vitro production of natural bioactive compounds, herbal preparation, and disease management (treatment and prevention). Therapeutic use of medicinal plants and their extracts. Volume 2: Phytochemistry and Bioactive Compounds 74, 585−664.

Ali, M.Y., Anuradha, V., Yogananth, N., Rajathilagam, R., Chanthuru, A., Mohamed Marzook, S., 2015. Green synthesis of silver nanoparticle by *Acanthus ilicifolius* mangrove plant against Armigeres subalbatus and Aedes aegypti mosquito larvae. International Journal of Nano Dimension 6, 197−204.

Alshehri, M.A., Trivedi, S., Alanazi, N.A., Panneerselvam, C., Baeshen, R., Alatawi, A., 2020. One-step synthesis of Ag nanoparticles using aqueous extracts from sundarbans mangroves revealed high toxicity on major mosquito vectors and microbial pathogens. Journal of Cluster Science 31, 177−184.

Arias, L.S., Pessan, J.P., Vieira, A.P.M., Lima, T.M.Td, Delbem, A.C.B., Monteiro, D.R., 2018. Iron oxide nanoparticles for biomedical applications: a perspective on synthesis, drugs, antimicrobial activity, and toxicity. Antibiotics 7, 46.

Asghar, M.A., Asghar, M.A., 2020. Green synthesized and characterized copper nanoparticles using various new plants extracts aggravate microbial cell membrane damage after interaction with lipopolysaccharide. International Journal of Biological Macromolecules 160, 1168−1176.

Audipudi, A.V., Pallavi, R., G, D.N.R.S., 2013. Characterization of L-Asparaginase producing bacteria from mangrove soil. International Journal of ChemTech Research 5,
109−112.

Babitha, S., 2009. Microbial pigments. In: S.n.N., P., P., A. (Eds.), Biotechnology for
Agro-Industrial Residues Utilisation. Springer, Dordrecht; Netherlands.

Bakshi, M., Ghosh, S., Chaudhuri, P., 2015. Green synthesis, characterization and antimicrobial potential of sliver nanoparticles using three mangrove plants from Indian
Sundarban. Bionanoscience 5, 162−170.

Balakrishnan, S., Srinivasan, M., Mohanraj, J., 2016. Biosynthesis of silver nanoparticles
from mangrove plant (*Avicennia marina*) extract and their potential mosquito larvicidal
property. Journal of Parasitic Diseases 40, 991−996.

Banerjee, K., Das, S., Choudhury, P., Ghosh, S., Baral, R., Choudhuri, S.K., 2017. A novel
approach of synthesizing and evaluating the anticancer potential of silver oxide nanoparticles in vitro. Chemotherapy 62, 279−289.

Behera, B.C., Mishra, R.R., Singh, S.K., Dutta, S.K., Thatoi, H., 2016. Cellulase from
Bacillus licheniformis and *Brucella* sp. isolated from mangrove soils of Mahanadi river
delta, Odisha, India. Biocatalysis and Biotransformation 34, 44−53.

Beolotto, V., Oliva, M., Marioli, J., Carezzano, M.M.D., 2016. Antimicrobial natural products against bacterial biofilms. In: Kon, K., M, R. (Eds.), Antibiotic Resistance.
Academic Press, London, United Kingdom.

Bhagat, C., Tank, S., Ghelani, A., Dudhagara, P., Patel, R., 2014. Bioremediation of CO2
and characterization of carbonic anhydrase from mangrove bacteria. Journal of
Environmental Science and Technology 7, 76−83.

Bhuvaneswari, R., Xavier, R.J., Arumugam, M., 2017. Facile synthesis of multifunctional
silver nanoparticles using mangrove plant Excoecaria agallocha L. for its antibacterial,
antioxidant and cytotoxic effects. Journal of Parasitic Diseases 41, 180−187.

Bialecka-Florjanczyk, E., Fabiszewska, A.U., Krzyczkowska, J., Kurylowicz, A., 2018. Synthetic
and natural lipase inhibitors. Mini-Reviews in Medicinal Chemistry 18, 672−683.

Bibi, F., Ullah, I., Alvi, S., Bakhsh, S., Yasir, M., Al-Ghamdi, A., et al., 2017. Isolation,
diversity, and biotechnological potential of rhizo-and endophytic bacteria associated
with mangrove plants from Saudi Arabia. Genetics and Molecular Research 16.

Boopathy, N.S., Kathiresan, K., 2010. Anticancer drugs from marine flora: an overview.
Journal of Oncology 2010.

Borm, P.J.A., Robbins, D., Haubold, S., Kuhlbusch, T., Fissan, H., Donaldson, K., et al.,
2006. The potential risks of nanomaterials: a review carried out for ECETOC. Particle
and fibre. Toxicology 3, 11.

Briskin, D.P., 2007. Biotechnological methods for selection of high-yielding cell lines and
production of secondary metabolites in medicinal plants. In: Kayser, O., Quax, W.J.
(Eds.), Medicinal Plant Biotechnology. From Basic Research to Industrial Applications.
Wiley-VCH, Weinheim, Germany.

Castro, R.A., Quecine, M.C., Lacava, P.T., Batista, B.D., Luvizotto, D.M., Marcon, J.,
et al., 2014. Isolation and enzyme bioprospection of endophytic bacteria associated
with plants of Brazilian mangrove ecosystem. SpringerPlus 3, 382.

Chakraborty, I., Redkar, P., Munjal, M., Kumar, S., Rao, B., 2015. Isolation and characterization of pigment producing marine actinobacteria from mangrove soil and applications
of bio-pigments. Der Pharmacia Lettre 7, 93−100.

Chantarasiri, A., 2015. Aquatic *Bacillus cereus* JD0404 isolated from the muddy sediments of mangrove swamps in Thailand and characterization of its cellulolytic activity. Egyptian Journal of Aquatic Research 41, 257–264.

Chiavaroli, A., Sinan, K.I., Zengin, G., Mahomoodally, M.F., Sadeer, N.B., Etienne, O. K., et al., 2020. Identification of chemical profiles and biological properties of Rhizophora racemosa G. Mey. extracts obtained by different methods and solvents. Antioxidants 9, 533.

Chidambaram, V., Rajamanickam, U., Ponnuswamy, R.D., 2020. Biotechnological potential of microbial pigments from mangrove ecosystems: a review. In: Patra, J.K., Mishra, R.R., Thatoi, H. (Eds.), Biotechnological Utilization of Mangrove Resources. Academic Press, Massachusetts; United States.

Chintapenta, L.K., Rath, C.C., Maringinti, B., Ozbay, G., 2014. Pigment production from a mangrove Penicillium. African Journal of Biotechnology 13.

Chugh, H., Sood, D., Chandra, I., Tomar, V., Dhawan, G., Chandra, R., 2018. Role of gold and silver nanoparticles in cancer nano-medicine. Artificial Cells, Nanomedicine, and Biotechnology 46, 1210–1220.

Das, S.K., Behera, S., Patra, J.K., Thatoi, H., 2019. Green synthesis of sliver nanoparticles using *Avicennia officinalis* and *Xylocarpus granatum* extracts and in vitro evaluation of antioxidant, antidiabetic and anti-inflammatory activities. Journal of Cluster Science 30, 1103–1113.

Das, A., Bhattacharya, S., Mohammed, A.Y.H., Rajan, S.S., 2014. In vitro antimicrobial activity and characterization of mangrove isolates of streptomycetes effective against bacteria and fungi of nosocomial origin. Brazilian Archives of Biology and Technology 57, 349–356.

Das, D., Goyal, A., 2014. Pharmaceutical enzymes. In: Kaur, S., Singh, G.D., Soccol, C.R. (Eds.), Biotransformation of Waste Biomass into High Value Biochemicals. Springer New York, United States.

Das, S.K., Thatoi, H., 2020. Mangrove plant: mediated green synthesis of nanoparticles and their pharmaceutical applications: an overview. In: Patra, J.K., Mishra, R.R., Thatoi, H. (Eds.), Biotechnological Utilzation of Mangrove Resources. Academic Press, Massachusetts; United States.

Davidson, M.B., 2014. Insulin analogs—is there a compelling case to use them? No! Diabetes Care 37, 1771–1774.

Dhas, S., Mukerjhee, A., Chandrasekaran, N., 2013. Phytosynthesis of silver nanoparticles using *Ceriops tagal* and its antimicrobial potential against human pathogens. International Journal of Pharmacy and Pharmaceutical Sciences 5, 349–352.

Dufossé, L., Fouillaud, M., Caro, Y., Mapari, S.A.S., Sutthiwong, N., 2014. Filamentous fungi are large-scale producers of pigments and colorants for the food industry. Current Opinion in Biotechnology 26, 56–61.

Gayathri, G.A., Mahalingam, G., 2020. Vaccines from mangrove microbes. In: Patra, J.K., Mishra, R.R., Thatoi, H. (Eds.), Biotechnological Utilization of Mangrove Resources. Academic Press, Massachusetts.

Ghizelini, A.M., Mendonça-Hagler, L.C.S., Macrae, A., 2012. Microbial diversity in Brazilian mangrove sediments: a mini review. Brazilian Journal of Microbiology 43, 1242–1254.

Gnanadesigan, M., Anand, M., Ravikumar, S., Maruthupandy, M., Ali, M.S., Vijayakumar, V., et al., 2012. Antibacterial potential of biosynthesised silver nanoparticles using *Avicennia marina* mangrove plant. Applied Nanoscience 2, 143–147.

Gopal, B., Chauhan, M., 2006. Biodiversity and its conservation in the Sundarban Mangrove Ecosystem. Aquatic Sciences 68, 338−354.

Gouda, S., Das, G., Sen, S.K., Thatoi, P., Patra, J.K., 2015. Mangroves, a potential source for green nanoparticle synthesis: a review. International Journal of Molecular Sciences 44, 635−645.

Grushevskaya, H.V., Krylova, N.G., 2018. Carbon nanotubes as a high-performance platform for target delivery of anticancer quinones. Current Pharmaceutical Design 24, 5207−5218.

Gunasekaran, B., Gothandam, K.M., 2020. A review on edible vaccines and their prospects. Brazilian Journal of Medical and Biological Research 53.

Gurudeeban, S., Satyavaniand, K., Ramanathan, T., 2011. Production of extra cellular-amylase using *Bacillus megaterium* isolated from white mangrove (*Avicennia marina*). Asian. Journal of Biotechnology 3, 310−316.

Immaculatejeyasanta, K., Madhanraj, P., Jamila, P., Panneerselvam, A., 2011. Case study on the extra cellular enzyme of marine fungi associated with mangrove driftwood of Muthupet Mangrove, Tamil Nadu, India. Journal of Pharmacy Research 4, 1385−1387.

Janeček, Š., Svensson, B., MacGregor, E.A., 2014. α-Amylase: an enzyme specificity found in various families of glycoside hydrolases. Cellular and Molecular Life Sciences 71, 1149−1170.

Jayaseelan, C., Rahuman, A.A., Rajakumar, G., Kirthi, A.V., Santhoshkumar, T., Marimuthu, S., et al., 2011. Synthesis of pediculocidal and larvicidal silver nanoparticles by leaf extract from heartleaf moonseed plant, Tinospora cordifolia Miers. Parasitology Research 109, 185−194.

Job, N., Manomi, S., Philip, R., 2015. Isolation and characterisation of endophytic fungi from *Avicennia officinalis*. International Journal of Biomedical Research 5, 4−8.

Joel, E.L., Bhimba, B.V., 2012. Production of alpha amylase by mangrove associated fungi Pestalotiopsis microspora strain VB5 and *Aspergillus oryzae* strain. International Journal of Molecular Sciences 41, 279−VB283.

Julsing, M.K., Quax, W.J., Kayser, O., 2007. The engineering of medicinal plants: prospects and limitations of medicinal plant biotechnology. In: Kayser, O., Quax, W.J. (Eds.), Medicinal Plant Biotechnology. From Basic Research to Industrial Applications. Wiley-VCH, Weinheim, Germany.

Kanchana, R., Correia, D., Sarkar, S., Gawde, P., Rodrigues, A., 2011. Production and partial characterization of cholesterol oxidase from Micrococcus sp. isolated from Goa, India. International Journal of Applied Biology and Pharmaceutical Technology 2, 393−398.

Karpagavinayagam, P., Prasanna, A.E.P., Vedhi, C., 2020. Eco-friendly synthesis of nickel oxide nanoparticles using *Avicennia Marina* leaf extract: morphological characterization and electrochemical application. Materials Today: Proceedings .

Kathiresan, K., Boopathy, N.S., Kavitha, S., 2006. Coastal vegetation—an underexplored source of anticancer drugs. Natural Product Reports 5, 115−119.

Kathiresan, K., Gomathi, V., Anburaj, R., Saravanakumar, K., 2014. Impact of mangrove vegetation on seasonal carbon burial and other sediment characteristics in the Vellar-Coleroon estuary. Indian Journal of Medical Research 25, 787−794.

Kathiresan, K., Manivannan, S., 2006. Alpha-Amylase production by Penicillium fellutanum isolated from mangrove rhizosphere soil. African Journal of. Biotechnology 5, 829−832.

Kathiresan, K., Saravanakumar, K., Anburaj, R., Gomathi, V., Abirami, G., Sahu, S.K., et al., 2011. Microbial enzyme activity in decomposing leaves of mangroves. International Journal of Advanced Biotechnology 2, 382−389.

Kayser, O., Warzecha, H., 2012. Pharmaceutical biotechnology and industrial applications – Learning lessons from molecular biology. In: Kayser, O., Warzecha, H. (Eds.), Pharmaceutical Biotechnology: Drug Discovery and Clinical Applications. Wiley-VCH, Weinheim, Germany.

Kharangate-Lad, A., Bhosle, S., 2016. Studies on siderophore and pigment produced by an adhered bacterial strain Halobacillus trueperi MXM-16 from the mangrove ecosystem of Goa, India. Indian Journal of Microbiology 56, 461−466.

Kiranmayi, M.U., Poda, S., Vijayalakshmi, M., 2014. Production and optimization of L-asparaginase by an actinobacterium isolated from Nizampatnam mangrove ecosystem. Journal of Environmental Biology 35, 799.

Kumaran, N.S., 2018. In vitro anti-inflammatory activity of silver nanoparticle synthesized *Avicennia marina* (Forssk.) Vierh.: a green synthetic approach. International Journal of Green Pharmacy 12.

Kumar, V.A., Ammani, K., Jobina, R., Parasuraman, P., Siddhardha, B., 2016. Larvicidal activity of green synthesized silver nanoparticles using *Excoecaria agallocha* L. (Euphorbiaceae) leaf extract against *Aedes aegypti*. IET Nanobiotechnology 10, 382−388.

Kumar, S., Rajeshkumar, S., 2018. Plant-based synthesis of nanoparticles and their impact. In: Tripathi, D.K., Ahmad, P., Sharma, S., Chauhan, D.K., Dubey, N.K. (Eds.), Nanomaterials in Plants, Algae, and Microorganisms. Academic Press, Massachusetts.

Lin, L.T., Hsu, W.C., Lin, C.C., 2014. Antiviral natural products and herbal medicines. Journal of Traditional and Complementary Medicine 4, 24−35.

Li, D.-L., Li, X.-M., Wang, B.-G., 2009. Natural anthraquinone derivatives from a marine mangrove plant-derived endophytic fungus *Eurotium rubrum*: structural elucidation and DPPH radical scavenging activity. Journal of Microbiology and Biotechnology 19, 675−680.

Luo, W., Lilian, L.P.V., Jones, E.B.G., 2005. Screening of marine fungi for lignocellulose-degrading enzyme activities. Botanica Marina 48, 379−386.

Mahomoodally, M.F., Sadeer, N., Edoo, M., Venugopala, K.N., 2020. The potential application of novel drug delivery systems for phytopharmaceuticals and natural extracts−current status and future perspectives. Mini Reviews in Medicinal Chemistry .

Maria, G.L., Sridhar, K.R., Raviraja, N.S., 2005. Antimicrobial and enzyme activity of mangrove endophytic fungi of southwest coast of India. Journal of Agricultural Science and Technology 1, 67−80.

Mauricio, M., Guerra-Ojeda, S., Marchio, P., Valles, S., Aldasoro, M., Escribano-Lopez, I., et al., 2018. Nanoparticles in medicine: a focus on vascular oxidative stress. Oxidative medicine and Cellular Longevity 2018.

Mayanglambam, C.S., Singh, A.K., Singh, S., Ngathem, T.C., Lukram, S., Yengkhom, D. S., et al., 2020. Enzymes from mangrove endophytes and their biotechnological/industrial applications. In: Patra, J.K., Mishra, R.R., Thatoi, H. (Eds.), Biotechnological Utilization of Mangrove Resources. Academic Press, Massachusetts.

Mtui, G., Masalu, R., 2008. Extracellular enzymes from brown-rot fungus Laetiporus sulphureus isolated from mangrove forests of coastal Tanzania. Scientific Research and Essays 3, 154−161.

Nabikhan, A., Rathinam, S., Kandasamy, K., 2017. Biogenic gold nanoparticles for reduction of 4-nitrophenol to 4-aminophenol: an eco-friendly bioremediation. IET Nanobiotechnology 12, 479−483.

Nagababu, P., Rao, V.U., 2017. Pharmacological assessment, green synthesis and characterization of silver nanoparticles of *Sonneratia apetala* buch.-ham. leaves. Journal of Applied Pharmaceutical Science 7, 175−182.

Naidu, K.S.B., Murugan, N., Adam, J., 2019. Biogenic synthesis of silver nanoparticles from *avicennia marina* seed extract and its antibacterial potential. Bionanoscience 9, 266−273.

Nair, S., 2007. *Vibrio rhizosphaerae* sp. nov., a red-pigmented bacterium that antagonizes phytopathogenic bacteria. International Journal of Systematic and Evolutionary Microbiology 57, 2241−2246.

Nathan, V.K., Ammini, P., Vijayan, J., 2018. Photocatalytic degradation of synthetic dyes using iron (III) oxide nanoparticles (Fe2O3-Nps) synthesised using *Rhizophora mucronata* Lam. IET Nanobiotechnology 13, 120−123.

Nicoletti, R., Salvatore, M.M., Andolfi, A., 2018. Secondary metabolites of mangrove-associated strains of Talaromyces. Marine Drugs 16, 12.

Numan, M., Bashir, S., Mumtaz, R., Tayyab, S., Rehman, N.U., Khan, A.L., et al., 2018. Therapeutic applications of bacterial pigments: a review of current status and future opportunities. 3 Biotech 8, 207-207.

Oksman-Caldentey, K.-M., Inzé, D., 2004. Plant cell factories in the post-genomic era: new ways to produce designer secondary metabolites. Trends in Plant Science 9, 433−440.

Patel, I., Kracher, D., Ma, S., Garajova, S., Haon, M., Faulds, C.B., et al., 2016. Salt-responsive lytic polysaccharide monooxygenases from the mangrove fungus *Pestalotiopsis* sp. NCi6. Biotechnology for Biofuels 9, 108.

Pierpont, T.M., Limper, C.B., Richards, K.L., 2018. Past, present, and future of Rituximab-The world's first oncology monoclonal antibody therapy. Frontiers in Oncology 8, 163-163.

Pillaiyar, T., Manickam, M., Namasivayam, V., 2017. Skin whitening agents: medicinal chemistry perspective of tyrosinase inhibitors. Journal of Enzyme Inhibition and Medicinal Chemistry 32, 403−425.

Pointing, S.B., Buswell, J.A., Jones, E.B.G., Vrijmoed, L.L.P., 1999. Extracellular cellulolytic enzyme profiles of five lignicolous mangrove fungi. Mycological Research 103, 696−700.

Prakash, M., 2013. Isolation and screening of degrading enzymes from mangrove derived fungi. International Journal of Current Microbiology and Applied Sciences 2, 127−129.

Purkait, R., Purkayastha, R., 1996. Pectolytic enzyme activities of some foliar fungi isolated from mangrove plants and their response to tannin. Indian Phytopathology 49, 366−372.

Raghukumar, C., Raghukumar, S., Chinnaraj, A., Chandramohan, D., D'Souza, T., Reddy, C., 1994. Laccase and other lignocellulose modifying enzymes of marine fungi isolated from the Coast of India. Botanica Marina 37, 515−524.

Rahman, M., Ahmed, A., Shahid, I., 1963. Phytochemical and pharmacological properties of Bruguiera gymnorrhiza roots extract. International Journal of Pharmaceutical Research 3, 63−67.

Rajeshkumar, S., Menon, S., Venkat Kumar, S., Tambuwala, M.M., Bakshi, H.A., Mehta, M., et al., 2019. Antibacterial and antioxidant potential of biosynthesized copper nanoparticles mediated through Cissus arnotiana plant extract. Journal of Photochemistry and Photobiology B: Biology 197, 111531.

Ramalingam, V., Dhinesh, P., Sundaramahalingam, S., Rajaram, R., 2019. Green fabrication of iron oxide nanoparticles using grey mangrove *Avicennia marina* for antibiofilm activity and in vitro toxicity. Surfaces and Interfaces 15, 70−77.

Ramteke, L., Jadhav, B., Gawali, P., 2018. Biogenic copper nanoparticles from the aqueous stem extract of Ceriops tagal. World Journal of Pharmaceutical Research 7, 933–947.

ReportLinker, 2021. Erythropoietin (EPO) global market report 2020-30: COVID-19 growth and change. Available from: <https://www.globenewswire.com/fr/new-release/2020/12/21/2148559/0/en/Erythropoietin-EPO-Global-Market-Report-2020-30-COVID-19-Growth-and-Change.html> (accessed 27.03.21).

Rohrmann, S., Molitoris, H.P., 1986. Morphological and physiological adaptions of the cyphellaceous fungus *Halocyphina villosa* (Aphyllophorales) to its marine habitat. Botinica Marina 29, 539–547.

Rudzik, R., Clancy, R., Perey, D., Day, R., Bienenstock, J., 1975. Repopulation with IgA-containing cells of bronchial and intestinal lamina propria after transfer of homologous Peyer's patch and bronchial lymphocytes. The Journal of Immunology 114, 1599–1604.

Sadeer, N.B., Fawzi, M.M., Gokhan, Z., Rajesh, J., Nadeem, N., Kannan, R.R.R., et al., 2019a. Ethnopharmacology, phytochemistry, and global distribution of mangroves-a comprehensive review. Marine Drugs 17 (9), 231.

Sadeer, N.B., Rocchetti, G., Senizza, B., Montesano, D., Zengin, G., Uysal, A., et al., 2019b. Untargeted metabolomic profiling, multivariate analysis and biological evaluation of the true mangrove (*Rhizophora mucronata* Lam.). Antioxidants 8, 489.

Sadeer, N.B., Sinan, K.I., Cziáky, Z., Jekő, J., Zengin, G., Jeewon, R., et al., 2020. Assessment of the pharmacological properties and phytochemical profile of *Bruguiera gymnorhiza* (L.) Lam using in vitro studies, in silico docking, and multivariate analysis. Biomolecules 10 (5), 731.

Sadeesh, K.R., Rajesh, R., Gokulakrishnan, S., Subramanian, J., 2015. Screening and characterization of fibrinolytic protease producing *Bacillus circulans* from mangrove sediments Pitchavaram, South East Coast of India. International Letters of Natural Sciences 1, 10–16.

Saha, M.L., Afrin, S., Sony, S.K., Islam, M.N., 2017. Pigment producing soil bacteria of Sundarban mangrove forest. Bangladesh Journal of Botany 46, 717–724.

Sahoo, K., Dhal, N., Das, R., 2014. Production of amylase enzyme from mangrove fungal isolates. African Journal of Biotechnology 13, 4338–4346.

Sahoo, A., Mandal, A.K., Dwivedi, K., Kumar, V., 2020. A cross talk between the immunization and edible vaccine: current challenges and future prospects. Life Sciences 261, 118343.

Salata, O.V., 2004. Applications of nanoparticles in biology and medicine. Journal of Nanobiotechnology 2, 1–6.

Sato, F., Hashimoto, T., Hachiya, A., Tamura, K.-i, Choi, K.-B., Morishige, T., et al., 2001. Metabolic engineering of plant alkaloid biosynthesis. Proceedings of the National Academy of Sciences 98, 367–372.

Satyavani, K., Gurudeeban, S., Ramanathan, T., 2014. Influence of leaf broth concentration of *Excoecaria agallocha* as a process variable in silver nanoparticles synthesis. Journal of Nanomedicine Research 1, 11.

Sengupta, A., Anwesha, B., Verma, S.K., Sarkar, A., 2020. Industrial applications of enzymes derived from Indian mangroves. In: Patra, J.K., Mishra, R.R., Thatoi, H. (Eds.), Biotechnological Utilization of Mangrove Resources. Academic Press, Massachusetts; United States.

Shakoor, S., Rao, A.Q., Shahid, N., Yaqoob, A., Samiullah, T.R., Shakoor, S., et al., 2019. Role of oral vaccines as an edible tool to prevent infectious diseases. Acta Virologica 63, 245–252.

Shome, R., Shome, B., 2001. Microbial L−asparaginase from mangroves of Andaman Islands. I.J.M.S 30, 183−184.

Singh, M., Kumar, M., Kalaivani, R., Manikandan, S., Kumaraguru, A., 2013. Metallic silver nanoparticle: a therapeutic agent in combination with antifungal drug against human fungal pathogen. Bioprocess and Biosystems Engineering 36, 407−415.

Soares, J.F.L., Dias, A.C.F., Fasanella, C.C., Taketani, R.G., Lima, A.Od.S., Melo, I.S., et al., 2013. *Endo*-and exoglucanase activities in bacteria from mangrove sediment. Brazilian Journal of Microbiology 44, 969−976.

Sohrab, S.S., 2020. An edible vaccine development for coronavirus disease 2019: the concept. Clinical and Experimental Vaccine Research 9, 164−168.

Sriramulu, M., Shanmugam, S., Ponnusamy, V.K., 2020. *Agaricus bisporus* mediated biosynthesis of copper nanoparticles and its biological effects: an in-vitro study. Colloid and Interface Science Communications 35, 100254.

Stapleton, P.A., Nurkiewicz, T.R., 2014. Vascular distribution of nanomaterials. Wiley Interdisciplinary Reviews: Nanomedicine and Nanobiotechnology 6, 338−348.

Syed Ali, M.Y., Anuradha, V., Yogananth, N., Rajathilagam, R., Chanthuru, A., Mohamed Marzook, S., 2015. Green synthesis of silver nanoparticle by *Acanthus ilicifolius* mangrove plant against Armigeres subalbatus and Aedes aegypti mosquito larvae. International Journal of Nano Dimension 6, 197−204.

Tan, B.L., Norhaizan, M.E., 2019. Carotenoids: how effective are they to prevent age-related diseases? Molecules (Basel, Switzerland) 24.

Thatoi, H., Behera, B.C., Mishra, R.R., Dutta, S.K., 2013. Biodiversity and biotechnological potential of microorganisms from mangrove ecosystems: a review. Annals of Microbiology 63, 1−19.

Thatoi, P., Kerry, R.G., Gouda, S., Das, G., Pramanik, K., Thatoi, H., et al., 2016. Photomediated green synthesis of silver and zinc oxide nanoparticles using aqueous extracts of two mangrove plant species, *Heritiera fomes* and *Sonneratia apetala* and investigation of their biomedical applications. Journal of Photochemistry and Photobiology B: Biology 163, 311−318.

Thenmozhi, C., Sankar, R., Karuppiah, V., Sampathkumar, P., 2011. L-asparaginase production by mangrove derived *Bacillus cereus* MAB5: optimization by response surface methodology. Asian Pacific Journal of Tropical Medicine 4, 486−491.

Tian, S., Saravanan, K., Mothana, R.A., Ramachandran, G., Rajivgandhi, G., Manoharan, N., 2020. Anti-cancer activity of biosynthesized silver nanoparticles using *Avicennia marina* against A549 lung cancer cells through ROS/mitochondrial damages. Saudi. Journal of Biological Sciences 27, 3018−3024.

Umashankari, J., Inbakandan, D., Ajithkumar, T.T., Balasubramanian, T., 2012. Mangrove plant, *Rhizophora mucronata* (Lamk, 1804) mediated one pot green synthesis of silver nanoparticles and its antibacterial activity against aquatic pathogens. Aquatic biosystems 8, 1−7.

Usha, R., Mala, K., Venil, C., Muthusamy, P., 2011. Screening of actinomycetes from mangrove ecosystem for L-asparaginase activity and optimization by response surface methodology. Polish Journal of Microbiology 60, 213−221.

Vartak, V., Shindikar, M., 2008. Micropropagation of a rare mangrove *Bruguiera cylindrica* L. towards conservation. Indian Journal of Biotechnology 7.

Varunkumar, K., Anusha, C., Saranya, T., Ramalingam, V., Raja, S., Ravikumar, V., 2020. *Avicennia marina* engineered nanoparticles induce apoptosis in adenocarcinoma lung cancer cell line through p53 mediated signaling pathways. Process Biochemistry 94, 349−358.

Venugopal, M., Saramma, A.V., 2008. An alkaline protease from *Bacillus circulans* BM15, newly isolated from a mangrove station: characterization and application in laundry detergent formulations. Indian Journal of Microbiology 47, 298.

Verpoorte, R., der Heijden, Van, Memelink, J., R., 2000. Engineering the plant cell factory for secondary metabolite production. Transgenic Research 9, 323−343.

Verpoorte, R., Memelink, J., 2002. Engineering secondary metabolite production in plants. Current Opinion in Biotechnology 13, 181−187.

Volesky, B., Luong, J.H.T., Aunstrup, K., 1984. Microbial enzymes: production, purification, and isolation. Critical Reviews in Biotechnology 2, 119−146.

Wink, M., 1999. Functions of Plant Secondary Metabolites and their Exploitation in Biotechnology. CRC Press, Boca Raton, FL.

Xie, L., Tang, H., Song, J., Long, J., Zhang, L., Li, X., 2019. Chrysophanol: a review of its pharmacology, toxicity and pharmacokinetics. Journal of Pharmacy and Pharmacology 71, 1475−1487.

Yasmeen, S., Muvva, V., Munaganti, R., 2017. Isolation and characterization of bioactive Streptomyces from mangrove eco-system of Machilipatnam, Krishna District, Andhra Pradesh. Asian Journal of Pharmaceutical and Clinical Research 9, 258.

Zangeneh, M.M., Ghaneialvar, H., Akbaribazm, M., Ghanimatdan, M., Abbasi, N., Goorani, S., et al., 2019. Novel synthesis of *Falcaria vulgaris* leaf extract conjugated copper nanoparticles with potent cytotoxicity, antioxidant, antifungal, antibacterial, and cutaneous wound healing activities under in vitro and in vivo condition. Journal of Photochemistry and Photobiology B: Biology 197, 111556.

Mangroves and their associated fungal endophytes: a prolific source of novel phytochemicals

4

4.1 Introduction

The use of medicinal plants leads to the detection and advancement of modernized therapeutics to treat different varieties of ailments, and they are the potential source for natural products (Venieraki et al., 2017). Plants are considered to be the "bio-factories" by pharmaceutical biology in generating potent compounds with therapeutic values. The coexistence of diverse microbes with plants can lead to both benefit and plague. As the inter organismal interaction continues, it results in the intense condition of the symbiotic and parasitic association (Baker and Satish, 2012). All over the world, the use of medicinal plants has rapidly increased due to the rising need for secondary metabolites, herbal drugs, and natural health products. From 1981 to 2014, more than 51% natural products based small molecule drugs were approved (Venieraki et al., 2017). For thousands of years, natural products such as metabolites and by-products of plants, animals and microbes are overworked to be used for human needs.

A special term is used when we refer to microorganisms present in plants; we use the term "endophyte". Endophytes are defined as microorganisms, classified as bacteria or fungi or actinomycetes, which spend their whole or part of their life cycle in the inter or intracellular tissues of different plant parts (stems, petioles, roots, leaves) without causing any diseases to their host plants (Singh, 2019; Tan and Zou, 2001). Importantly, like any other living organism, plants are flexible and can adapt themselves and integrate with a different environment by strategically facing external stresses. For instance, the healthy growth and complex adaptative response of plants, often categorized as an intelligent response by a few authors (Chamovitz, 2018; Trewavas, 2005), is associated with this world of microbes. This exquisite and complex way of adapting to an ever-changing environment has attracted the attention of several scientists. It is intriguing to notice that even after 500 million years of evolution, plants still need the assistance of the endophytic community to be able to resist stress toler-ance, including climate change and adapt themselves to their continuously changing environments (Deng and Cao, 2017) (Fig. 4.1). This adaptation behav-ior is directly buttressed by the production of bioactive compounds known as sec-ondary metabolites (Singh, 2019). The endophytes survive on the nutrients produced by the plants and in return, these endophytes yielded functional metabo-lites for their host plants. There is a positive linear relationship between endophytes and their host plants in terms of the production of these bioactive compounds (Palanichamy et al., 2018). The presence of secondary metabolites in plants has interested many researchers for many years due to the influential pharmacological properties that they possess.

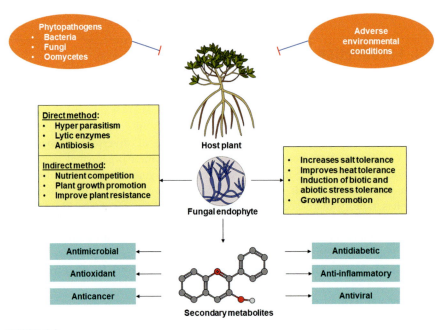

FIGURE 4.1

A representation of endophytic fungal association with mangrove plant as their host. The different roles that endophytes have toward their host are in terms of plant growth, defense system, salt and heat tolerance. Endophytes produce secondary metabolites that exhibit potential pharmacological activity.

Ever since the landmark discovery of paclitaxel from endophytic *Taxomyces andreanae*, plant endophytes have been the fountainheads of bioactive second-ary metabolites with potential application in medicine, agriculture, and food industry. In the last two decades, lead molecules with antimicrobial, anticancer, antioxidant, and antiinflammatory properties have been successfully discovered from endophytic microorganisms. Many researchers started to select medicinal plants having ethnobotanical importance and to target their fungal endophytes and investigate the set of phytochemicals present (Verma et al., 2011), as it is believed that these endophytes could produce phytochemicals having medicinal abilities similar to their host plants (Schulz et al., 2002). Strikingly, although endophytes are acknowledged for their biological potentialities, they are recognized as a poorly explored group of microorganisms (Bhardwaj and Agrawal, 2014). Microbiological research in mangroves has received relatively little attention, in comparison with the classical ecological, hydrological and biogeochemical studies.

Various mangrove species are traditionally used as a remedy against a wide array of diseases, namely, diabetes, hypertension, snake bites, gastrointestinal disorders (diarrhea, constipation, dysentery, dyspepsia), rheumatism, fever, hematuria, hepatitis, toothache, oral infection, among others. There are a considerable number of pharmacological studies conducted on mangroves with antioxidant, antimicrobial and antidiabetic reported as the most common assays (Sadeer et al., 2019). However, it is acknowledged that there is a paucity of studies on endophytic fungi associated with mangrove plants (Chaeprasert et al., 2010). Research showed that only 1%−2% of the plant species have been investigated for their associated endophytic fungi, mostly in terrestrial hosts and neglecting aquatic plants like mangroves (Khare et al., 2018). The mangrove community is recognized as a wealthy storehouse of novel fungal endophytes and they represent the second-largest ecological subgroup of marine fungi and more than 200 species have already been isolated and identified (Chaeprasert et al., 2010; Debbab et al., 2013; Li and Weng, 2017). Interestingly, the symbiotic relationship that exists between endophytes and their host plants or environments triggers the production of further bioactive compounds. The environment in which a plant survives affects the endophytes population (Tan and Zou, 2001). Since mangroves thrive in a harsh coastal condition it is vital to probe into these plant species to discover what type of functional metabolites they possess. Therefore, in the current chapter, we will discuss the various fungal endophytes as a novel bioresource of pharmacologically important phytochemicals.

4.2 Natural products from endophytes

Endophytic fungi represent one of the virtual prolific sources of new natural products. Discovery of novel natural products from marine organisms, including plants is an ongoing challenge and a continuing need as long as diseases are not being alleviated significantly. The bioactive metabolites produced by endophytes represent a goldmine of information for our health. Sharma et al. (2018) stated that the compounds yielded by endophytes have economic importance toward human beings as antibiotics. Marine fungi are considered as a storehouse of peptides (Sun et al., 2019). Along the same line, mangrove endophytic fungi have attracted much attention solely due to its ability to produce a unique and unprecedented plethora of secondary metabolites. Generally, endophytes are known to produce several bioactive potentialities, including phenols, steroids, xanthones, tetralones, terpenoids, isocoumarins, benzopyrones, phenols, enniatines, and ergosterol. The metabolites are recognized as vital compounds for the plants since they are produced to compete with neighboring pathogens which consequently explained why these phytocompounds displayed significant antimicrobial properties (Singh, 2019).

In the past few years, studies related to the isolation and characterization of phytocompounds have significantly increased. Interestingly, mangrove-derived fungi have attracted the attention of the pharmaceutical community since it is acknowledged that metabolites yield by mangrove endophytes are structurally unique and pharmacologically important (Wang et al., 2014b). Liu et al. (2018a) isolated a new 10-membered macrolactone, hypoxylide, from the fungal endophyte *Annulohypoxylon* sp. originated from the mangrove species, *Rhizophora racemosa* G. Mey. Similarly, in another study, Liu et al. (2018b) isolated two new 2, 3-diaryl indone derivatives such as (+)-ascomindone D and (-)-ascomindone D and two prenylated polyketides, namely, ascomfurans C and ascomarugosin A isolated from the endophytic fungus *Ascomycota* sp. SK2YWS-L of *Kandelia candel* (L.) Druce. Wu et al. (2015) isolated two novel phytochemicals, namely, (Z)-7, 40-dimethoxy-6-hydroxy-aurone-4-O-b-glucopyranoside and (1S, 3R, 4S)-1-(40-hydroxyl-phenyl)-3,4-dihydro-3,4,5-trimethyl-1H-2-benzopyran-6,8-diol. These compounds showed good neuroprotective activity in PC12 cells. Furthermore, Bai et al. (2014) recovered *Aspergillus flavipes* AIL8 from *Acanthus ilicifolius* L. and isolated two novel aromatic butyrolactones, namely, flavipesins A and B. These results showed that mangrove endophytic fungi are potential sources of novel compounds and need further exploration for other possibilities. Table 4.1 summarizes other fungal strains isolated till date from different parts of mangrove species. The chemical structures of compounds isolated from mangrove fungal endophytes are illustrated in Figs. 4.2—4.25. The following section elaborates on the biological activities exhibited by different fungal endophytes identified in various mangrove species.

Table 4.1 Phytochemical profiles of endophytic fungi from different mangrove species.

Mangrove species (Family)	Region/ country	Plant part (s)	Endophytic fungi	Phytochemical constituents	References
Acanthus ilicifolius L. (Acanthaceae)	Southwest coast of India	L	*Alternaria chlamydosporus, Aspergillus*	NI	Lobo et al. (2005)
		St	*Aspergillus*	NI	
		R	*Pestalotiopsis*, sterile isolate (MSI 1)	NI	
	Guangdong Province, China	L	*Aspergillus flavipes* AIL8	Flavipesins A (**1**) and B (**2**), phenyl dioxolanone (**3**), meroterpenoids	Bai et al. (2014)
	NI	NI	*Aspergillus flavipes*	Cytochalasins Z_{16}-Z_{20} (**4**–**8**)	Lin et al. (2009)
	Thailand	L	*Phyllosticta, Cladosporium, Colletotrichum, Phomopsis, Xylaria*	NI	Chaeprasert et al. (2010)
	Guangdong Province, China	L	*Lasiodiplodia*	β-resorcylic acid derivatives	Chen et al. (2015)
	Guangxi Province, China	L	*Talaromyces stipitatus* SK-4	Tararomyones A (**9**) and B (**10**)	Cai et al. (2017)
	South China	NI	*Penicillium*	Penicinoline (**11**)	Salini (2014)
		B	*Diaporthe phaseolorum*	10H-chromeno[3,2-c] pyridine (**12**), diaporphasines A-D (**13**–**16**), isoindolinone (**17**), meyeroguillines C (**18**) and D (**19**), meyeroguilline A (**20**), 5-deoxybostrycoidin (**21**), fusaristatin A (**22**)	Cui et al. (2017)

(Continued)

Table 4.1 Phytochemical profiles of endophytic fungi from different mangrove species. *Continued*

Mangrove species (Family)	Region/ country	Plant part (s)	Endophytic fungi	Phytochemical constituents	References
	NI	NI	Cumulospora marina, Pestalotiopsis	Flavonoids, terpenes steroids, triterpenoidal saponins (stigmasterol)	Eldeen and Effendy (2013)
Acanthus ebracteatus Vahl (Acanthaceae)	West Kalimantan, Indonesia	B	Pseudocosmospora sp. Bm-1–1	Cosmosporin A (**23**), 6-carboxy-cosmosporin A (**24**), rel-(6aS,10aR)-Δ⁹-tetrahydrocannabiorcolic acid B (**25**), cannabiorcichromenic acid (**26**), decarboxy-cannabiorcichromenic acid (**27**), rel-(6aS,10aR)-decarboxy-Δ⁹-tetrahydrocannabiorcolic acid B (**28**)	Nakamura et al. (2019)
Aegiceras corniculatum (L.) Blanco (Aegicerataceae)	Beibu Gulf, China	L	Colletotrichum, Alternaria, Phomopsis, Pestalotiopsis, Guignardia, Cladosporium, Glamerella	NI	Bin et al. (2014)
	Fujian Province, China	L	Fusarium incarnatum HKI00504	Pyrrole alkaloids: N-[4-(2-formyl-5-hydroxymethyl-pyrrol-1-yl)-butyl]-acetamide (**29**), N-[5-(2-formyl-5-hydroxymethyl-pyrrol-1-yl)-pentyl]-acetamide (**30**), Indole derivative: (3aR,8aR)-3a-acetoxyl-1,2,3,3a,8,8a-hexahydropyrrolo-[2,3-b]indole (**31**), N-acetyltryptamine A (**32**)	Li et al. (2008)
	Southern China	L, Tw	Pestalotiopsis humus, Leptosphaerulina chartarum, Phomopsis, Hortaea weneckii, Cladosporium perangustum, Lophiostoma, Alternaria	NI	Li et al. (2016)

	NI	alternate, Mycosphaerella, Phyllosticta, Dothideomycetes, Leptosphaerulina, Passalora, Phomopsis, Phyllosticta capitalensis, Phomopsis azadirachtae, Pseudopletania, Creosphaeria sassafras, Fusarium striatum, Hypoxylon investiens, Neofusicoccum parvuum, Phomopsis, Rhizopycnis, Sporormiaceae, Xylaria		
South China	NI	Streptomyces sp. (gt-20026114), Penicillium	Cyclopentenone derivatives, polyketides	Lin et al. (2010)
Fujian Province, China	NI	Norcardiopsis sp. a00203	Norcardiatones A-C (**33–35**)	
NI	NI	Streptomyces	p-aminoacetophenonic acids: (E)-11-(4′-aminophenyl)-5, 9-dihydroxy-4,6,8-trimethyl-11-oxo-undec-2-enoic acid (**36**), 9-(4′-aminophenyl)-3,7-dihydroxy-2,4,6-trimethyl-9-oxo-nonoic acid (**37**), (2E)-11-(4′-aminophenyl)-5, 9-O-cyclo-4,6,8-trimethyl-11-oxo-undec-2-enoic acid (**38**), 9-(4′-aminophenyl)-3,7-O-cyclo-2,4,6-trimethyl-9-oxo-nonoic acid (**39**)	Salini (2014)
NI	NI	Cladosporium sphaerospermum	Amino acids, benzoquinones, carbohydrates, carotenoids, tannins, coumarins, flavonoids, polyphenols, proteins, sugars,	Eldeen and Effendy (2013)

(Continued)

Table 4.1 Phytochemical profiles of endophytic fungi from different mangrove species. *Continued*

Mangrove species (Family)	Region/ country	Plant part (s)	Endophytic fungi	Phytochemical constituents	References
Acrostichum aureum L. (Pteridaceae)	Southwest coast of India	NI	*Acrenaonium, Aspergillus, Fusarium, Nigrospora oryzae, Penicillium, Trichoderma, Tritrachium*	saponins, triterpenes glycosides, p-aminoacetophenonic acids, citrinin (**40**), quinolactacin	Lobo et al. (2005)
	Guangxi Province, China	NI	*Aspergillus ustus*	Drimane sesquiterpene	Salini (2014)
	NI	L, P, Rh, R	*Acremonium, Alternaria chlamydosporus, Alternaria, Aspergillus, Cumulospora marina Schmidt, Cytospora, Dicyma, Fusarium oxysporum, Nigrospora oryzae, Schl. ex Fries, Paecilomyces puntoni, Paecilomyces, Penicillium, Phoma, Pestalotiopsis, Trichoderma*	NI	Lobo et al. (2005)
Avicennia marina (Forssk.) Vierh. (Acanthaceae)	NI	NI	*Xylaria, Hypocrea lixii*	Alcohols, amino acids, carbohydrates, fatty acids, hydrocarbons, inorganic salts, minerals, phytoalexins, carboxylic acids, steroids, tannins, triterpenes, vitamins, n-hexadecanoic acid, cyclic peptides: xyloketals, xyloallenolides	Eldeen and Effendy (2013)

Location	L	Species	Compounds	Reference
Oman	L	Unidentified	Farinomaleins C–E (**41**–**43**)	El Amrani et al. (2012)
Hainan Province, China	NI	*Aspergillus niger* MA-132	Nigerapyrones A–H (**44**–**51**), asnipyrones A (**52**) and B (**53**)	Liu et al. (2011)
Jiulong river estuary, Fujian Province, China	NI	*Dothiorella* sp. HTF3	Cytosporone B (**54**)	Salini (2014)
Southern China	L, Tw	*Phomopsis, Phomopsis azadirachtae, Leptosphaerulina chartarum, Phyllostica capitalensis, Pyronema, Fusarium equiseti, Hypoxylon investiens, Alternaria alternate, Cladosporium perangustum, Hortaea werneckii, Leptosphaeruline, Sordariomycetes*	NI	Li et al. (2016)
Mai Po, Hong Kong	S	*Xylaria*	Xyloketals A-I (**55**–**63**), Xyloallendide A (**64**) and B (**65**), steroids, esters, lactones	Zhu et al. (2009)
NI	NI	*Penicillium brocae* MA-231	Brocazines A-F (**66**–**71**)	Meng et al. (2015)
Hainan Island, China	NI	*Penicillium brocae* MA-231	Penicibrocazine A-E (**72**–**76**), epicoccin A (**77**), phomazine A (**78**), Hexahydro-2-hydroxy-1-phenyl-1*H*-pyrrolizin-3-one (**79**)	Meng et al. (2017)

(Continued)

Table 4.1 Phytochemical profiles of endophytic fungi from different mangrove species. *Continued*

Mangrove species (Family)	Region/ country	Plant part (s)	Endophytic fungi	Phytochemical constituents	References
	Karankadu, India	L	*Aspergillus awamari, Aspergillus favipes, Aspergillus chevalieri, Aspergillus flavus, Aspergillus clavatus, Aspergillus fumigates, Penicillium candidum, Penicillium japonicum, Penicillium purpurogenum, Phomopsis*	NI	Bharathidasan and Panneerselvam (2015)
	Hong Kong	S	Endophytic fungus no. 2106	No. 2106A (**80**), cyclo-(N-MeVal-N-MeAla) (**81**)	Wang et al. (2008)
	NI	NI	*Penicillium citrinum*	(Z)-7,4′-dimethoxy-6-hydroxyaurone-4-O-β-glucopyranoside (**82**), (-)-4-O-(4-O-β-D-glucopyranosylcaffeoyl) quinic acid (**83**)	Liu et al. (2015)
	Fujian Province, China	NI	*Penicillium* sp. FJ-1	4-(20,30-dihydroxy-30-methyl butanoxy)-phenethanol (**84**), 15-hydroxyl-6α,12-epoxy-7b,10aH,11bH-spiroax-4-ene-12-one (**85**)	Zheng et al. (2014)
Avicennia officinalis L. (Acanthaceae)	Ernakulam, Kerala, India	L, St	*Aspergillus, Penicillium, Acremonium, Curumlaria, Cladosporium, Phoma, Fusarium, Sterile mycelia, Candida*	NI	Job et al. (2015)
	NI	NI	*Hypocrea lixii* VB1	NI	Salini (2014)

Bruguiera sexangula var. rhynchopetala W. C. Ko (Rhizophoraceae)	Hainan Island, China	NI	Nigrospora	Anthraquinones	Salini (2014)
	Qinglan Port, Hainan Province, China	R	Penicillium sp. 091402	(3R*,4S*)-6,8-dihydroxy-3,4,7-trimethylisocoumarin (86), (3R,4S)-6,8-dihydroxy-3,4,5-trimethylisocoumarin (87), (3R,4S)-6,8-dihydroxy-3,4,5,7-tetramethylisochroman (88), (S)-3-(3',5'-dihydroxy-2',4'-methylphenyl) butan-2-one (89), Phenol A (90), 3,4,5-trimethyl-1,2-benzenediol (91)	Han et al. (2009)
	Dong Zhai Gang, Hainan Province, China	L	Penicillium sp. B21	Penicitrinone acetate	Deng and Cao (2017)
	South China sea	NI	Penicillium citrinum HL-5126	4-chloro-1-hydroxy-3-methoxy-6-methyl-8-methoxycarbonyl-xanthen-9-one (92), 2'-acetoxy-7-chlorocitreorosein (93)	He et al. (2017)
	Hainan, China	B	Pestalotiopsis foedan	[(3R,4R,6R,7S)-7-hydroxyl-3,7-dimethyl-oxabicyclo [3.3.1] nonan-2-one (94), (3R, 4R)-3-(7-methylcyclohexenyl)-propanoic acid (95)	Xu et al. (2016)

(Continued)

Table 4.1 Phytochemical profiles of endophytic fungi from different mangrove species. *Continued*

Mangrove species (Family)	Region/ country	Plant part (s)	Endophytic fungi	Phytochemical constituents	References
	South China sea	NI	*Penicillium citrinum* HL-5126	(2R*,4R*)-3,4-dihydro-5-methoxy-2-methyl-2H-1-benzopyran-4-ol (**96**)	Zheng et al. (2014)
	South China sea	NI	*Stemphylium* sp. 33231	Infectopyrones A (**97**) and B (**98**)	Zhou et al. (2014)
	Dong Zhai, Hainan province, China	NI	*Pestalotiopsis clavispora*	(15α)-15-hydroxysoyasapogenol B (**99**), (7β,15α)-7,15-dihydroxysoyasapogenol B (**100**), (7β)-7,29-dihydroxysoyasapogenol B (**101**)	Luo et al. (2011)
	South coast of China	NI	*Pestalotiopsis, Phomopsis*	NI	Xing and Guo (2011)
Bruguiera sexangula (Lour.) Poir. (Rhizophoraceae)	Chaung Tha, Myanmar	NI	*Chalaropsis*	NI	Phyo (2011)
	NI	NI	NI	Phenolics, steroids, alkaloids, tannins	Salini (2014)
	NI	NI	*Streptomyces*	Xiamycin (**102**)	Salini (2014)
Bruguiera gymnorhiza (L.) Lam. (Rhizophoraceae)	NI	St	*Streptomyces* sp. GT2002/1503	Xiamycin (**102**), methyl ester (**103**)	Ding et al. (2010)
	NI	NI	*Penicillium citrinum*	(Z)-7,4'-dimethoxy-6-hydroxy-aurone-4-O-β-glucopyranoside	Wu et al. (2015)

Host plant	Location	Tissue	Fungal species	Compounds	References
Ceriops tagal (Perr.) C. B. Rob. (Rhizophoraceae)	Fujian province, China	St, B	*Penicillium* sp. GD6	(82), (1S, 3R,4S)-1-(4'-hydroxyl-phenyl)-3,4-dihydro-3,4,5-trimethyl-1H-2-benzopyran-6,8-diol (104)	Jiang et al. (2018)
	Zhanjiang, China	B	*Penicillium sclerotiorum*	2-deoxy-sohirnone C (105), 5S-hydroxynorvalineS-Ile (106), 3S-hydroxylcyclo(S-Pro-S-Phe) (107), cyclo(S-Phe-S-Gln) (108)	Li et al. (2014)
	Zhanjiang, Guangdong, China	NI	*Penicillium* sp. GD6	(+)-cyclopenol (109), 3-(dimethylaminomethyl)-1-(1,1-dimethyl-2-propenyl) indole (110), anacine (111), aurantiomide C (112), viridicatin (113), 3-O-methylviridicatin (114), verrucosidin (115), ergosterol (116), ergosterol peroxide (117)	Zhou et al. (2014)
	Zhanjiang, China	L	*Aspergillus*	Penibruguieramine A (118), scalusamide A (119), meleagrin (120), roquefortine F (121)	Li et al. (2012)
	South China sea	NI	*Penicillium* sp. FJ-1	Aspergillumarins A (122) and B (123)	Jin et al. (2013)
	NI	NI	*Fusarium*	7-hydroxy-deoxytalaroflavone (124), deoxytalaroflavone (125)	Lv et al. (2015)
	Hainan Island, China	B	*Coriolopsis* sp. J5	Cyclic depsipeptides: W493 A (126), B (127), C (128) and D (129), 5-(3-methoxy-3-oxopropyl)-furan-2-carboxylic acid (130), 1-(5-(2-hydroxypropanoyl)-furan-2-yl)-pentan-3-one (131),	Chen et al. (2017)

(Continued)

Table 4.1 Phytochemical profiles of endophytic fungi from different mangrove species. *Continued*

Mangrove species (Family)	Region/country	Plant part (s)	Endophytic fungi	Phytochemical constituents	References
	Dong Zhai Gang, Hainan province, China	L	Endophytic fungus J3	2-hydroxy-1-(5-(1-hydroxypentyl)-furan-2-yl)-propan-1-one (**132**), 1-(5-(1,2-dihydroxypropyl)-furan-2-yl)-pentan-1-one (**133**), 5-(1-hydroxypent-4-en-1-yl)-furan-2-carboxylic acid (**134**), 5-(3-hydroxypentyl)-furan-2-carboxylic acid (**135**), 5-(1-hydroxypentyl)-furan-2-carboxylic acid (**136**), (E)-5-(2-carboxyvinyl)-furan-2-carboxylic acid (**137**)	Zeng et al. (2015)
Excoecaria agallocha L. (Euphorbiaceae)	Wenchang, Hainan, China	St	*Cladosporium* sp. OUCMDZ-302	2α-hydroxyxylaranol B (**138**), 4β-hydroxyxylaranol B (**139**), 3, 4-seco-sonderianol (**140**)	Wang et al. (2018)
	NI	NI	*Penicillium expansum*	Polyketides	Salini (2014)
	Guangxi province, China	B	*Aspergillus versicolor* SYSU-SKS025	Expansols A (**141**) and B (**142**) 3-arylisoindolinone enantiomers: (+)-asperglactam A (**143**), (−)-asperglactam A (**144**), nor-bisabolane enantiomers: (+)-1-hydroxyboivinianic acid (**145**), (−)-1-hydroxyboivinianic acid (**146**)	Cui et al. (2018)

Host plant (family)	Plant part	Location	Endophytic fungus	Secondary metabolites	References
	St	South China sea	*Phomopsis* sp. ZSU-H76	Phomopsin A (**147**), B (**148**) and C (**149**), cytosporone B (**150**) and C (**151**), 5-hydroxy-6,8-dimethoxy-2-benzyl-4H-naphtho[2,3-β]-pyran-4-one (**152**), 5,7-dihydroxy-2-methylbenzopyran-4-one (**153**), 3,5-dihydroxy-2,7-dimethylbenzopyran-4-one (**154**), cyclo (Tyr-Tyr) (**155**)	Huang et al. (2008); Huang et al. (2010)
	NI	NI	*Lasiodiplodia* sp. 318	(R)-ethyl 35-dihydroxy-7-(8-hydroxynonyl) benzoate (**156**), ethyl-2,4-dihydroxy-6-(8-oxononyl) benzoate (**157**), (R)-Zearalane (**158**), 2,4-dihydroxy-6-nonylbenzoate (**159**), (R)-de-O-methyllasiodiplodin (**160**)	Huang et al. (2017)
Heritiera littoralis Aiton (Sterculiaceae)	NI	NI	*Penicillium expansum* 091006	Expansols C–F (**161–164**), 3-O-methyldiorcinol (**165**)	Wang et al. (2012)
	R	Samut Sakhon province, Thailand	*Penicillium chermesinum*	TMC-264 (**166**), penicilliumolide B (**167**)	Darsih et al. (2015)
Heritiera fomes Buch.-Ham. (Sterculiaceae)	NI	Sundarbans, Bangladesh	*Pestalotia*	Xylitol (**168**), oxysporone (**169**)	Nurunnabi et al. (2018)
Lumnitzera racemosa Willd. (Combretaceae)	R	WenChang in Hainan Island, China	*Penicillium sumatrense* MA-92	Sumalarins A (**170**), B (**171**), C (**172**)	Meng et al. (2013)

(Continued)

Table 4.1 Phytochemical profiles of endophytic fungi from different mangrove species. *Continued*

Mangrove species (Family)	Region/ country	Plant part (s)	Endophytic fungi	Phytochemical constituents	References
Kandelia candel (L.) Druce (Rhizophoraceae)	Q'iao island, Zhuhai, China	NI	*Talaromyces*	7-epiaustdiol (**173**), 8-O-methylepiaustdiol stemphyperylenol (**174**), secalonic acid A (**175**)	Salini (2014)
	Hong Kong	L	Endophytic fungus 1962	Cyclic depsipeptides: cyclo-(Leu-Tyr) (**176**), cyclo-(Phe-Gly) (**177**), cyclo-(Leu-Leu) (**178**)	Huang et al. (2007)
	South China Sea	Ba	*Sporothrix* sp. KAC-1985	Sporothrin A (**179**), B (**180**) and C (**181**), 3-methoxy-6-methyl-1,2-benzenediol (**182**), 5-hydroxy-2-methyl-4-chromanone (**183**), 5-carboxymellein (**184**), diaporthin (**185**), 7-chloro-2',5,6-trimethoxy-6'-methylspiro[benzofuran-2(3*H*),1'-(2) cyclohexene]-3,4'-dione (**186**), 7-methylbenzofuran-2-carboxylate (**187**), cerevisterol (**188**), peroxyergosterol (**189**), 1,8-dihydroxy-4-methylanthraquinone (**190**), cytochalasin IV (**191**), 3,5-dimethylphenol (**192**), 1,8-dimethoxynaphthalene (**193**), 1-hydroxy-8-methoxynaphthalene (**194**), 1,8-dihydroxy-5-methoxy-3-methyl-9*H*-xanthen-9-one (**195**), ergosterol (**196**), cyclo(L-Leu-L-Pro) (**197**,	Wen et al. (2013)

Location	Type	Source	Compounds	Reference
			cyclo-L-phenylalanyl-L-alanine (**198**), 2,4-dihydroxypyrimidine (**199**)	
Southern China	B	*Pestalotiopsis vaccinii* cgmcc3.9199	Vaccinols J–S (**200–209**)	Wang et al. (2017)
Daya Bay, Shenzhen, Guangdong Province, China	F	*Botryosphaeria* sp. SCSIO KcF6	Botryosphaerin A (**210**) and B (**211**), botryoisocoumarin A (**212**)	Ju et al. (2015)
Nl	St	*Streptomyces* sp. HKI0595	Kandenols A – E (**213–217**)	Ding et al. (2012)
South China Sea	R	*Nigrospora* sp. strain No. 1403	Methyl 3-chloro-6-hydroxy-2-(4-hydroxy-2-methoxy-6-methylphenoxy)-4-methoxybenzoate (**218**), (2S,5'R,E)-7-hydroxy-4,6-dimethoxy-2-(1-methoxy-3-oxo5-methylhex-1-enyl)-benzofuran-3(2H)-one (**219**), griseofulvin (**220**), dechlorogriseofulvin (**221**), bostrycin (**222**), deoxybostrycin (**223**)	Xia et al. (2011)
South China Sea	L	Endophytic fungus ZZF13, *Guignardia* sp. 4382	(+)-(**224**) and (-)-ascomindone D (**225**), ascomfurans C (**226**), ascomarugosin A (**227**)	Liu et al. (2018b)
Fujian Province, China	L	*Phomopsis* sp. A123	Phomopsidone A (**228**)	Zhang et al. (2014b)
South China Sea	Nl	*Diaporthe phaseolorum* var. *sojae*	Lactones: 1893A (**229**), 1893B (**230**)	Cheng et al. (2008)

(Continued)

Table 4.1 Phytochemical profiles of endophytic fungi from different mangrove species. *Continued*

Mangrove species (Family)	Region/ country	Plant part (s)	Endophytic fungi	Phytochemical constituents	References
	Fujian Province, China	St	*Streptomyces griseus* subsp.	7-(4-aminophenyl)-2,4-dimethyl-7-oxo-hept-5-enoic acid (**231**), 9-(4-aminophenyl)-7-hydroxy-2,4,6-trimethyl-9-oxo-non-2-enoic acid (**232**), 12-(4-aminophenyl)-10-hydroxy-6-(1-hydroxyethyl)-7,9-dimethyl-12-oxo-dodeca-2,4-dienoic acid (**233**)	Guan et al. (2005)
	Guangxi Province, China	L	*Penicillium sp.* sk5GW1L	Arigsugacin I (**234**), arigsugacin F (**235**), territrem B (**236**)	Huang et al. (2013)
	Hong Kong	L	Isolate 1850	Sterigmatocystin (**237**), dihydrosterigmatocystin (**238**), secosterigmatocystin (**239**)	Zhu and Lin (2007)
	South China Sea	L	*Penicillium sp.* ZH58	4-(methoxymethyl)-7-methoxy-6-methyl-1(3H)-isobenzofuranone (**240**), lumichrome (**241**), curvulari (**242**), 5,5'-oxy-dimethylene-bis(2-furaldehyde) (**243**), chromone (**244**), harman(1-methyl-β-carboline) (**245**), N9-methyl-1-methyl-β-carboline (**246**)	Yang et al. (2013)
Kandelia obovata Sheue, H. Y. Liu and J. Yong (Rhizophoraceae)	NI	NI	*Aspergillus terreus* H010	Aspterpenacids A (**247**) and B (**248**)	Liu et al. (2016)

Plant (family)	Location		Fungal source	Compounds	References
Rhizophora annamalayana Kathiresan (Rhizophoraceae)	Vellar estuary, India	L	*Fusarium oxysporum*	Taxol (**249**)	Elavarasi et al. (2012)
Rhizophora mucronata Lam. (Rhizophoraceae)	NI	NI	*Pestalotiopsis* sp. JCM2A4	Pestalotiopyrones A–H (**250**–**257**), pestalotiopisorin A (**258**), pestalotiollides A–B (**259**–**260**), pestalotiopin A (**261**), pestalotiopamides A–D (**262**–**265**), nigrosporapyrone D (**266**), *p*-hydroxy benzaldehyde (**267**), cytosporones J–L (**268**–**270**)	Xu et al. (2011); Xu et al. (2009)
	Hainan Island, China	L	*Pestalotiopsis* sp. JCM2A4	Tetradecanoic acid (**271**), nonanoic acid (**272**), pentadecanoic acid (**273**), suberic acid monomethyl ester (**274**), tetrahydroedulan (**275**)	Li et al. (2013)
Rhizophora racemosa G. Mey, (Rhizophoraceae)	NI	NI	*Phomopsis* sp. IM 41–1	Phomoxanthone A (**276**), 12-*O*-deacetyl-phomoxanthone A (**277**)	Shiono et al. (2013)
	NI	NI	*Annulohypoxylon*	Hypoxylide (**278**)	Liu et al. (2018b)
Rhizophora stylosa Griff. (Rhizophoraceae)	NI	L	*Aspergillus nidulans* MA-143	Aniquinazolines A–D (**279**–**282**)	Chun-Yan et al. (2013)
	Hainan Island, China	L	*Penicillium oxalicum* EN-201	Penioxamide A (**283**), 18-hydroxydecaturin B (**284**)	Zhang et al. (2015)

(Continued)

Table 4.1 Phytochemical profiles of endophytic fungi from different mangrove species. *Continued*

Mangrove species (Family)	Region/ country	Plant part (s)	Endophytic fungi	Phytochemical constituents	References
	China	L	*Aspergillus nidulans* MA-143	Isoversicolorin C (**285**), isosecosterigmatocystin (**286**) and glulisine A (**287**)	Yang et al. (2018)
Sonneratia laba Sm. (Lythraceae)	China	L	*Alternaria*	Xanalteric acids I (**288**) and II (**289**)	Kjer et al. (2009)
Xylocarpus granatum J. Koenig (Meliaceae)	Hainan Province, China	L	*Trichoderma* sp. Xy24	(9R, 10R)-dihydro-harzianone (**290**), harzianelactone (**291**)	Zhang et al. (2014a); Zhang et al. (2016)
	Thailand	L	Endophytic fungus XG8D	Merulinols A—G (**292**—**298**)	Choodej et al. (2016)
	Thailand	L	*Phomopsis* sp. xy21	Phomoxanthones F-K (**299**—**304**)	Hu et al. (2018)

B, Branch; *Ba*, bark; *F*, fruit; *L*, leaf; *NI*, not indicated; *R*, root; *Rh*, rhizome; *S*, seed; *St*, stem; *St B*, stem bark; *Tw*, twig.

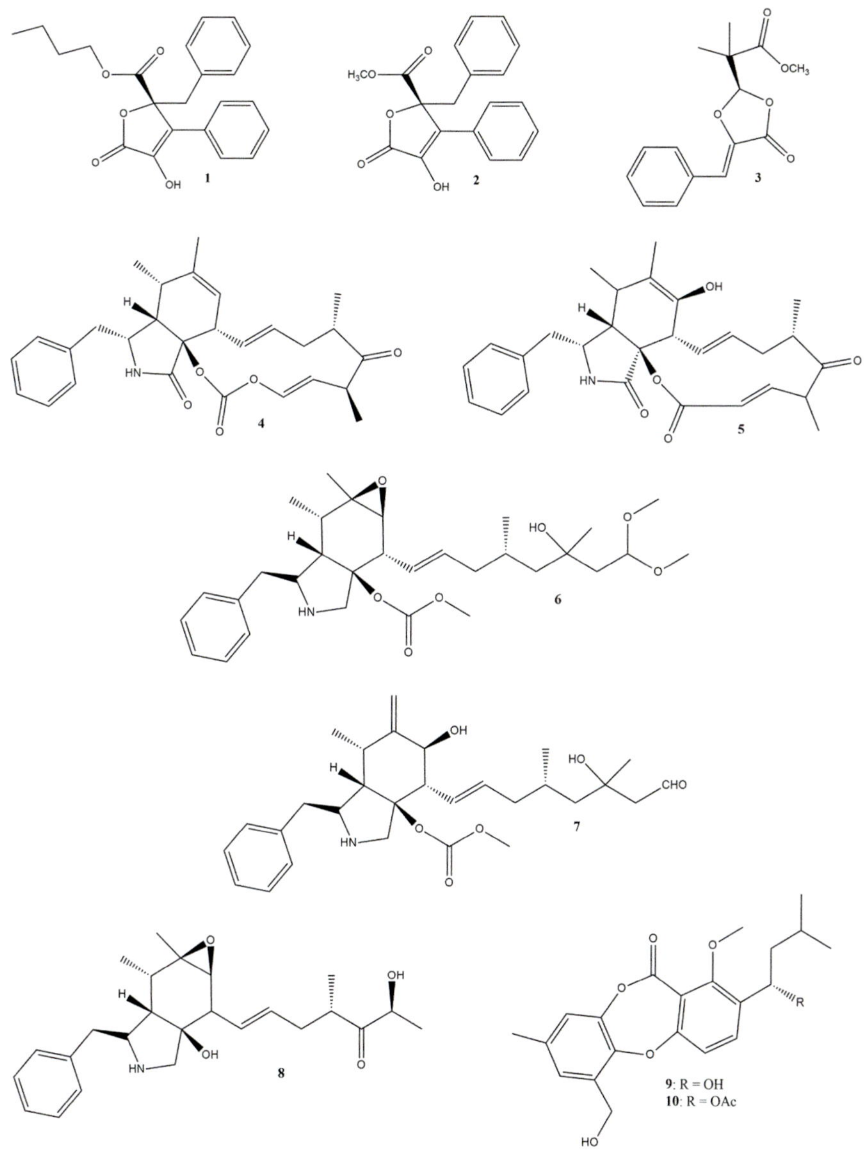

FIGURE 4.2

Chemical structures of compounds 1−10 isolated from fungal endophytes of mangroves.

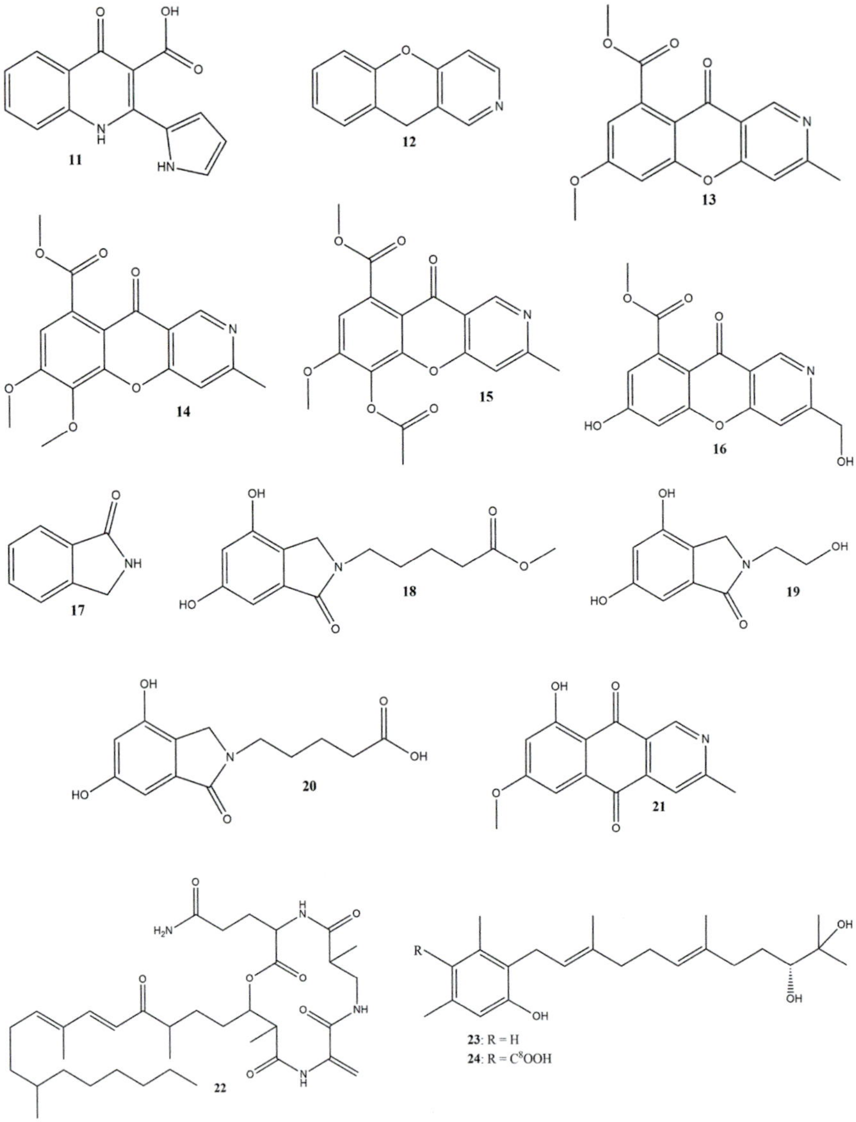

FIGURE 4.3

Chemical structures of compounds 11–24 isolated from fungal endophytes of mangroves.

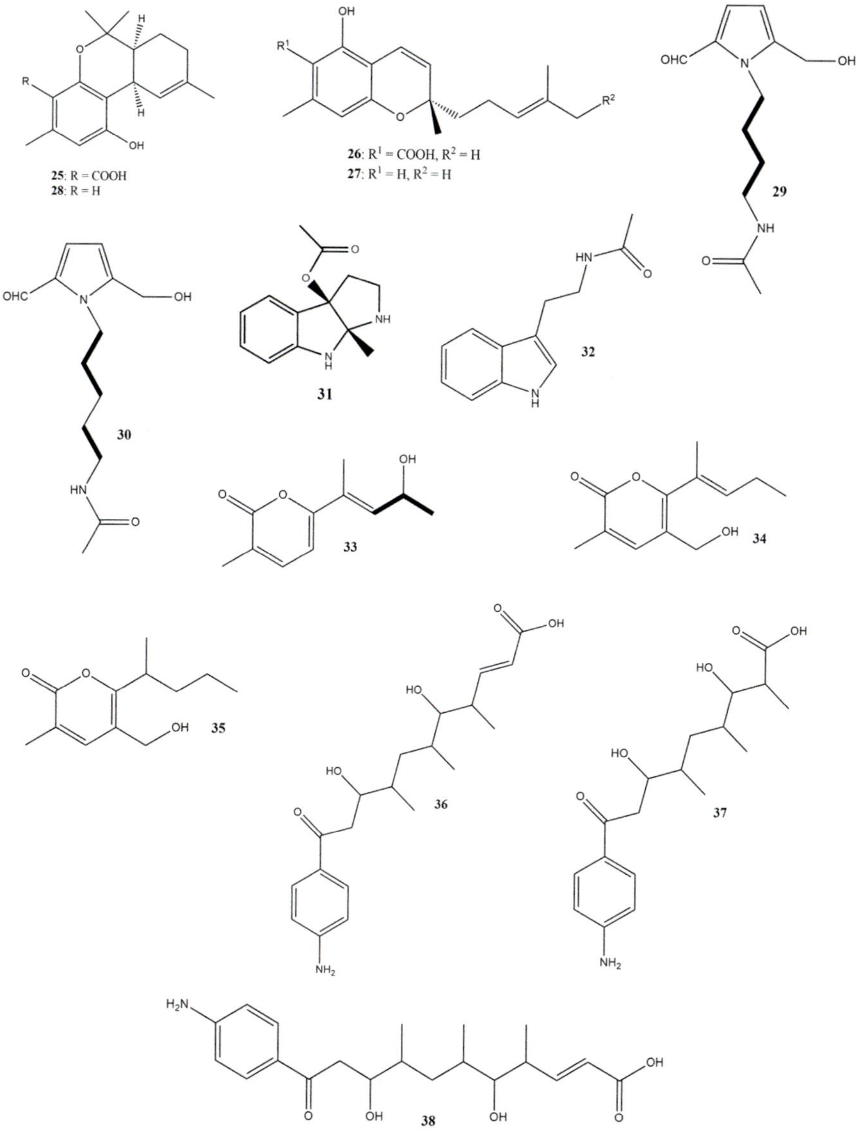

FIGURE 4.4

Chemical structures of compounds 25–38 isolated from fungal endophytes of mangroves.

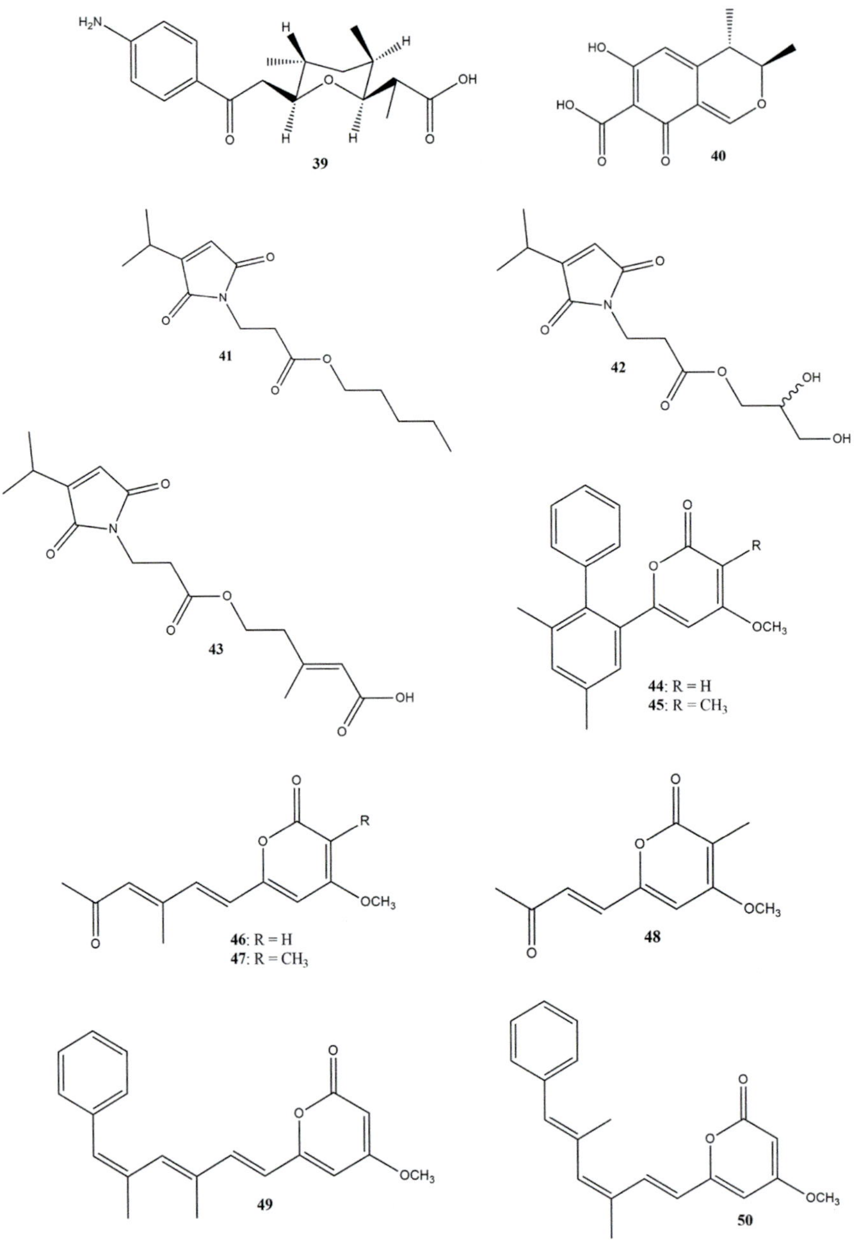

FIGURE 4.5

Chemical structures of compounds 39–50 isolated from fungal endophytes of mangroves.

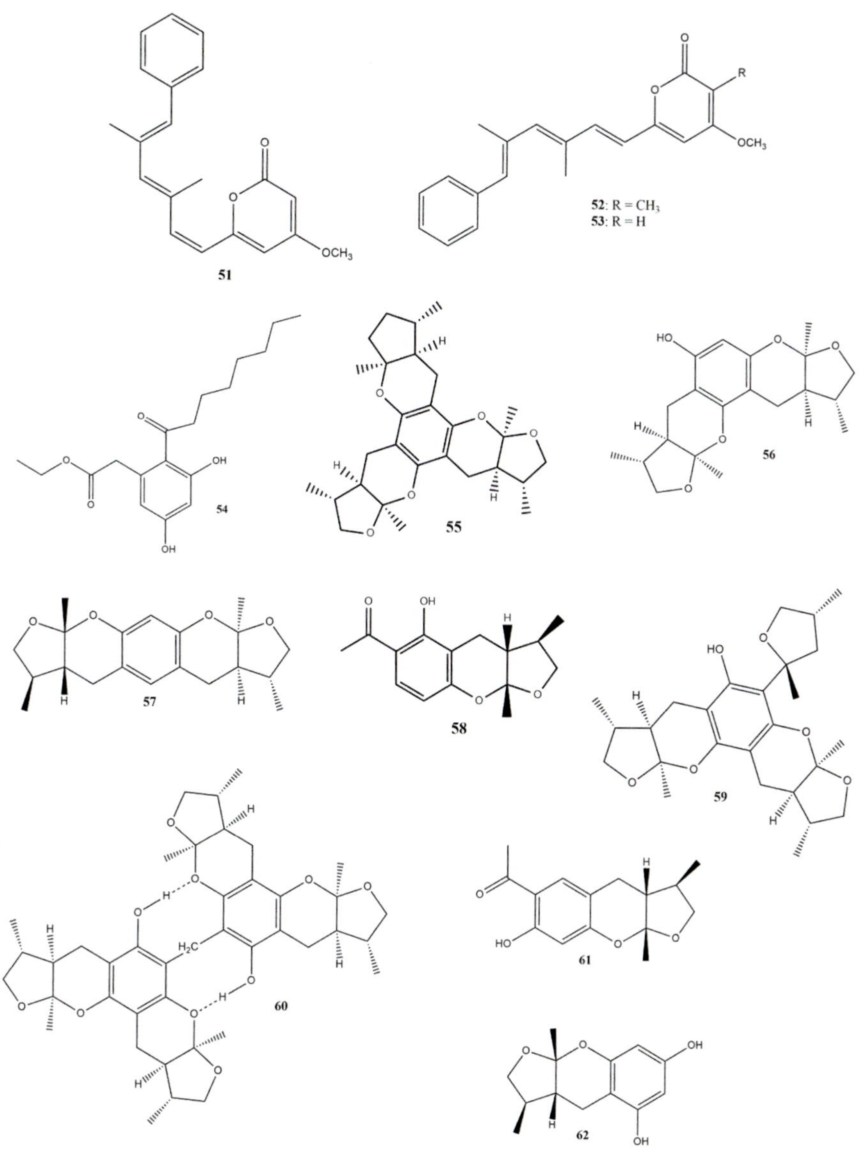

FIGURE 4.6

Chemical structures of compounds 51−62 isolated from fungal endophytes of mangroves.

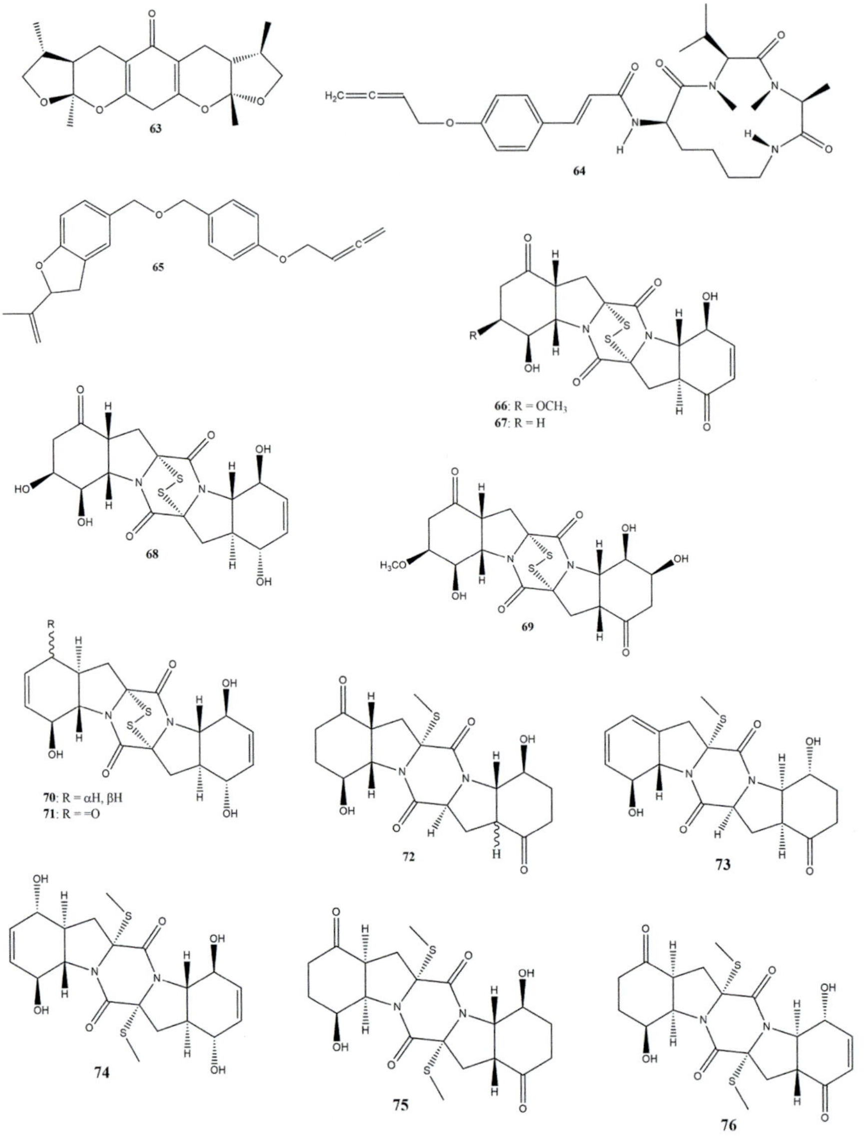

FIGURE 4.7

Chemical structures of compounds 63–76 isolated from fungal endophytes of mangroves.

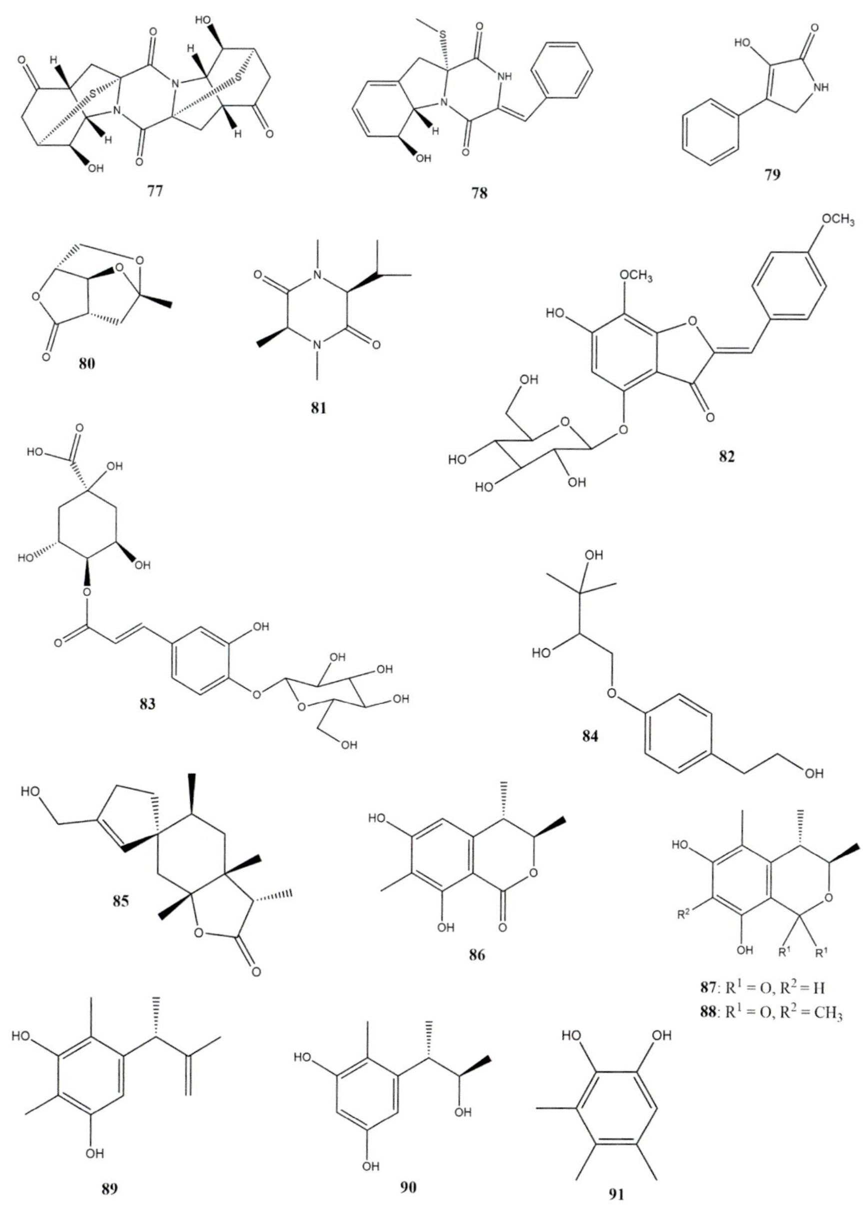

FIGURE 4.8

Chemical structures of compounds 77−91 isolated from fungal endophytes of mangroves.

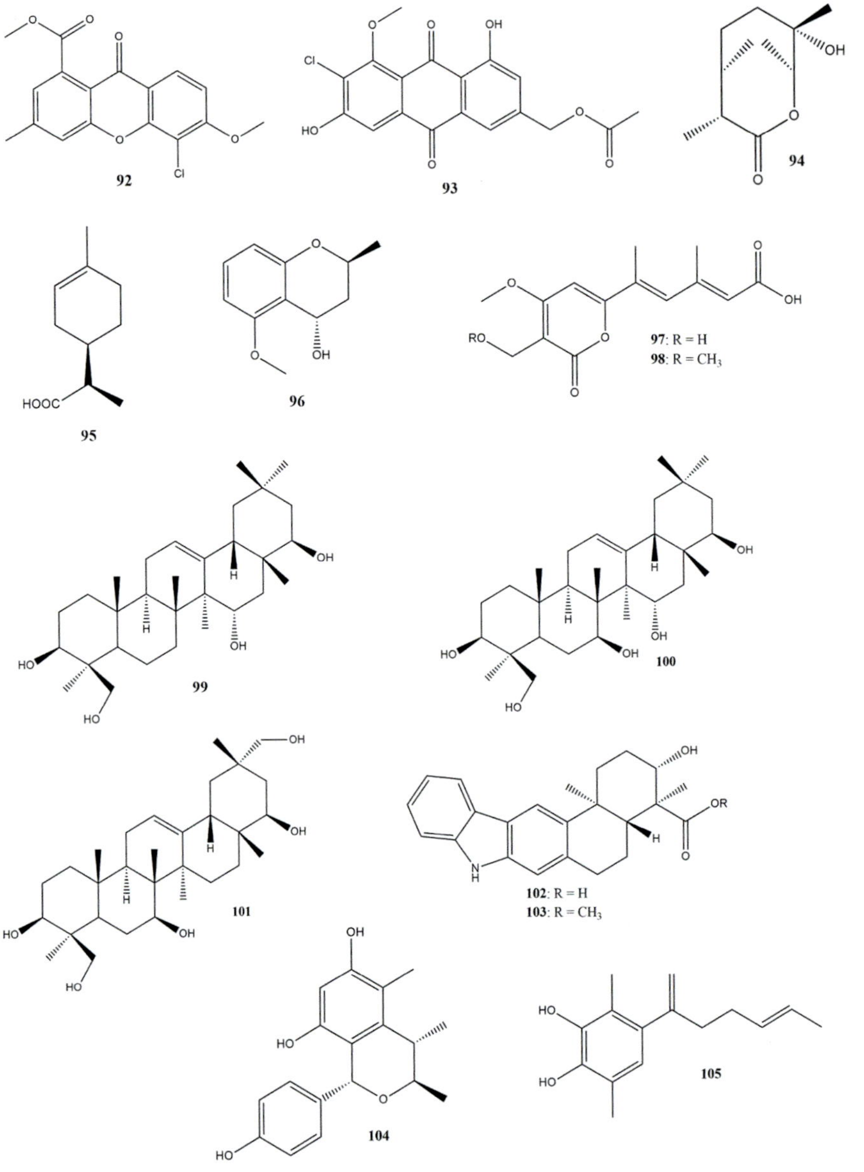

FIGURE 4.9

Chemical structures of compounds 92–105 isolated from fungal endophytes of mangroves.

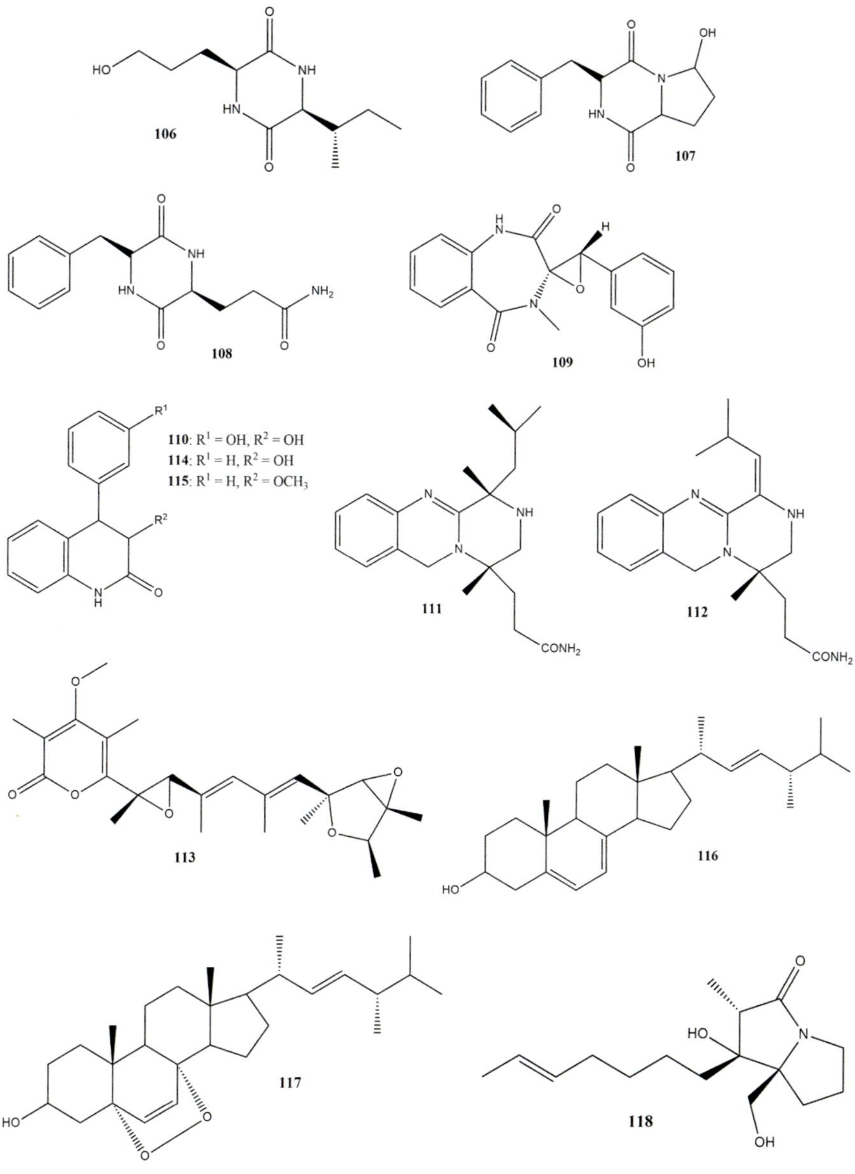

FIGURE 4.10

Chemical structures of compounds 106–118 isolated from fungal endophytes of mangroves.

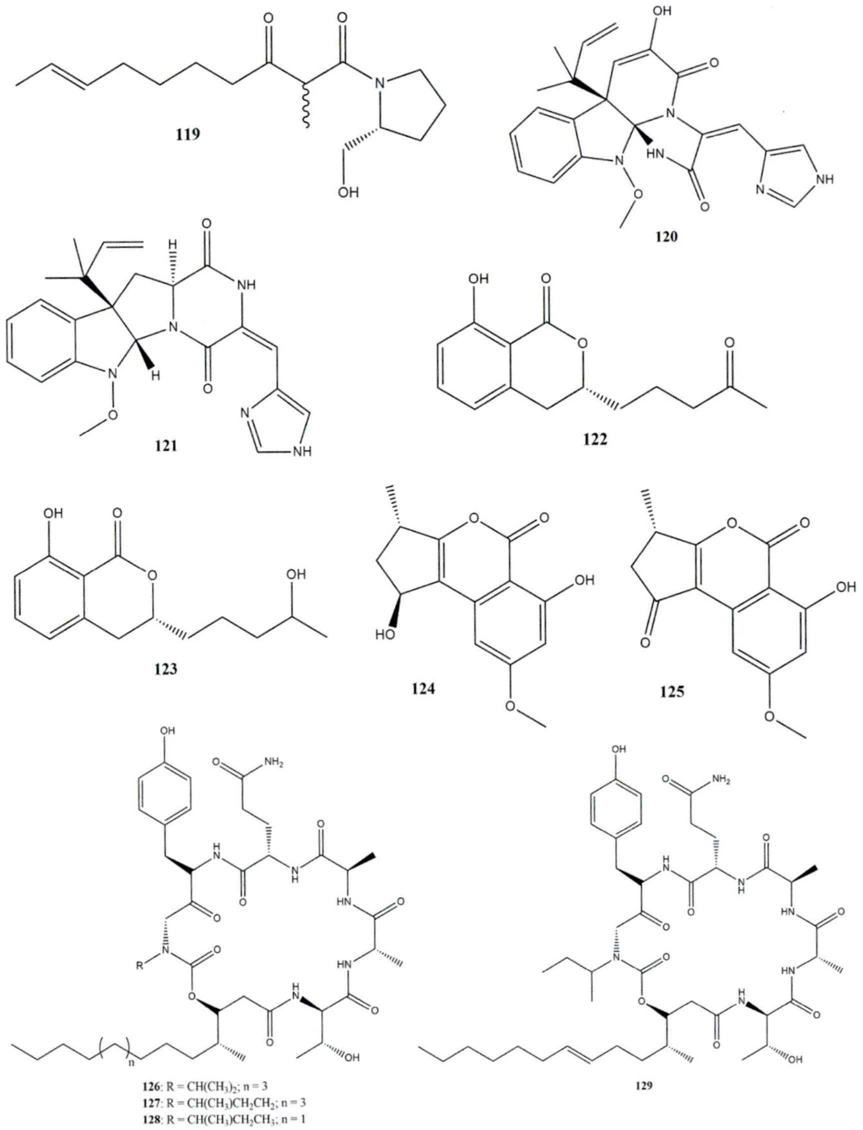

FIGURE 4.11

Chemical structures of compounds 119–129 isolated from fungal endophytes of mangroves.

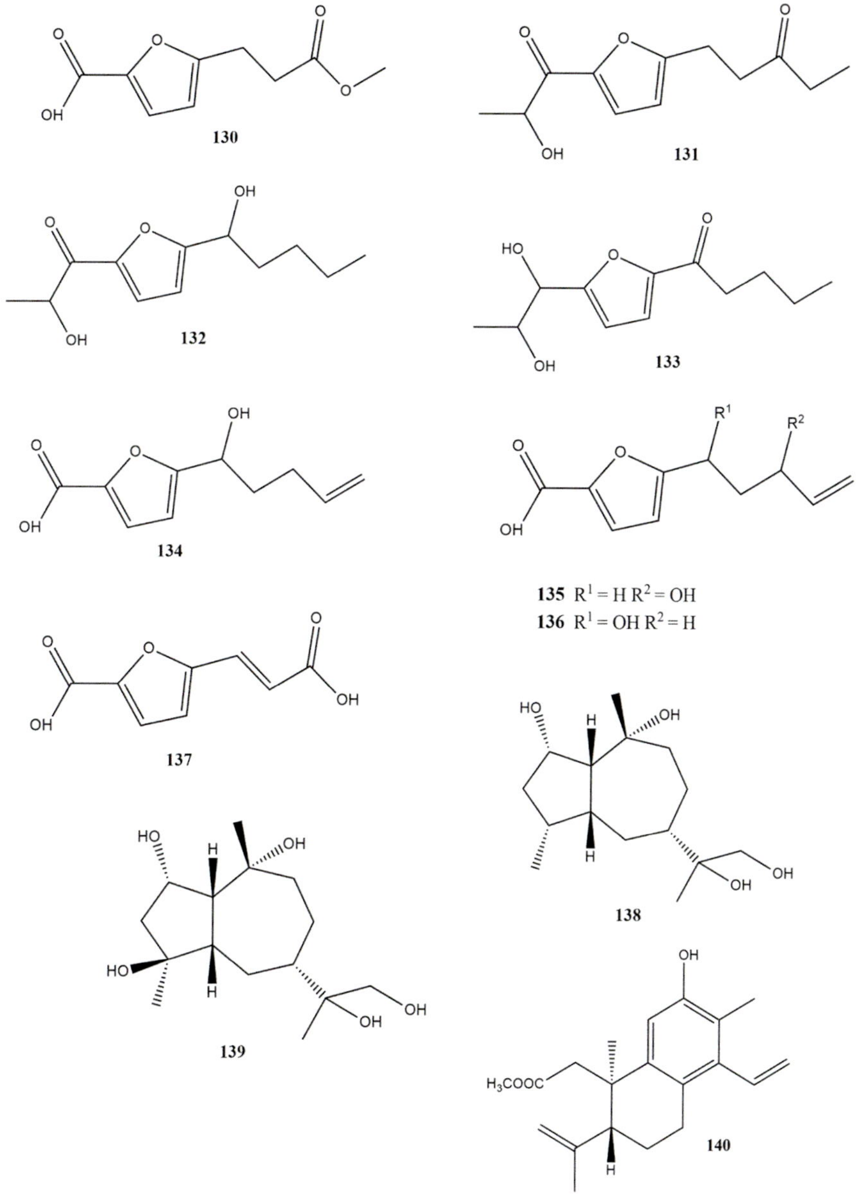

FIGURE 4.12

Chemical structures of compounds 130–140 isolated from fungal endophytes of mangroves.

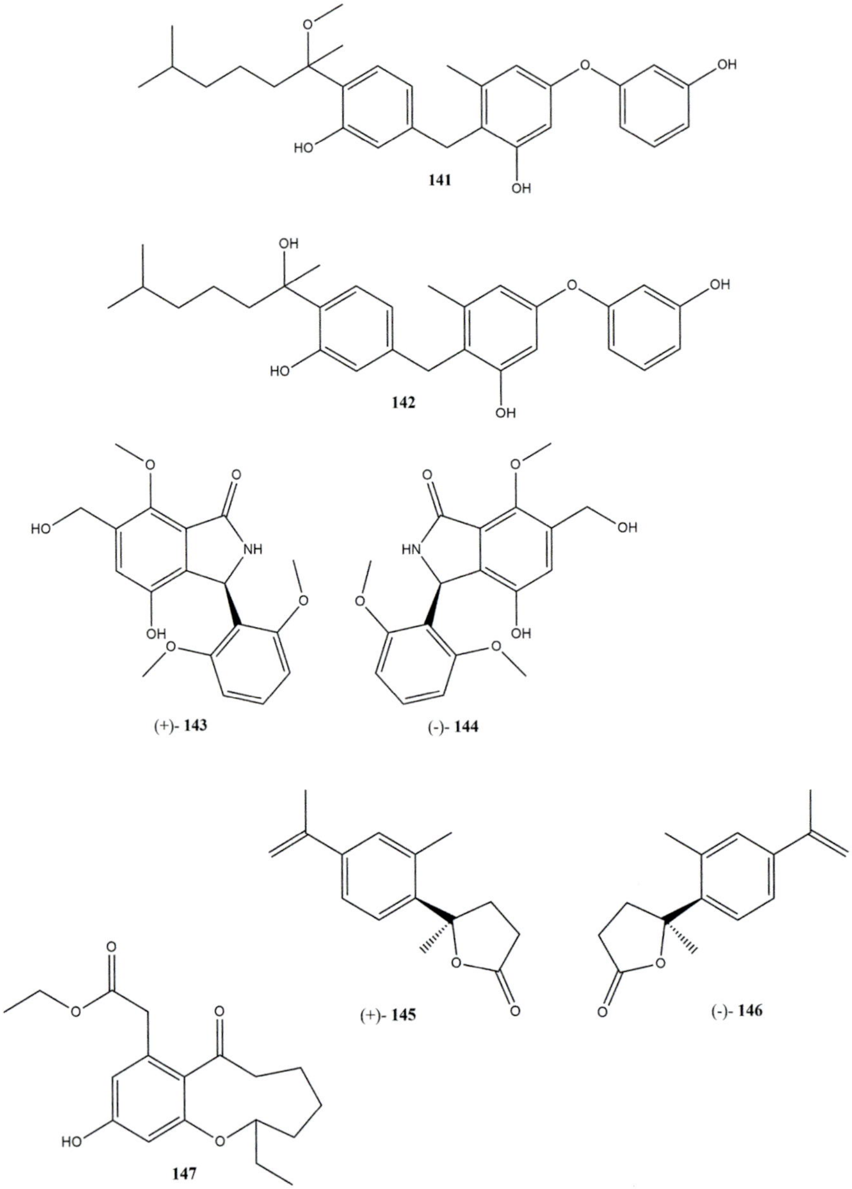

FIGURE 4.13

Chemical structures of compounds 141−147 isolated from fungal endophytes of mangroves.

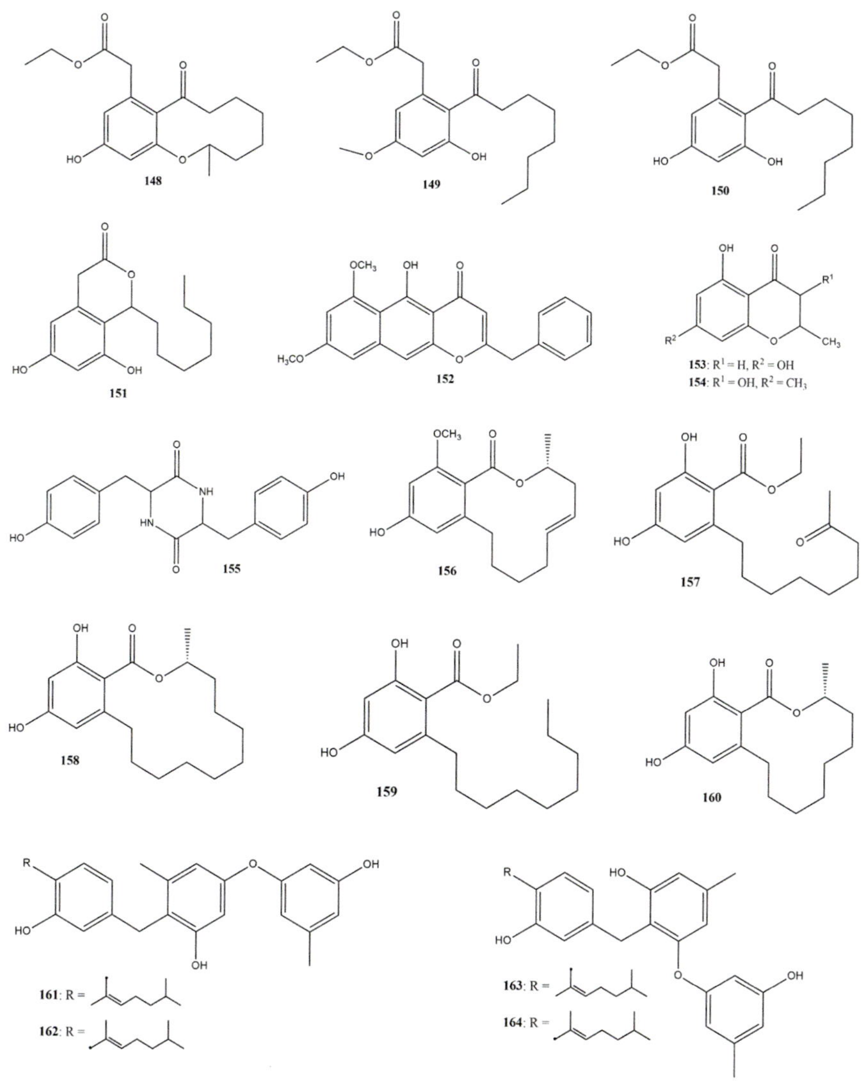

FIGURE 4.14

Chemical structures of compounds 148–164 isolated from fungal endophytes of mangroves.

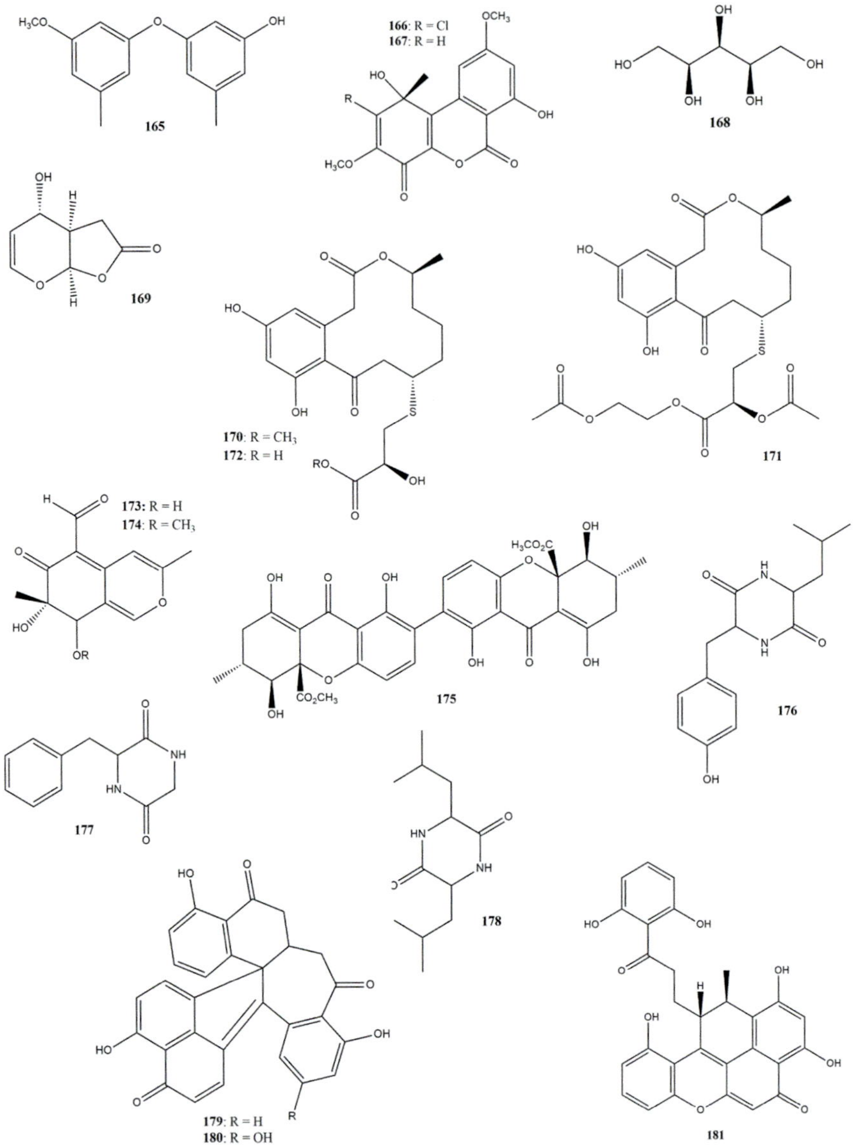

FIGURE 4.15

Chemical structures of compounds 165–181 isolated from fungal endophytes of mangroves.

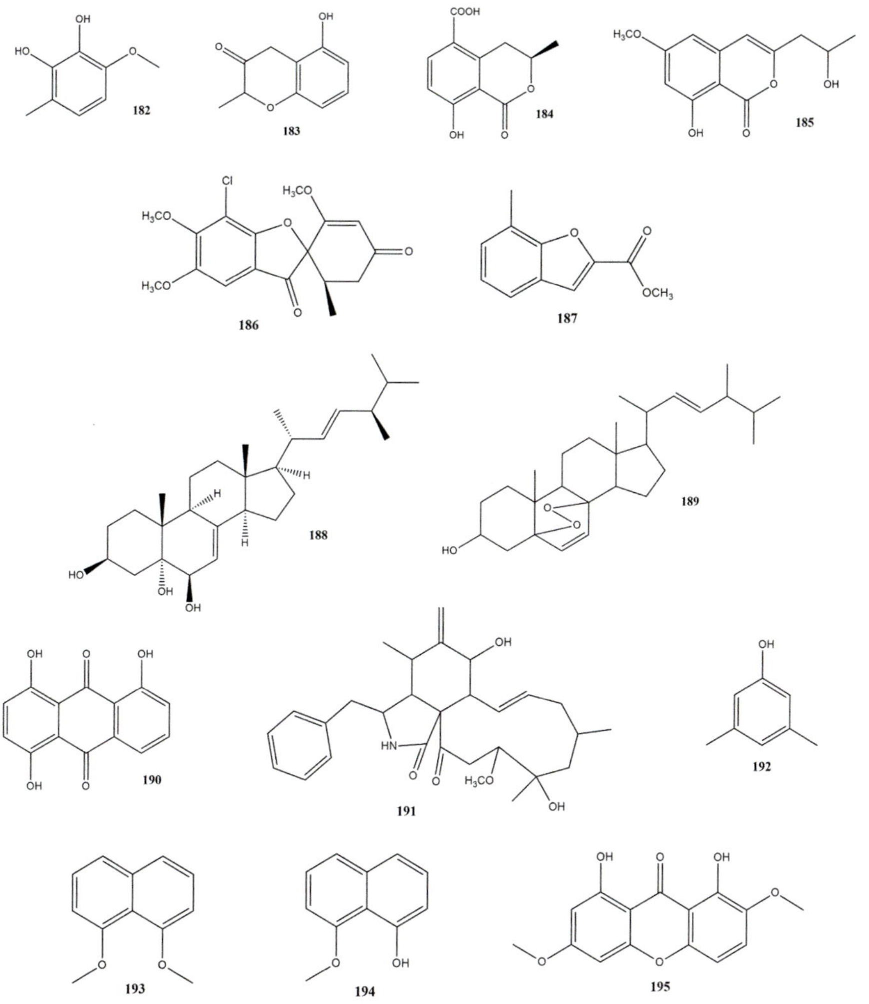

FIGURE 4.16

Chemical structures of compounds 182–195 isolated from fungal endophytes of mangroves.

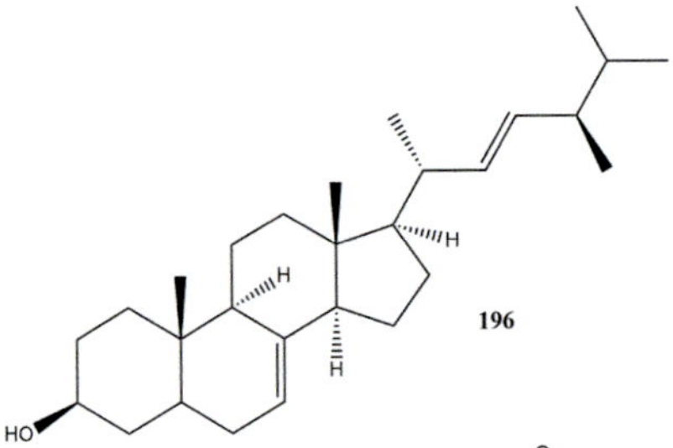

196

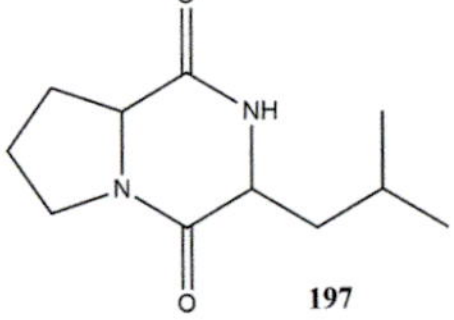

197

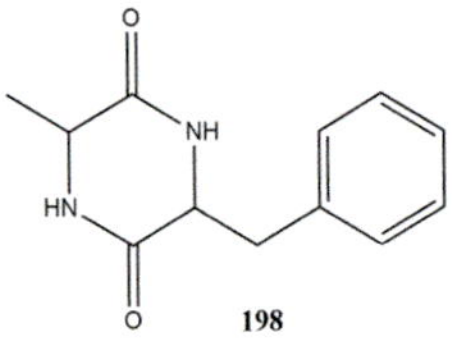

198

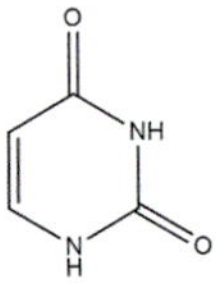

199

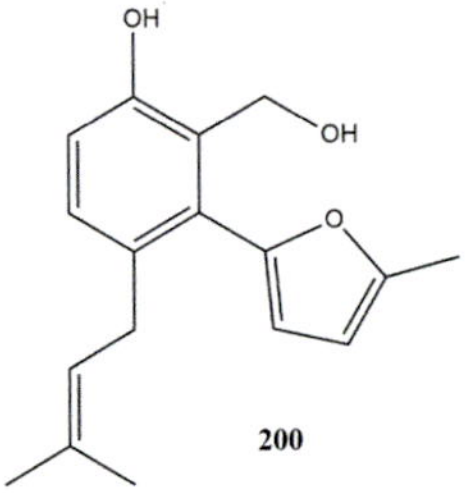

200

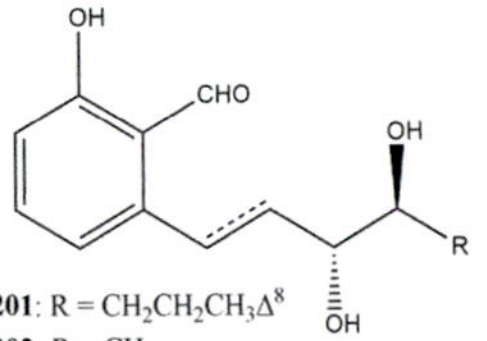

201: R = $CH_2CH_2CH_3\Delta^8$
202: R = CH_3

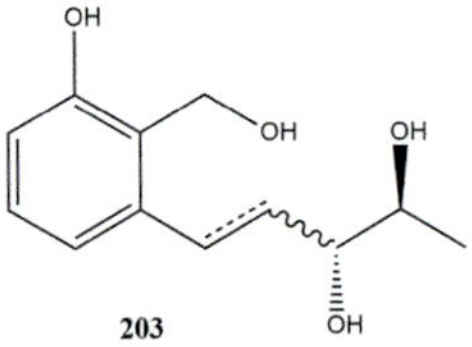

203

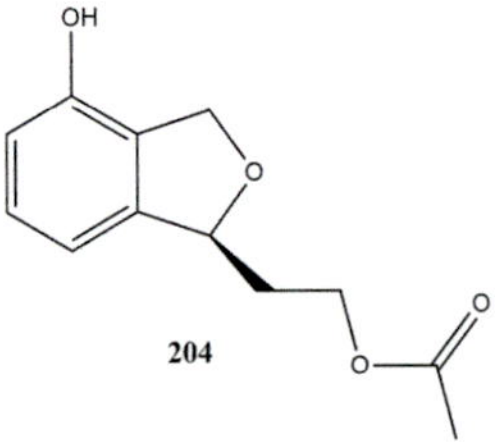

204

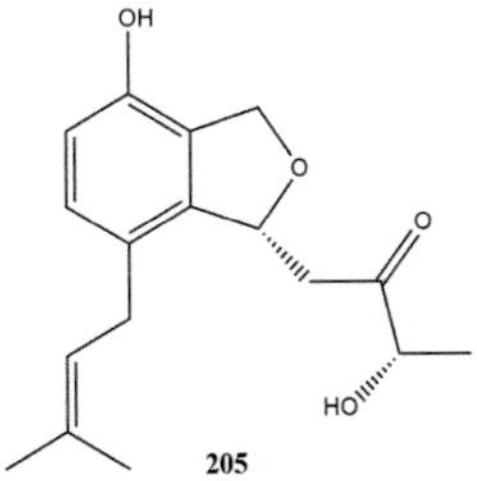

205

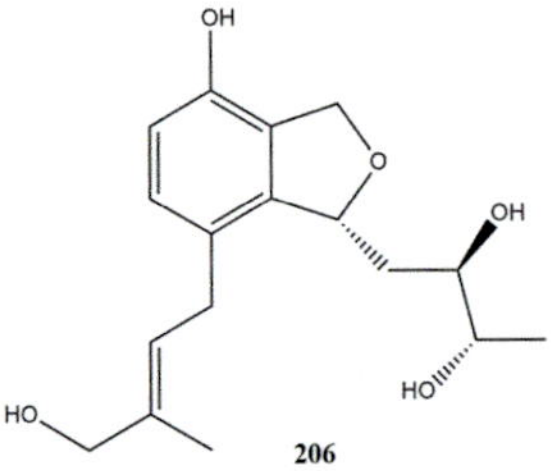

206

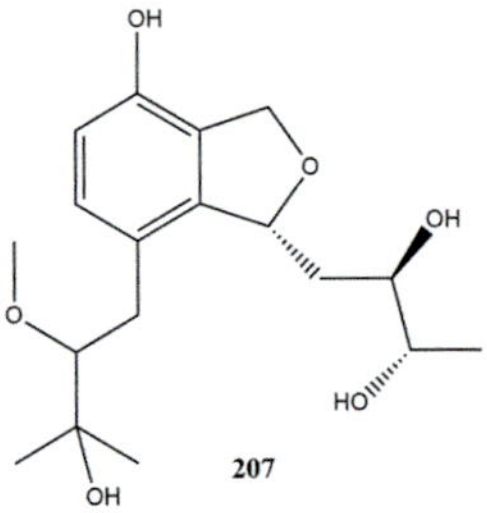

207

FIGURE 4.17

Chemical structures of compounds 196–207 isolated from fungal endophytes of mangroves.

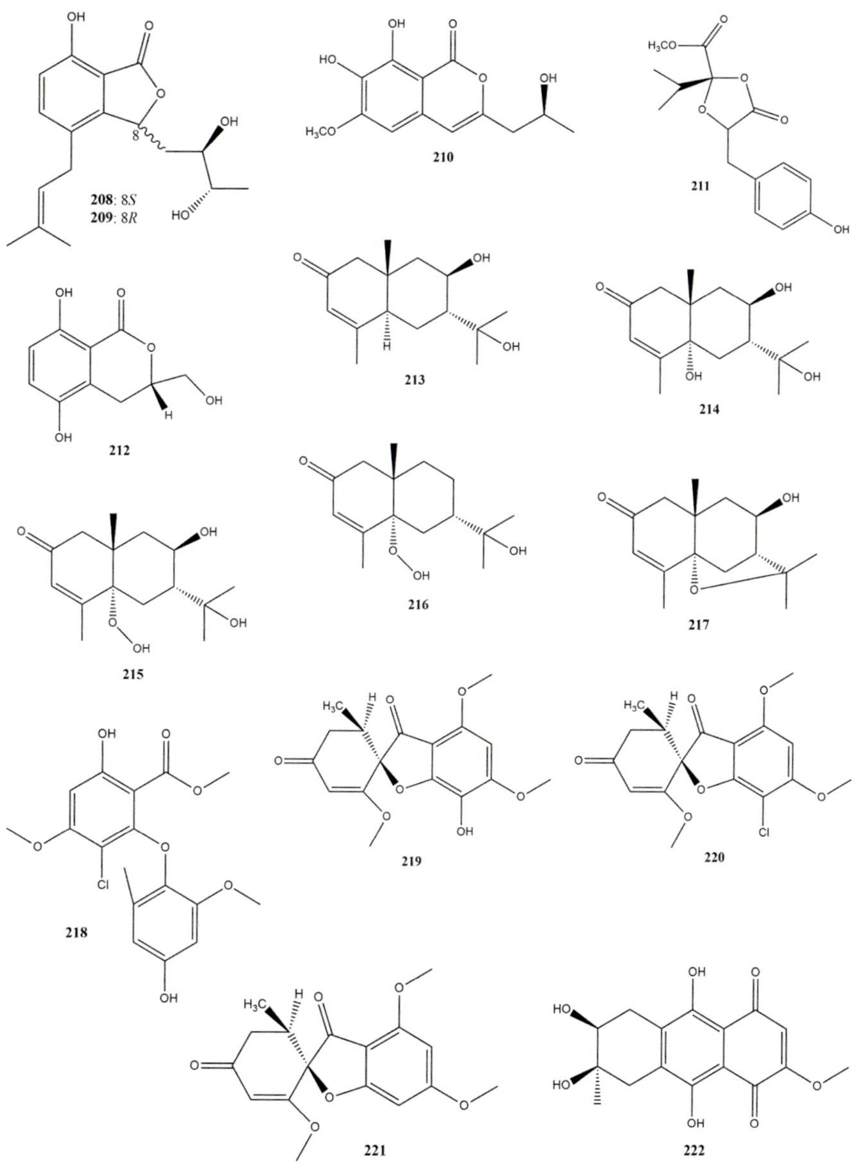

FIGURE 4.18

Chemical structures of compounds 208–222 isolated from fungal endophytes of mangroves.

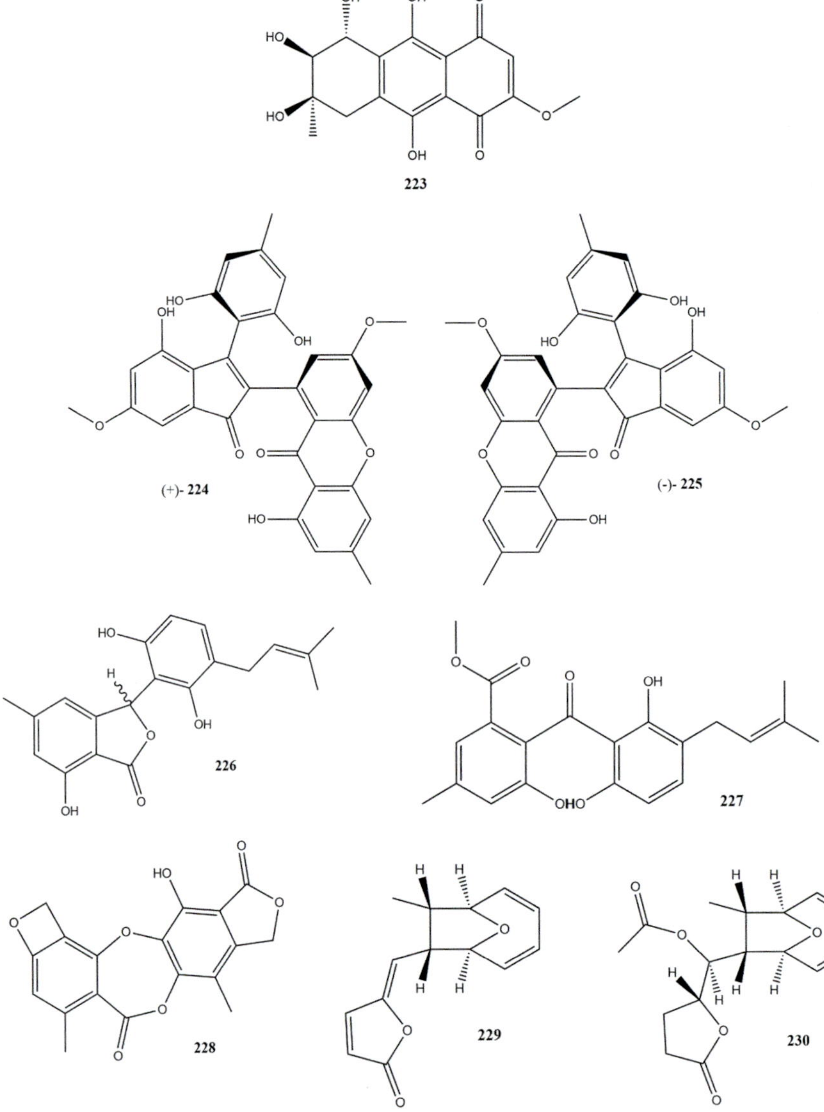

FIGURE 4.19

Chemical structures of compounds 223–230 isolated from fungal endophytes of mangroves.

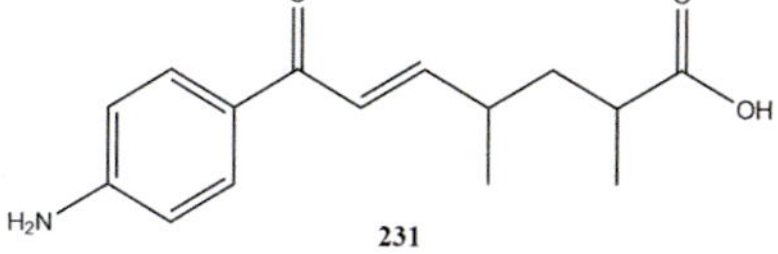

231

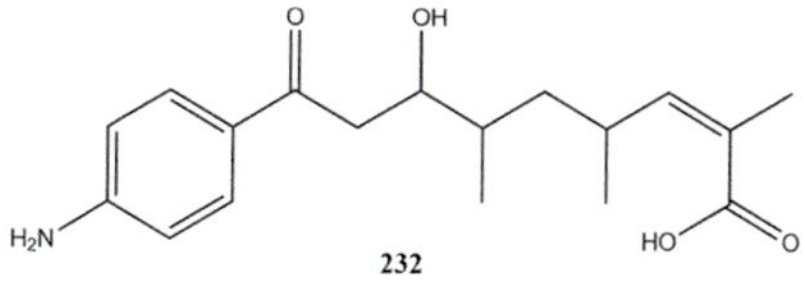

232

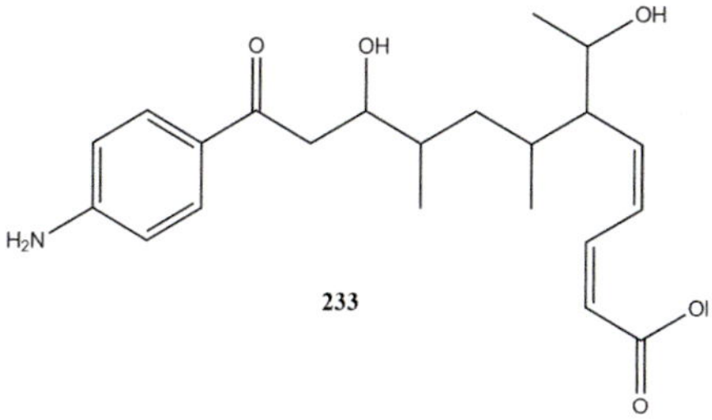

233

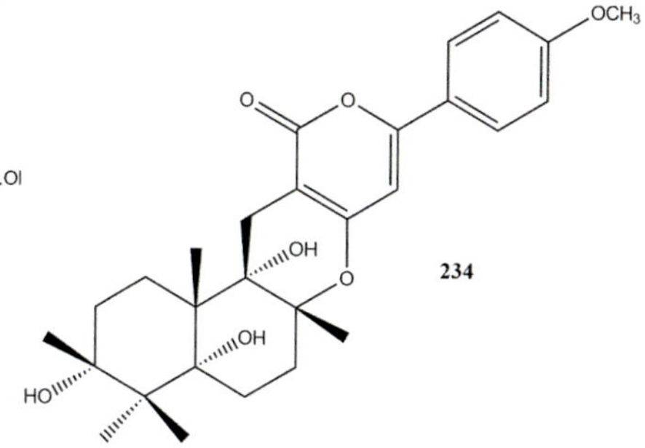

234

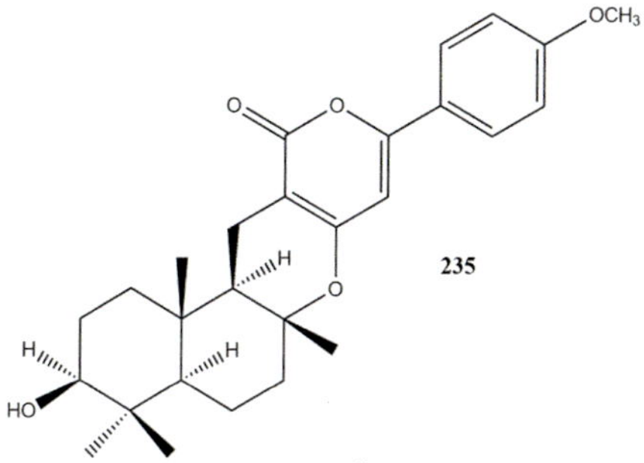

235

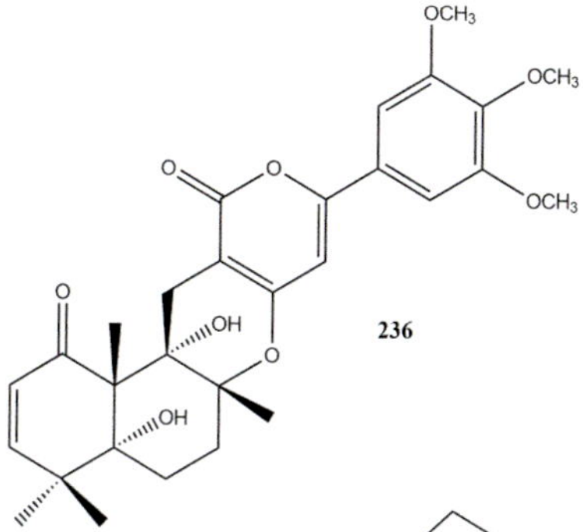

236

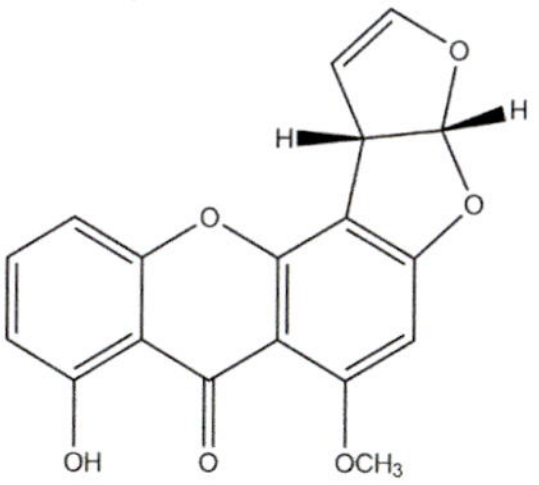

237

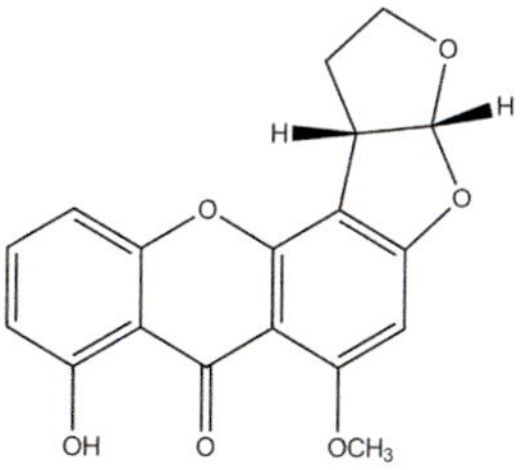

238

FIGURE 4.20

Chemical structures of compounds 231–238 isolated from fungal endophytes of mangroves.

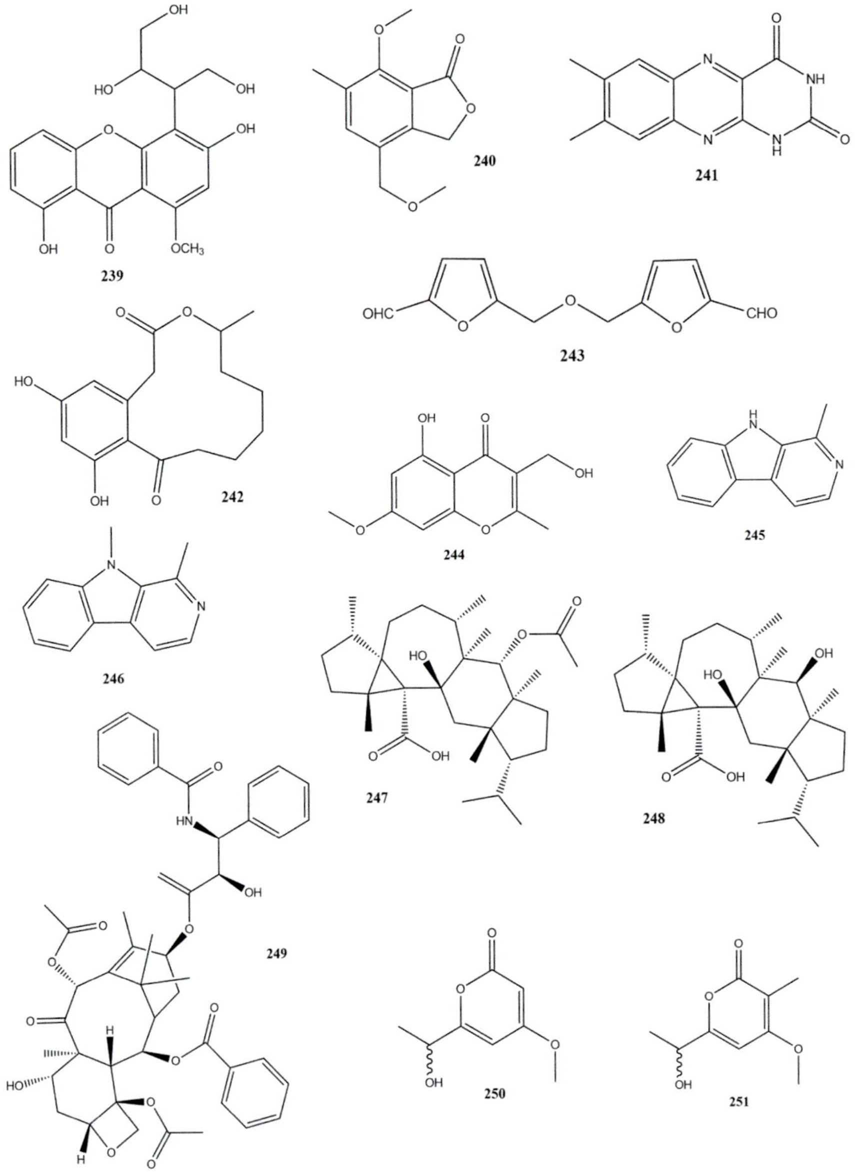

FIGURE 4.21
Chemical structures of compounds 239–251 isolated from fungal endophytes of mangroves.

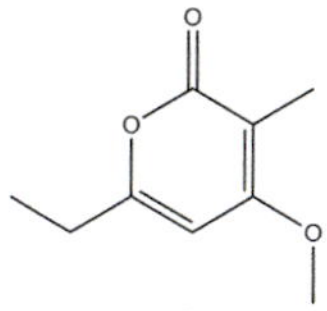
252

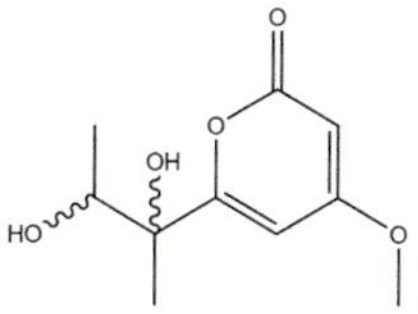
253

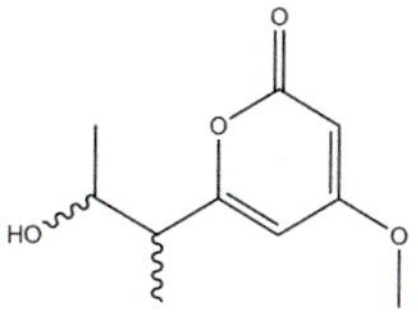
254

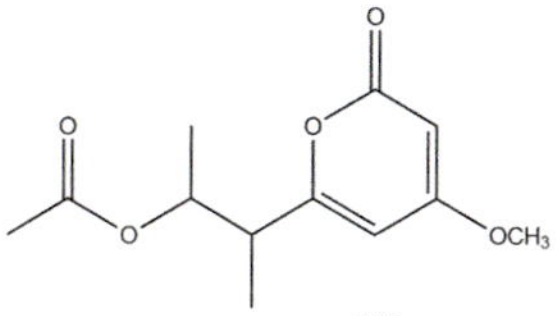
255

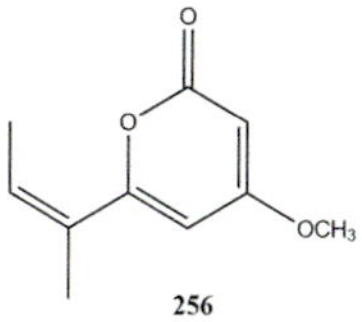
256

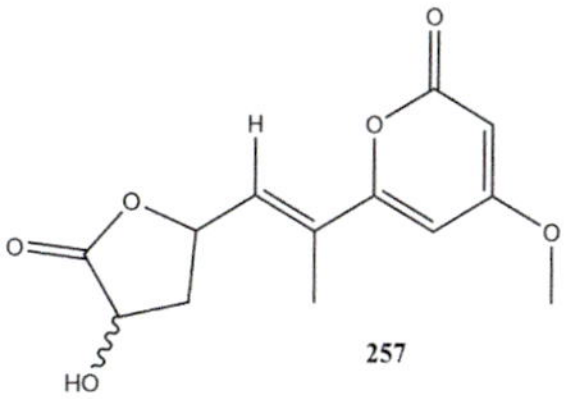
257

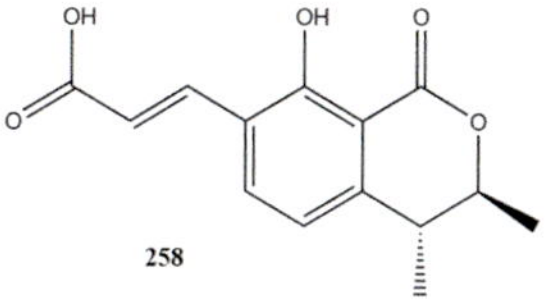
258

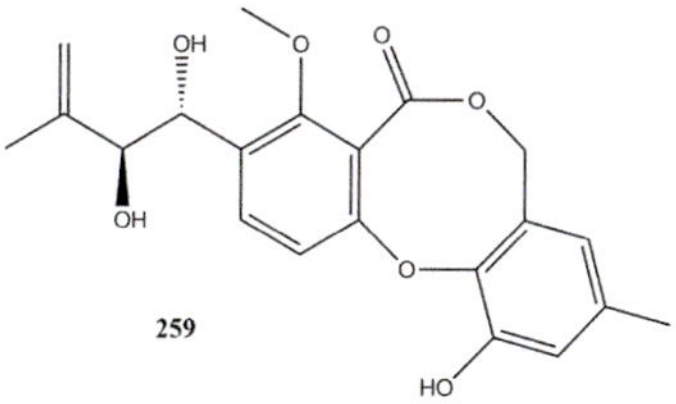
259

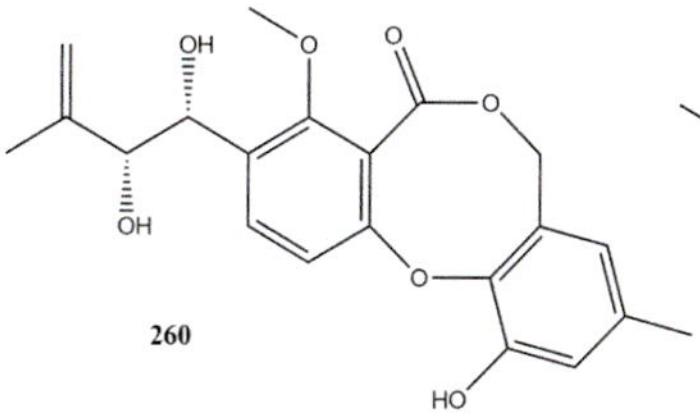
260

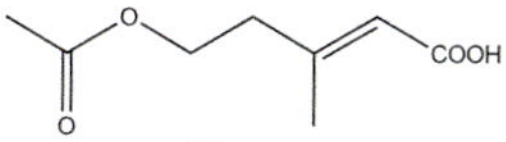
261

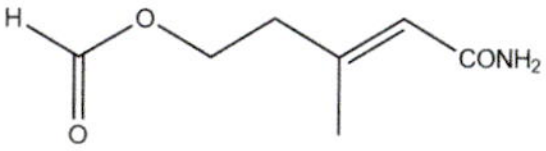
262

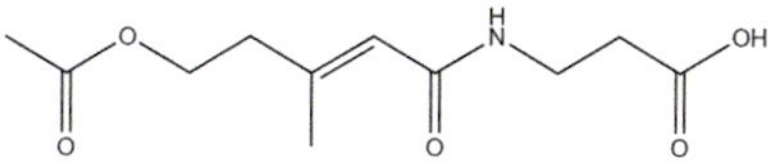
263

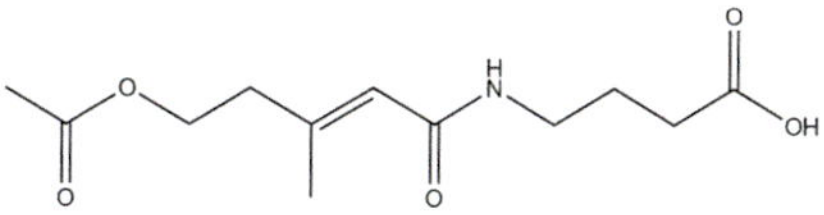
264

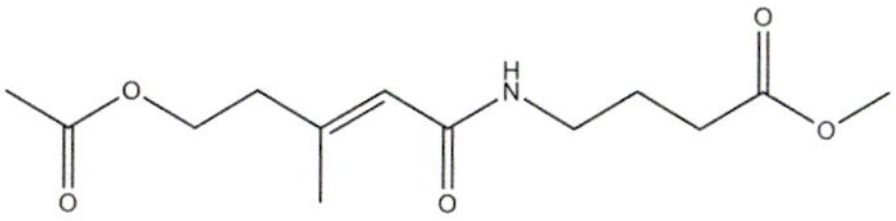
265

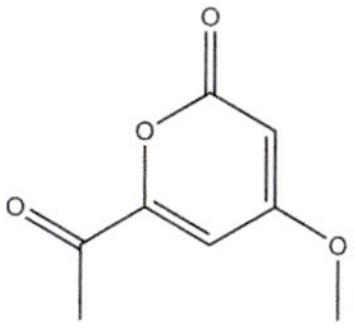
266

FIGURE 4.22

Chemical structures of compounds 252–266 isolated from fungal endophytes of mangroves.

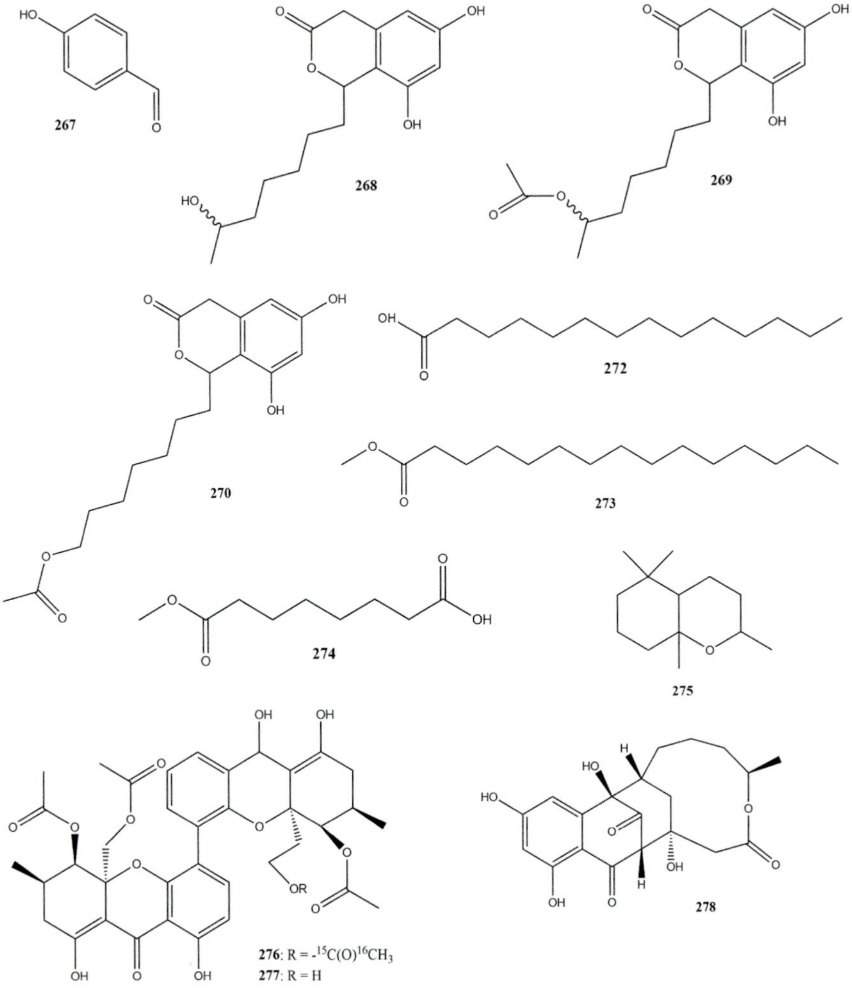

FIGURE 4.23

Chemical structures of compounds 267–278 isolated from fungal endophytes of mangroves.

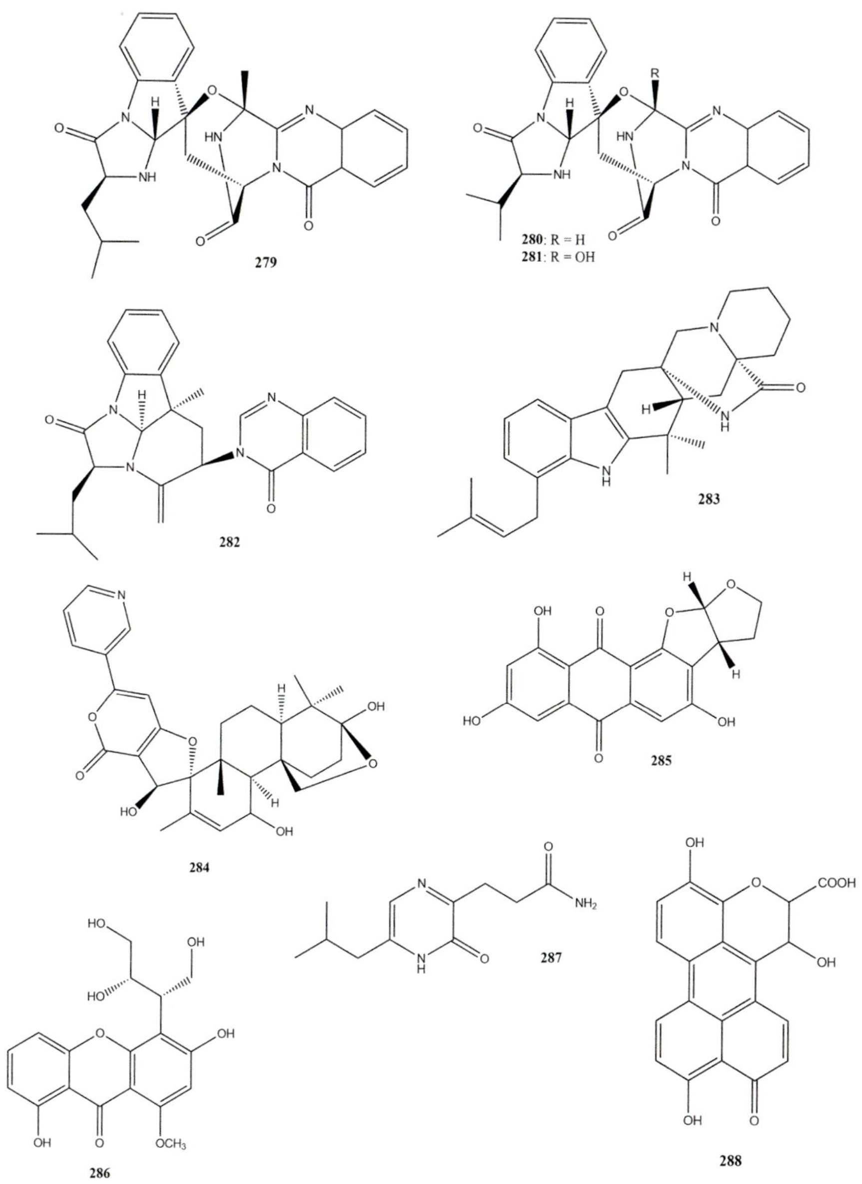

FIGURE 4.24

Chemical structures of compounds 279–288 isolated from fungal endophytes of mangroves.

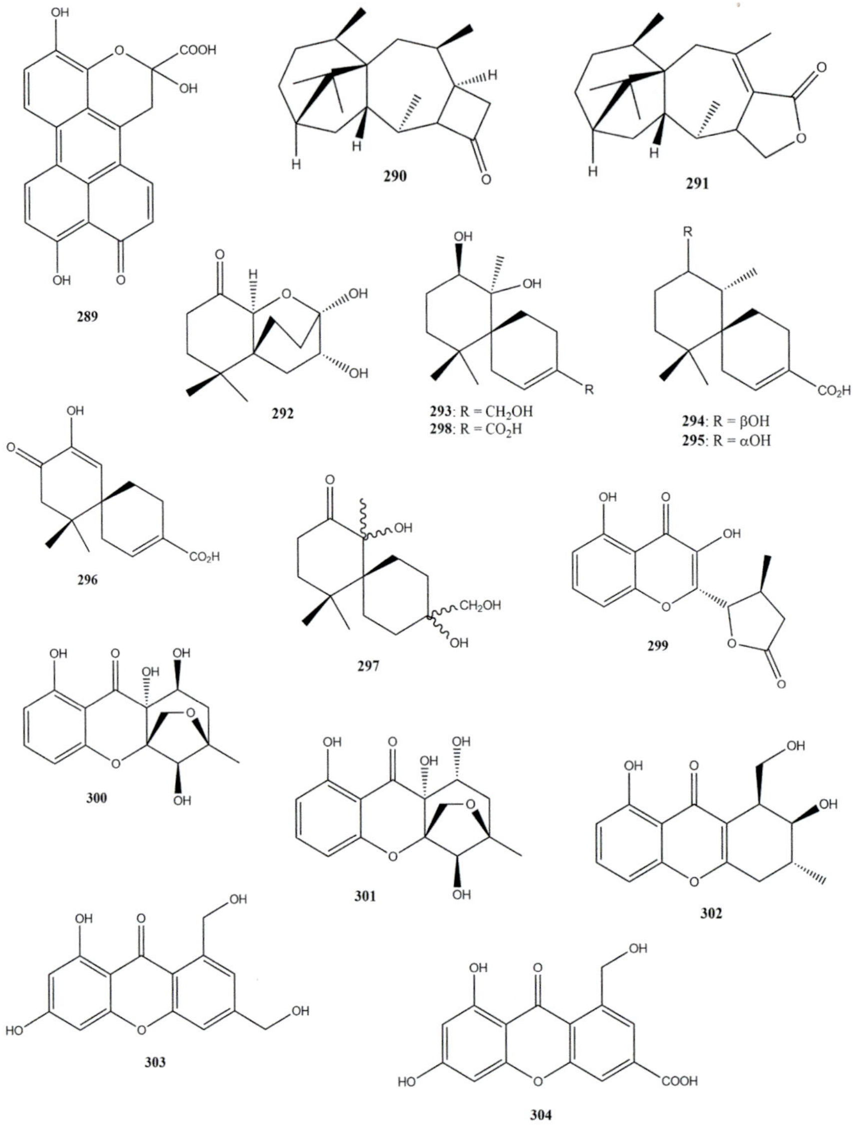

FIGURE 4.25

Chemical structures of compounds 289–304 isolated from fungal endophytes of mangroves.

4.3 Biological activities of mangrove endophytic fungi

4.3.1 Antioxidant

An antioxidant inhibits or delays oxidation of biological molecules either by scavenging noxious free radicals or chelating metal ions (Flora et al., 2015). Numerous antioxidant compounds possess multiple biological activities, namely, antiinflammatory, antitumor, antimutagenic, antimicrobial and anticarcinogenic (Joseph and Priya, 2011). Antioxidants are potential agents found in medicinal plants, vegetables, fruits with the ability to prevent oxidative stress diseases, namely, cancer, cardiovascular and inflammatory diseases, diabetes mellitus and neurodegenerative (Alzheimer's and Parkinson's) diseases (Salini, 2014). Huang et al. (2007) mentioned that the presence of phenolic contents in endophytes were the primary contributors to antioxidant activity. Strobel et al. (2004) emphasized that the strong antioxidant activity exhibited by some medicinal plants reflect on their endophytes with the same activity.

Mangroves are the storehouses of scads of endophytes. A study conducted by Bharathidasan and Panneerselvam (2012) showed that the endophyte *Phomopsis amygdale* isolated from a mangrove plant in India exhibits significant antioxidant activity against 2,2-diphenyl-1-picrylhydrazyl (DPPH) and 2,2'-azino-bis(3-ethylbenzothiazoline)-6-sulfonic acid (ABTS) radicals (Bharathidasan and Panneerselvam, 2012). The endophytic fungus *Trichoderma* sp. isolated from the leaves of the mangrove species *Aegiceras corniculatum* (L.) Blanco showed potent activity against DPPH and hydroxyl radicals (Saravanakumar, 2014). The two new resveratrol derivatives isolated from the root of a semimangrove species, *Myoporum bontioides* A. Gray (Siebold and Zucc.), demonstrated moderate antioxidant activity against DPPH (Dong et al., 2018). Another study conducted by Wang et al. (2014a,b) isolated three other resveratrol derivatives, namely, resveratrodehydes A−C from the fungus *Alternaria* sp. R6 obtained from the root of *M. bontioides*. The half maximal inhibitory concentration (IC50) values of the three resveratrol derivatives from DPPH assay were 447.62 ± 5.00, >900.00 and 572.68 ± 6.41 μM, respectively. The collected data showed that resveratrodehyde A and C showed moderate activity while resveratrodehyde B exhibited marginal activity (Wang et al., 2014a). The mangrove endophytic fungus *Aspergillus* sp. Y16 produced a bioactive compound, exopolysaccharide As1−1, showing good antioxidant activity against DPPH and superoxide radicals (Chen et al., 2011). Among the four mangroves screened, namely, *Avicennia officinalis* L., *K. candel* (L.) Druce, *Excoecaria agallocha* L. and *Rhizophora mucronata* Lam, the fungus *Aspergillus flavus* was found to be dominant and was thus subjected to a series of antioxidant assays (DPPH, hydroxyl radicals, reducing power, metal chelating, hydrogen peroxide, β-carotene-linoleate model system). The isolated fungus exhibited a good overall antioxidant activity (Ravindran et al., 2012). A novel metabolite identified as phomopyrone A along with two known metabolites were isolated from the endophytic fungi *Phomopsis* sp. HNY29−2B. The isolated compounds were assessed for their antioxidant properties using DPPH radical scavenging assay. Nonetheless, the compounds exhibited considerable antioxidative activities since IC50 values were above 100 μM (Cai et al., 2017).

Out of the 46 isolated fungal strains obtained from *Rhizophora stylosa* Griff. and *R. mucronata*, 39 of them exhibited antioxidant activity against DPPH and ABTS radicals (Zhou et al., 2018). The fungal isolate *Phomopsis* sp. A123 isolated from the leaf of *K. candel* produced a novel depsidone metabolite, phomopsidone A (228). Results from antioxidant assay from the latter compound revealed weak activity against DPPH radicals (Zhang et al., 2014b). A recent study conducted by Rahmawati et al. (2019), demonstrated that the endophytic microbes present in the fruit of *Xylocarpus granatum* J. Koenig exhibited highest antioxidant activity against DPPH radicals compared to that of the extracts. It was observed that the antioxidant activities of the endophytes were superior to the crude extracts. On that ground, the author concluded that endophytic microbes could represent a potential source of future antioxidant agents.

4.3.2 Antimicrobial and cytotoxicity properties

Drug resistance microorganism is a major concern and the search for novel antibacterial or antifungal drugs remains challenging. It is believed that endophytes could represent a potential source of natural products with notable antimicrobial activities based on previous scientific evidence. Antimicrobial bioactive compounds produced by endophytes belong to a diverse structural phytochemical class, namely, alkaloids, phenols, terpenoids, peptides, steroids, flavonoids and quinines (Yu et al., 2010). A study conducted by Cui et al. (2008) isolated an endophytic fungus *Penicillium* sp. 0935030 from *Acrostichum aureum* L. which produced peptides effective against *Staphylococcus aureus* and *Candida albicans*. Recently, Chi et al. (2019) isolated 168 endophytic fungi from the leaves of *A. ilicifolius var. xiamenensis* (R.T. Zhang) Y.F. Deng, N.H. Xia and Heng B. Chen. Out of 168, 28 fungal strains showed antimicrobial activity against potential pathogens such as *Escherichia coli*, *Bacillus subtilis*, *S. aureus*, *C. albicans* and *Cryptococcus neoformans*. The 14 endophytic fungi isolated from both *A. ilicifolius* and *A. aureum* were tested against a panel of bacteria (*B. subtilis, Enterococcus sp., Klebsiella pneumoniae, Pseudomonas aeruginosa, Salmonella typhi* and *S. aureus*) and fungal pathogens (*C. albicans* and *Trichophyton metagrophytes*). Results showed that *Cumulospora marina* and *Pestalotiopsis* sp. showed significant activity against Gram-positive and Gram-negative bacteria and *C. albicans* (Lobo et al., 2005). The antibacterial activity of the aforementioned fungi was attributed to the metabolites they produced, namely, flavonoids, terpenes steroids and triterpenoidal saponins (Eldeen and Effendy, 2013). *Aspergillus* sp. 3 showed considerable inhibition against *C. albicans* while the inhibition of *Aspergillus* sp. 2 was limited only to bacteria (Lobo et al., 2005). The meroterpenoids produced by the endophytic fungus *A. flavipes* AIL8 isolated from *A. ilicifolius* did not show any antibacterial and cytotoxicity activity. This lack of activity was attributed to the structural differences in the isoprenoid side chains compared to tricycloalternarenes (Bai et al., 2014). Another study conducted on *A. ilicifolius* successfully isolated 71 fungal endophytes and were subjected to bacterial analysis. The fungal *Xylaria* showed effective activity against both Gram-positive and Gram-negative bacteria (Chaeprasert et al., 2010). Cai et al. (2017) isolated two novel depsidones identified as talaromyones A (9) and B (10) which displayed good antibacterial activity against *B. subtilis* with MIC value of 12.5 μg/mL. Recently, a study isolated an endophytic fungus *Pseudocosmospora* sp. Bm-1−1 from the branch of *Acanthus ebracteatus* Vahl collected in Indonesia. Three novel terpenoids, namely, cosmosporin A (23), 6-carboxy-cosmosporin A (24) and rel-(6aS,10aR)-Δ9-tetrahydrocannabiorcolic acid B (25) together with four known compounds cannabiorcichromenic acid (26), decarboxy-cannabiorcichromenic acid (27), and rel-(6aS,10aR)-decarboxy-Δ9-tetrahydrocannabiorcolic acid B (28) were extracted from the rice culture of the fungus. Compounds 25 and 28 were observed to inhibit human cancer HL-60 cell line with IC50 values 24.1 and 1.6 μM, respectively (Nakamura et al., 2019).

Furthermore, Meng et al. (2017) isolated five new sulfide diketopiperazine derivatives, namely, penicibrocazines A−E (72−76) from the fungus *Penicillium brocae* MA-231 derived from the mangrove plant *Avicennia marina*. The identified compounds were tested for their antimicrobial and cytotoxicity activities. Compounds 73−75 showed inhibition against *S. aureus* with MIC values ranging from 0.25 to 32.0 μg/mL and *Gaeumannomyces graminis* with MIC values of 0.25 to 64.0 μg/mL. However, compound 72 did not show activity against *S. aureus*. Compounds 72−76 were also screened for cytotoxicity activities nevertheless, none of the compounds showed notable activity since the IC50 value was above 10 μM. Later in 2017, the same group of researchers tested the isolated penicibrocazines A−E (72−76) against a plethora of bacteria, including *E. coli, Micrococcus luteus, S. aureus, Aeromonas hydrophilia, Edwardsiella tarda, Vibrio anguillarum, Vibrio harveyi*, and *Vibrio parahaemolyticus*. Compound 76 exhibited higher activity compared to other compounds and this is because compound 76 possessed S-methyl groups and these groups were attributed to an increase in antibacterial activity (Meng et al., 2017). Amrani and coworkers isolated an unidentified fungus from the leaves of *A. marina* collected in Oman. The fungus produced three novel metabolites characterized as farinomalein C−E (41−43) and a new congener. Cytotoxicity results demonstrated that only compound 42 displayed activity against the mouse lymphoma cell line L5178Y resulting in an IC50 value of 4.4 μg/mL. The isolated compounds were also assessed for their antimicrobial activities however, none of them showed any activity (El Amrani et al., 2012).

Eight new α-pyrone derivatives together with two known compounds were successfully isolated from *Aspergillus niger* MA-132 from *A. marina* using shake-flask fermentation. The novel compounds were characterized by HPLC and identified as nigerapyrones A−H (44−51). The isolated compounds were tested for their biological activities in terms of antimicrobial and cytotoxicity. Data revealed that compounds 45, 47, 48 and 50 did not show any potential activity against the tested microbes which are *Alternaria brassicae, Fusarium oxysporum, Coniella diplodiella, Physalospora piricola, S. aureus* and *E. coli.* Interestingly, the same compounds showed weak cytotoxicity activities against a few tumor cell lines, namely, HEPG2 (human hepatocellular liver carcinoma) and MCF-7 (human breast adenocarcinoma). However, compound 48 was the least active and exhibited weak activity against a wider set of cell lines, including MCF-7, HepG2, Du145, NCI-H460, and MDA-MB-231 cell lines with IC50 values of 105, 86, 86, 43 and 48 μM, accordingly (Liu et al., 2011).

A study conducted by Zheng et al. (2014), isolated two novel compounds, namely, 4-(2′,3′-dihydroxy-3′-methyl-butanoxy)-phenethanol and 15-hydroxy-6α,12-epoxy-7β,10-αH,11-βH-spiroax-4-ene-12-one (84−85) based on the spectroscopic analysis. These compounds were isolated from *Penicillium* sp. FJ-1 from the mangrove species *A. marina.* Anti-tumoral activity was evaluated on both compounds using both in vitro and animal models. After the administration of compound 85 to mice for six days, a drastic decline in the tumor growth of osteosarcoma was observed. On the other hand, compound 84 exhibited weak antitumor activity against MG-63 cell lines with IC50 value 35 μM while compound 85 proved to be more potent with an IC50 of 55 nM (Zheng et al., 2014).

The isolated fungal endophytes *Penicillium citrinum* HL-5126 extracted from the mangrove plant *Bruguiera sexangula* (Lour.) Poir. produced two novel compounds, namely, 4-chloro-1-hydroxy-3-methoxy-6-methyl-8-methoxycarbonyl-xanthen-9-one and 2′-acetoxy-7-chlorocitreorosein (92−93). The identified compounds were evaluated for their antimicrobial activity. Results demonstrated the bacterial growth of *V. parahaemolyticus* was successfully inhibited by compound 93 with a MIC value of 10 μM (He et al., 2017).

Another well-known mangrove species scrutinized for its antimicrobial and cytotoxicity activities is *Bruguiera gymnorhiza* (L.) Lam. (family Rhizophoraceae). Jiang et al. (2018) collected the stems and barks of the mangrove plant in Fujian Province, China. The endophytic fungus *Penicillium* sp. GD6 isolated was found to produce one new sorbicillin derivatives (48) and one new alkaloid, namely, 2-deoxy-sohirnone C (105) and 5S-hydroxynorvaline-S-Ile (106) respectively and two other compounds, 3S-hydroxylcyclo(S-Pro-S-Phe) and cyclo(S-Phe-S-Gln) (107−108). The identified compounds were screened for their antibacterial activities. However, only compound 105 moderately inhibited the growth of methicillin-resistant *S. aureus* (MRSA) with an MIC value of 80 μg/mL (Jiang et al., 2018). Interestingly, Li et al. (2012) isolated the marine endophytic fungus *Aspergillus* sp. from the leaves of *B. gymnorhiza.* Two new coumarins, namely, aspergillumarins A (122) and B (123) were identified from the fungus using 1H and 13C NMR techniques. The two compounds demonstrated weak antibacterial activity against *S. aureus* and *B. subtiltis* (Li et al., 2012). Two compounds, namely, xiamycin (168) and oxysporone (169) isolated from *Streptomyces* sp. GT2002/1503 of *B. gymnorhiza.* Compound 169 displayed better and significant inhibitory effects compared to compound 168 against MRSA strains, including SA1199B and EMRSA-15, both giving MIC values of 32 μM

(Nurunnabi et al., 2018). A series of endophytes were isolated from *B. gymnorhiza* identified as *Hypocreales, Fusarium, Ascomycota, Stemphylium, Phomopsis, Alternaria* and *Diaporthe*. The ethyl acetate extracts of each fungus were prepared and assessed for their cytotoxicity activities against KB and KBv200 cell lines resulting in IC50 values ranging from 8 to 98.80 μg/mL (Xiaoling et al., 2010).

Jin et al. (2013) conducted research on a different mangrove species, *Ceriops tagal* and successfully isolated the fungus *Penicillium* sp. FJ-1 from the plant and extracted two flavones, namely, 7-hydroxy-deoxytalaroflavone (124) and deoxytalaroflavone (125) using column chromatography on silica gel. Both compounds exhibited weak antibacterial activity against *S. aureus* and MRSA (Jin et al., 2013). Two new peptides coded as W493 C (128) and D (129) and two known compounds W493 A (126) and B (127) were extracted from the ethyl acetate extract of *Fusarium* sp. derived from *C. tagal*. Compound 126 and 127 showed a moderate antifungal activity against *Cladosporium cladosporiodes* and exhibited a weak antitumor activity against the tested human ovarian cancer cell line A2780 using 3-(4,5)-dimethylthiahiazo (-z-y1)-3,5-di-phenytetrazoliumromide (MTT) assay (Lv et al., 2015). Another fungus *Coriolopsis* sp. J5 isolated from the branches of *C. tagal* produced eight new metabolites among which six are new furan derivatives 5-(3-methoxy-3-oxopropyl)-furan-2-carboxylic acid, 1-(5-(2-hydroxypropanoyl)-furan-2-yl)-pentan-3-one, 2-hydroxy-1-(5-(1-hydroxypentyl)-furan-2-yl)-propan-1-one, 1-(5-(1,2-dihydroxypropyl)-furan-2-yl)-pentan-1-one, 5-(1-hydroxypent-4-en-1-yl)-furan-2-carboxylic acid and 5-(3-hydroxypentyl)-furan-2-carboxylic acid (130−135) and two are new natural products 5-(1-hydroxypentyl)-furan-2-carboxylic acid (136) and (E)-5-(2-carboxyvinyl)-furan-2-carboxylic acid (137). All identified compounds were evaluated for their antimicrobial and cytotoxicity activities (K562, SGC-7901 and BEL-7402 cell lines). A wide spectrum of microbes involving *S. aureus* (ATCC51650), *Ralstonia solanacearum, F. oxysporum* f. sp. *cubense* race 4, *F. oxysporum* f. sp. *niveum, F. oxysporum* f. sp. *vasinfectum* and *C. albicans* (ATCC 10231) were selected. However, none of the identified compounds showed considerable antimicrobial and cytotoxic activities (Chen et al., 2017). Furthermore, two new sesquiterpenoids, namely, 2α-hydroxyxylaranol B (138) and 4β-hydroxyxylaranol B (139) and one known terpenoid 3,4-seco-sonderianol (140) were derived from the fungus J3 of *C. tagal*. Among the three isolated compounds, only compound 140 demonstrated cytotoxic activities against the following cell lines: K562, SGC-7901 and BEL-7402 (Zeng et al., 2015).

Another mangrove plant well studied is *E. agallocha*, also known as Blind-your-eye mangrove. Huang and coworkers isolated a new compound, 5-hydroxy-6,8-dimethoxy-2-benzyl-4H-naphtho[2,3-b]-pyran-4-one (152) together with three known compounds (153−155) from the same fungal strain *Phomopsis* sp. ZSU-H76 of *E. agallocha* (Huang et al., 2008, 2010). In this study, cytotoxicity activities were investigated on the isolated compounds (i.e. 152−155). Results reported that compound 152 demonstrated activity against Hep-2 and HepG2 cell lines resulting in IC50 values of 10 and 8 μg/mL, respectively (Huang et al., 2010).

Four new polyphenols, expansols C-F (161−164), one new diphenyl ether derivative, 3-O-methyldiorcinol (165), together with 12 known compounds were isolated from the fungus *Penicillium expansum* 091006 hosted by the mangrove plant *E. agallocha*. Cytotoxicity results showed that compounds 161 and 163 exhibited weak activity against HL-60 cell lines resulting in IC50 values 18.2 and 20.8 μM, respectively (Wang et al., 2012).

Another underexplored mangrove species is *Lumnitzera racemosa*. Six metabolites, namely, sumalarins A-C (170−172) were isolated from the marine-derived fungus *Penicillium sumatrense* MA-92 hosted by *L. racemosa*. Interestingly, all compounds (170−172) exhibited significant cytotoxicity activity against some tumor cell lines (Meng et al., 2013).

Huang et al. (2007) also conducted research on another mangrove species which is *K. candel* apart from *E. agallocha*. For instance, a fungal endophyte coded No. 1962 was isolated from the foliage of *K. candel*. Several metabolites were successfully extracted through maceration and separated using column chromatography with silica gel. Three known cyclodipeptides cyclo-(Leu-Tyr) (176), cyclo-(Phe-Gly) (177), and cyclo-(Leu-Leu) (178) were identified from the fungus. Using MTT assay, compound 176 exhibited weak cytotoxicity activity against the human cancer cell line MCF-7 with a high IC50 value of 100 μg/mL (Huang et al., 2007). Wen et al. (2013) isolated a fungus *Sporothrix* sp. 4335 from the bark of *K. candel* collected in the South China Sea. A total of 19 bioactive compounds (179−199) were identified from the ethyl acetate extract using 1H and 13C NMR. The successfully isolated compounds are listed in Table 4.1. All identified compounds were evaluated for their cytotoxicity activities against the human liver cancer cell line HepG2 and results showed that only compound 180, 181 and 189 exhibited activity, however weak, resulting in IC50 values 20, 23 and 23 μg/mL, respectively (Wen et al., 2013). Wang et al. (2015) isolated two novel prenylated phenols, vaccinol H and I, along with three known phenols. Nevertheless, none of the characterized compounds displayed cytotoxic effects. Later, the same research group isolated a great number of metabolites from the same fungus *Pestalotiopsis vaccinii* cgmcc3.9199. A total of 15 compounds were identified among which ten are reported as new compounds, namely, vaccinols J-S (200−209) as listed in Table 4.1. Similarly, with the results reported in their previous study with different metabolites, this study also did not report any cytotoxicity activity with the isolated compounds against the cell lines K562, MCF-7 and SGC7901 (Wang et al., 2017). Five new sesquiterpenes, namely, kandenols A-E (213−217) were isolated from the mangrove-derived fungus *Streptomyces* sp. HK10595 obtained from *K. candel*. The compounds showed weak antimicrobial activity against *B. subtilis* ATCC 6633 and *Mycobacterium vaccae* MET 10670 and did not exhibit any cytotoxicity against 12 tested human cell tumor lines (Ding et al., 2012). Two new compounds, methyl 3-chloro-6-hydroxy-2-(4-hydroxy-2-methoxy-6-methylphenoxy)-4-methoxybenzoate (218) and (2S,5′ R,E)-7-hydroxy-4,6-dimethoxy-2-(1-methoxy-3-oxo-5-methylhex-1-enyl)-benzofuran-3(2H)-one (219) along with four known metabolites, namely, griseofulvin (220), dechlorogriseofulvin (221), bostrycin (222), and deoxybostrycin (223) isolated from the fungal endophyte

Nigrospora sp. 1403 derived from *K. candel*. Compounds 222 and 223 significantly inhibit the growth of six human cancer cell lines, namely, A549, Hep-2, HepG2, KB, MCF-7 and MCF-7/Adr resulting in IC50 values at 2.64, 5.39, 5.90, 4.19, 6.13 and 6.68 μg/mL. Similarly, compound 223 displayed strong cytotoxicity activity against the same panel of cell lines resulting in IC50 values 2.44, 3.15, 4.41, 3.15, 4.76 and 5.46 μg/mL. In terms of antimicrobial screening, only compound 222 and 223 showed activity against *S. aureus* (ATCC 27154), *E. coli* (ATCC 25922), *P. aeruginosa* (ATCC 25668), *Sarcina ventriculi* (ATCC 29068), *C. albicans* (ATCC 10231) and *B. subtilis* (ATCC 6633) while the other identified compounds did not inhibit any microbial growth (Xia et al., 2011). A new depsidone, phomopsidone A (228), and four known compounds (184−187) were identified from the crude extract of *Phomopsis* sp. A123 isolated from the leaf of *K. candel*. Using MTT bioassay, the new compound, phomopsidone A, displayed activity against the cell line MDA-MB-435 resulting in an IC50 value of 63 μM (Zhang et al., 2014b). The marine-derived fungus, *Talaromyces* sp. ZH-154 isolated from the stem bark of *K. candel* collected in South China Sea was found to produce two bioactive compounds, 7-epiaustdiol (173) and 8-O-methylepiaustdiol (174), along with a known metabolite secalonic acid A (175). The identified compounds were assessed for their antimicrobial and cytotoxicity effects. The new compound, 7-epiaustdiol (173), displayed potent inhibitory effect to the growth of *P. aeruginosa* giving a MIC value of 6.25 μg/mL. In terms of cytotoxicity effects, compound 175 exhibited the highest activity against two human cancer cell lines, namely, KB and KBv200, resulting in IC50 values of 0.63 and 1.05 μg/mL, respectively, in contrast to the other isolated metabolites (Liu et al., 2010). On the other hand, Yang et al. (2013) isolated a new ketone known as 4-(methoxymethyl)-7-methoxy-6-methyl-1(3H)-isobenzofuranone (194), characterized by nuclear magnetic resonance spectrometry (1H and 13C) along with seven known metabolites: lumichrome (241), curvularin (242), 5,5′-oxy-dimethylene-bis(2-furaldehyde) (243), chromone (244), harman(1-methyl-β-carboline) (245) and N9-methyl-1-methyl-β-carboline (246) from the mangrove endophytic fungus *Penicillium* sp. ZH58. The derived metabolites were evaluated for their cytotoxicity effects. Among the eight bioactive compounds isolated, compound 240 displayed toxic effects toward the human cell lines KB and KBv200 resulting in IC50 values 6 and 10 μg/mL, respectively (Yang et al., 2013).

Shiono et al. (2013) conducted an experiment on a different species of mangrove, *R. mucronata* collected in Jakarta, Indonesia. Two tetrahydroxanthones, namely, phomoxanthone A (276) and 12-O-deacetyl-phomoxanthone A (277) were extracted from the fungus *Phomopsis* sp. IM41−1. The isolated metabolites were evaluated for their antimicrobial properties using disk diffusion method. Results demonstrated that both compounds displayed moderate inhibitory activity against *Botrytis cinerea, Sclerotinia sclerotiorum, Diaporthe citri* (=*Diaporthe medusaea*), and *S. aureus* at a concentration of 30 μg per disk (Shiono et al., 2013). *Rhizophora mucronata* hosted an endophytic fungus *Hypocrea lixii* VB1 which was found to be significantly potent against Hep2 cell line resulting in low IC50 value (< 10 μg/mL). Additionally, the ethyl acetate extract of the fungus showed antibacterial activity against *Proteus vulgaris*, *B. subtilis*, *P. aeruginosa*, *E. coli*, and *S. aureus* with a zone of inhibition ranging from 10 to 25 mm (Bhimba et al., 2012).

Buatong et al. (2011) successfully isolated the following endophytic fungi from six genera: *Acremonium, Diaporthe, Hypoxylon, Pestalotiopsis, Phomopsis*, and *Xylaria* from the leaves and branches of *Rhizophora apiculata* Blume. Using agar diffusion method, the antimicrobial activities of the fungi were evaluated. However, results showed that *Phomopsis* sp. MA194 displayed inhibitory activity against Gram-positive bacteria, yeast and *Microsporum gypseum* with the lowest MIC values ranging from 8 to 32 µg/mL (Buatong et al., 2011). The three metabolites aniduquinolones A − C (279−282) derived from the fungus *Aspergillus nidulans* MA-143 isolated from the leaves of *R. stylosa* were assessed for their antibacterial and toxicity activity using human cancer cell lines and brine shrimp lethality test. Results showed that none of the identified metabolites displayed antibacterial and cytotoxicity activities. Nevertheless, compounds 280 and 282 exhibited toxicity effects on brine shrimp resulting in LD50 values of 7.1, 4.5 and 5.5 µg/mL, respectively (Chun-Yan et al., 2013). The mangrove species, *R. stylosa* produced an endophyte fungus *Penicillium oxalicum* EN-201 from which two novel alkaloids penioxamide A (283) and 18-hydroxydecaturin B (284) were isolated from the ethyl acetate extract of the fungus. The isolated metabolites were evaluated in terms of toxicity using the brine shrimp lethality test. Compounds 283 and 284 demonstrated lethality to brine shrimp (Artemia salina) with LD50 values of 5.6 and 2.3 µg/mL respectively (Zhang et al., 2015). The group of Yang et al. (2018) successfully identified three compounds, namely, Isoversicolorin C (285), isosecosterigmatocystin (286) and glulisine A (287) from the endophytic fungus *Aspergillus nidulans* MA-143 of *R. stylosa*. The isolated metabolites were evaluated for their antibacterial properties and tested against *E. coli*, *M. luteus*, and *V. vulnificus*. However, only compound 285 exhibited a potent inhibitory effect (Yang et al., 2018). Five endophytic fungi from different species, namely, *Aspergillus* sp., *Acremonium* sp., *Fusarium* sp., *Penicillium* sp. and *Ampelomyces* sp. were isolated from three different parts (leaf, root, stem) of *R. mucronata*. The isolated fungi were evaluated for their antimicrobial activities. Results demonstrated that only *Penicillium* sp. showed a broader bacterial resistance against *S. aureus* (ATCC 9144) and *E. coli* (ATCC 8739) resulting in inhibition zone of 12.13 and 11.82 mm, respectively (Prihanto et al., 2011).

Nurrunabi et al. (2018) isolated the fungal endophyte *Colletotrichum gloeosporioides* from a poorly studied mangrove species, *Sonneratia apetala* Buch.-Ham. The ethyl acetate extract of the fungus displayed good antimicrobial activities against *P. aeruginosa* and *M. luteus* giving MIC values of 2.4×10^{-4} and 0.125 mg/mL, respectively (Nurunnabi et al., 2018). Another poorly studied mangrove species is *Sonneratia alba* Sm. The isolated endophytic fungus *Alternaria* sp. was found to yield two new carboxylic acids characterized as xanalteric acids I (230) and II (231). The two-novel mangrove-derived metabolites displayed weak inhibitory activity to *S. aureus* (Kjer et al., 2009). Similarly, to *R. stylosa*, *X. granatum* is another underexplored species. The fungal endophyte *Trichoderma* sp. Xy24 yielded two novel terpenoids identified (9R,10R)-dihydro-harzianone (290) and harzianelactone (291) using extensive spectroscopic techniques. Cytotoxicity screening showed that compound 290 displayed activity against HeLa and MCF-7 cell line resulting in IC50 values of 30.1 and 30.7 μmol/L, respectively (Zhang et al., 2016). In another study conducted by Choodej et al. (2016), the endophytic fungus Basidiomycetous fungus XG8D yielded a greater number of compounds compared to the previous study by Zhang et al. (2016). Six novel sesquiterpenes identified as merulinols A-F (292–298) together with four known metabolites. All isolated compounds were evaluated for their cytotoxicity effects however, only compounds 292 and 295 displayed cytotoxicity activity against the gastric KATO-3 cells resulting in IC50 values of 35.0 and 25.3 μM, respectively (Choodej et al., 2016). The same mangrove species hosted the fungus *Phomopsis* sp. xy21 yielding six novel polyketides, namely, phomoxanthones F-K (299–304) and three known metabolites. However, none of them displayed cytotoxicity effects against the eight tested human cell lines (A375, AGS, HCT-8, HCT-8/T, A549, MDA-MB-231, SMMC-7721, and A2780) (Hu et al., 2018).

4.4 Conclusion

It is hoped that the findings presented in this chapter provide readers with useful information for understanding the potential of endophytes hosted by mangroves in producing bioactive compounds for pharmaceutical and industrial applications, and therefore motivate scientists to undertake projects that may result in the development of novel natural drugs. Fungal endophytes associated with mangrove plants are strongly considered as a crucial and viable constituent of microbial diversity which explores a plethora of reward to the host via the biosynthesis of secondary metabolites. A perusal of research literature highlights that several mangrove plants are well known to harbor potent endophytic fungi which exhibit biologically secondary metabolites. Hence, it is more important to bio prospect fungal endophytes inhabiting mangroves for bioactive compounds. Biodiscovery of natural products derived from fungal endophytes provides an alternative solution to the current situation in the era of emerging new diseases that are resistant to available drugs. Therefore, it is important to understand the hidden mechanism underlying in plant-microbe interactions. Advanced integral approaches to study plant endophyte positive interactions are a matter of concern. Taking all of this into account, extensive research on various fungal endophytes shows a bright future for effective output in pharmaceutical industries and sustainable agriculture.

References

Bai, Z.-Q., Lin, X., Wang, Y., Wang, J., Zhou, X., Yang, B., et al., 2014. New phenyl derivatives from endophytic fungus *Aspergillus flavipes* AIL8 derived of mangrove plant *Acanthus ilicifolius*. Fitoterapia 95, 194–202.

Baker, S., Satish, S., 2012. Endophytes: natural warehouse of bioactive compounds. Drug invention today 4, 548−553.

Bharathidasan, R., Panneerselvam, A., 2012. Antioxidant activity of the endophytic fungi isolated from mangrove environment of Karankadu, Ramanathapuram district. International Journal of Pharmaceutical Sciences and Research 3, 2866−2869.

Bharathidasan, R., Panneerselvam, A., 2015. Antibacterial activity of endophytic fungi extracts from the mangrove plant *Avicennia marina* (Forsk) Vierh. International Journal of Advanced Research in Biological Sciences 2, 145−148.

Bhardwaj, A., Agrawal, P., 2014. A review fungal endophytes: as a store house of bioactive compound. World Journal of Pharmaceutical Sciences 3, 228−237.

Bhimba, B.V., Agnel Defora Franco, D.A., Mathew, J.M., Jose, G.M., Joel, E.L., Thangaraj, M., 2012. Anticancer and antimicrobial activity of mangrove derived fungi *Hypocrea lixii* VB1. Chinese Journal of Natural Medicines 10, 77−80.

Bin, G., Yanping, C., Hong, Z., Zheng, X., Yanqiu, Z., Huaiyi, F., et al., 2014. Isolation, characterization and anti-multiple drug resistant (MDR) bacterial activity of endophytic fungi Isolated from the mangrove plant, *Aegiceras corniculatum*. Tropical Journal of Pharmaceutical Research 13, 593−599.

Buatong, J., Phongpaichit, S., Rukachaisirikul, V., Sakayaroj, J., 2011. Antimicrobial activity of crude extracts from mangrove fungal endophytes. World Journal of Microbiology Biotechnology 27, 3005−3008.

Cai, R., Chen, S., Long, Y., Li, C., Huang, X., She, Z., 2017. Depsidones from *Talaromyces stipitatus* SK-4, an endophytic fungus of the mangrove plant *Acanthus ilicifolius*. Phytochemistry Letters 20, 196−199.

Chaeprasert, S., Piapukiew, J., Whalley, A.J.S., Sihanonth, P., 2010. Endophytic fungi from mangrove plant species of Thailand: their antimicrobial and anticancer potentials. Botanica Marina 53, 555−564.

Chamovitz, D.A., 2018. Plants are intelligent; now what? Nature Plants 4, 622−623.

Cheng, Z.-S., Tang, W.-C., Xu, S.-L., Sun, S.-F., Huang, B.-Y., Yan, X., et al., 2008. First report of an endophyte (*Diaporthe phaseolorum* var. sojae) from *Kandelia candel*. Journal of Forestry Research 19, 277−282.

Chen, S., Liu, Z., Li, H., Xia, G., Lu, Y., He, L., et al., 2015. β-Resorcylic acid derivatives with α-glucosidase inhibitory activity from *Lasiodiplodia* sp. ZJ-HQ1, an endophytic fungus in the medicinal plant *Acanthus ilicifolius*. Phytochemistry Letters 13, 141−146.

Chen, Y., Mao, W., Tao, H., Zhu, W., Qi, X., Chen, Y., et al., 2011. Structural characterization and antioxidant properties of an exopolysaccharide produced by the mangrove endophytic fungus *Aspergillus* sp. Y16. Bioresource Technology 102, 8179−8184.

Chen, L.L., Wang, P., Chen, H.Q., Guo, Z.K., Wang, H., Dai, H.F., et al., 2017. New furan derivatives from a mangrove-derived endophytic fungus *Coriolopsis* sp. Molecules 22.

Chi, W.-C., Pang, K.-L., Chen, W.-L., Wang, G.-J., Lee, T.-H., 2019. Antimicrobial and iNOS inhibitory activities of the endophytic fungi isolated from the mangrove plant *Acanthus ilicifolius* var. xiamenensis. Botanical Studies 60, 4-4.

Choodej, S., Teerawatananond, T., Mitsunaga, T., Pudhom, K., 2016. Chamigrane sesquiterpenes from a basidiomycetous endophytic fungus XG8D associated with Thai mangrove *Xylocarpus granatum*. Marine drugs 14, 132.

Chun-Yan, A., Xiao-Ming, L., Han, L., Chun-Shun, L., Ming-Hui, W., Gang-Ming, X., et al., 2013. 4-Phenyl-3,4-dihydroquinolone derivatives from *Aspergillus nidulans* MA-

143, an endophytic fungus isolated from the mangrove plant *Rhizophora stylosa*. Journal of Natural Products 76, 1896—1901.

Cui, H., Liu, Y., Li, T., Zhang, Z., Ding, M., Long, Y., et al., 2018. 3-Arylisoindolinone and sesquiterpene derivatives from the mangrove endophytic fungi *Aspergillus versicolor* SYSU-SKS025. Fitoterapia 124, 177—181.

Cui, H., Mei, W., Miao, C., Lin, H., Hong, K., Dai, H., 2008. Antibacterial constituents from the endophytic fungus *Penicillium* sp. 0935030 of mangrove plant *Acrostichum aureum*. Chinese Journal of Antibiotics 33, 407—410.

Cui, H., Yu, J., Chen, S., Ding, M., Huang, X., Yuan, J., et al., 2017. Alkaloids from the mangrove endophytic fungus *Diaporthe phaseolorum* SKS019. Bioorganic & Medicinal Chemistry Letters 27, 803—807.

Darsih, C., Prachyawarakorn, V., Wiyakrutta, S., Mahidol, C., Ruchirawat, S., Kittakoop, P., 2015. Cytotoxic metabolites from the endophytic fungus *Penicillium chermesinum*: discovery of a cysteine-targeted Michael acceptor as a pharmacophore for fragment-based drug discovery, bioconjugation and click reactions. RSC Advances 5, 70595—70603.

Debbab, A., Aly, A.H., Proksch, P., 2013. Mangrove derived fungal endophytes—a chemical and biological perception. Fungal Diversity 61, 1—27.

Deng, Z., Cao, L., 2017. Fungal endophytes and their interactions with plants in phytoremediation: a review. Chemosphere 168, 1100—1106.

Ding, L., Maier, A., Fiebig, H.-H., Lin, W.-H., Peschel, G., Hertweck, C., 2012. Kandenols A—E, eudesmenes from an endophytic *Streptomyces* sp. of the mangrove tree *Kandelia candel*. Journal of Natural Products 75, 2223—2227.

Ding, L., Münch, J., Goerls, H., Maier, A., Fiebig, H.-H., Lin, W.-H., et al., 2010. Xiamycin, a pentacyclic indolosesquiterpene with selective anti-HIV activity from a bacterial mangrove endophyte. Bioorganic and Medicinal Chemistry Letters 20, 6685—6687.

Dong, L.-M., Huang, L.-L., Dai, H., Xu, Q.-L., Ouyang, J.-K., Jia, X.-C., et al., 2018. Anti-MRSA sesquiterpenes from the semi-mangrove plant *Myoporum bontioides* A. Gray. Marine drugs 16, 438.

El Amrani, M., Debbab, A., Aly, A.H., Wray, V., Dobretsov, S., Müller, W.E.G., et al., 2012. Farinomalein derivatives from an unidentified endophytic fungus isolated from the mangrove plant *Avicennia marina*. Tetrahedron Letters 53, 6721—6724.

Elavarasi, A., Rathna, G.S., Kalaiselvam, M., 2012. Taxol producing mangrove endophytic fungi Fusarium oxysporum from *Rhizophora annamalayana*. Asian Pacific Journal of Tropical Biomedicine 2, S1081—S1085.

Eldeen, M., Effendy, A.W.M., 2013. Antimicrobial agents from mangrove plants and their endophytes. In: Mendez-Vilas, A. (Ed.), Microbial Pathogens and Strategies for Combating them: Science, Technology and Education. Formatex, Spain, pp. 872—882.

Flora, G., Mittal, M., Flora, S.J.S., 2015. 26—Medical countermeasures—chelation therapy. In: Flora, S.J.S. (Ed.), Handbook of Arsenic Toxicology. Academic Press, Oxford, pp. 589—626.

Guan, S.-h, Sattler, I., Lin, W.-h, Guo, D.-a, Grabley, S., 2005. p-Aminoacetophenonic acids produced by a mangrove endophyte: *Streptomyces* griseus subsp. Journal of Natural Products 68, 1198—1200.

Han, Z., Mei, W., Zhao, Y., Deng, Y., Dai, H., 2009. A new cytotoxic isocoumarin from endophytic fungus *Penicillium* sp. 091402 of the mangrove plant *Bruguiera sexangula*. Chemistry of Natural Compounds 45, 805—807.

He, K.-Y., Zhang, C., Duan, Y.-R., Huang, G.-L., Yang, C.-Y., Lu, X.-R., et al., 2017. New chlorinated xanthone and anthraquinone produced by a mangrove-derived fungus *Penicillium citrinum* HL-5126. The Journal of Antibiotics (Tokyo) 70, 823.

Huang, Z., Cai, X., Shao, C., She, Z., Xia, X., Chen, Y., et al., 2008. Chemistry and weak antimicrobial activities of phomopsins produced by mangrove endophytic fungus *Phomopsis* sp. ZSU-H76. Phytochemistry 69, 1604–1608.

Huang, H., She, Z., Lin, Y., Vrijmoed, L.L., Lin, W., 2007. Cyclic peptides from an endophytic fungus obtained from a mangrove leaf (*Kandelia candel*). Journal of Natural Products 70, 1696–1699.

Huang, X., Sun, X., Ding, B., Lin, M., Liu, L., Huang, H., et al., 2013. A new anti-acetylcholinesterase α-pyrone meroterpene, arigsugacin I, from mangrove endophytic fungus *Penicillium* sp. sk5GW1L of *Kandelia candel*. Planta Medica 79, 1572–1575.

Huang, J., Xu, J., Wang, Z., Khan, D., Niaz, S.I., Zhu, Y., et al., 2017. New lasiodiplodins from mangrove endophytic fungus *Lasiodiplodia* sp. 318#. Natural product research 31, 326–332.

Huang, Z., Yang, R., Guo, Z., She, Z., Lin, Y., 2010. A new naphtho-γ-pyrone from mangrove endophytic fungus ZSU-H26. Chemistry of Natural Compounds 46, 15–18.

Hu, H.B., Luo, Y.F., Wang, P., Wang, W.J., Wu, J., 2018. Xanthone-derived polyketides from the Thai mangrove endophytic fungus *Phomopsis* sp. Fitoterapia 131, 265–xy271.

Jiang, C.-S., Zhou, Z.-F., Yang, X.-H., Lan, L.-F., Gu, Y.-C., Ye, B.-P., et al., 2018. Antibacterial sorbicillin and diketopiperazines from the endogenous fungus *Penicillium* sp. GD6 associated Chinese mangrove *Bruguiera gymnorrhiza*. Chin J Nat Med 16, 358–365.

Jin, P.F., Zuo, W.J., Guo, Z.K., Mei, W.L., Dai, H.F., 2013. Metabolites from the endophytic fungus *Penicillium* sp. FJ-1 of *Ceriops tagal*. Yao Xue Xue Bao 48, 1688–1691.

Job, N., Manomi, S., Philip, R., 2015. Isolation and characterization of endophytic fungi from *Avicennia officinalis*. International Journal of Biological and Medical Research 5, 4–8.

Joseph, B., Priya, M., 2011. Bioactive compounds from endophytes and their potential in pharmaceutical effect: a review. American Journal of Biochemistry and Molecular Biology 1, 291–309.

Ju, Z., Lin, X., Lu, X., Tu, Z., Wang, J., Kaliyaperumal, K., et al., 2015. Botryoisocoumarin A, a new COX-2 inhibitor from the mangrove *Kandelia candel* endophytic fungus *Botryosphaeria* sp. KcF6. The Journal of Antibiotics (Tokyo) 68.

Khare, E., Mishra, J., Arora, N.K., 2018. Multifaceted interactions between endophytes and plant: developments and prospects. Frontiers in Microbiology 9, 2732.

Kjer, J., Wray, V., Edrada-Ebel, R., Ebel, R., Pretsch, A., Lin, W., et al., 2009. Xanalteric acids I and II and related phenolic compounds from an endophytic *Alternaria* sp. isolated from the mangrove plant *Sonneratia alba*. Journal of Natural Products 72, 2053–2057.

Lin, C., Chunhua, L., Yuemao, S., 2010. Three new 2-pyranone derivatives from mangrove endophytic actinomycete strain *Nocardiopsis* sp. A00203. Records of Natural Products 4.

Lin, Z.J., Zhang, G.J., Zhu, T.J., Liu, R., Wei, H.J., Gu, Q.Q., 2009. Bioactive cytochalasins from *Aspergillus flavipes*, an endophytic fungus associated with the mangrove plant *Acanthus ilicifolius*. Helvetica 92.

Liu, F., Cai, X.L., Yang, H., Xia, X.K., Guo, Z.Y., Yuan, J., et al., 2010. The bioactive metabolites of the mangrove endophytic fungus *Talaromyces* sp. ZH-154 isolated from *Kandelia candel* (L.) Druce. Planta Medica 76, 185–189.

Liu, Z., Chen, Y., Chen, S., Liu, Y., Lu, Y., Chen, D., et al., 2016. Aspterpenacids A and B, two sesterterpenoids from a mangrove endophytic fungus *Aspergillus terreus* H010. Organic Letters 18, 1406–H1409.

Liu, Y., Kurtán, T., Mándi, A., Weber, H., Wang, C., Hartmann, R., et al., 2018a. A novel 10-membered macrocyclic lactone from the mangrove-derived endophytic fungus *Annulohypoxylon* sp. Tetrahedron Letters 59, 632−636.

Liu, D., Li, X.-M., Meng, L., Li, C.-S., Gao, S.-S., Shang, Z., et al., 2011. Nigerapyrones A−H, α-pyrone derivatives from the marine mangrove-derived endophytic fungus *Aspergillus niger* MA-132. Journal of Natural Products 74, 1787−1791.

Liu, Z., Qiu, P., Li, J., Chen, G., Chen, Y., Liu, H., et al., 2018b. Anti-inflammatory polyketides from the mangrove-derived fungus *Ascomycota* sp. SK2YWS-L. Tetrahedron 74, 746−751.

Liu, J., Xu, M., Zhu, M.Y., Feng, Y., 2015. Chemoreversal metabolites from the endophytic fungus *Penicillium citrinum* isolated from a mangrove *Avicennia marina*. Natural Products Communication 10, 1203−1205.

Li, L.-Y., Ding, Y., Groth, I., Menzel, K.-D., Peschel, G., Voigt, K., et al., 2008. Pyrrole and indole alkaloids from an endophytic *Fusarium incarnatum* (HKI00504) isolated from the mangrove plant *Aegiceras corniculatum*. Journal of Asian Natural Products Research 10, 765−770.

Li, J.-L., Sun, X., Chen, L., Guo, L.-D., 2016. Community structure of endophytic fungi of four mangrove species in southern China. Mycology 7, 180−190.

Li, J., Wang, J., Jiang, C.S., Li, G., Guo, Y.W., 2014. (+)-Cyclopenol, a new naturally occurring 7-membered 2,5-dioxopiperazine alkaloid from the fungus *Penicillium sclerotiorum* endogenous with the Chinese mangrove *Bruguiera gymnorrhiza*. Journal of Asian Natural Products Research 16, 542−548.

Li, S., Wei, M., Chen, G., Lin, Y., 2012. Two new dihydroisocoumarins from the endophytic fungus *Aspergillus* sp. collected from the south china sea. Chemistry of Natural Compounds 48, 371−373.

Li, F.-S., Weng, J.-K., 2017. Demystifying traditional herbal medicine with modern approach. Nature Plants 3, 1−7.

Li, D., Yan, S., Proksch, P., Liang, Z., Li, Q., Xu, J., 2013. Volatile metabolites profiling of a Chinese mangrove endophytic *Pestalotiopsis* sp. strain. African Journal of Biotechnology 12.

Lobo, M., Sridhar, K., Seetharam, R., 2005. Antimicrobial and enzyme activity of mangrove endophytic fungi of southwest coast of India. Journal of Agricultural Technology 1 (1), 67−80.

Luo, D.Q., Deng, H.Y., Yang, X.L., Shi, B.Z., Zhang, J.Z., 2011. Oleanane-type triterpenoids from the endophytic fungus *Pestalotiopsis clavispora* isolated from the Chinese mangrove plant *Bruguiera sexangula*. Helvetica 94, 1041−1047.

Lv, F., Daletos, G., Lin, W., Proksch, P., 2015. Two new cyclic depsipeptides from the endophytic fungus *Fusarium* sp. Natural Product Communication 10, 1667−1670.

Meng, L.-H., Li, X.-M., Liu, Y., Xu, G.-M., Wang, B.-G., 2017. Antimicrobial alkaloids produced by the mangrove endophyte *Penicillium brocae* MA-231 using the OSMAC approach. RSC Advances 7, 55026−55033.

Meng, L.-H., Li, X.-M., Lv, C.-T., Li, C.-S., Xu, G.-M., Huang, C.-G., et al., 2013. Sulfur-containing cytotoxic curvularin macrolides from *Penicillium sumatrense* MA-92, a fungus obtained from the rhizosphere of the mangrove *Lumnitzera racemosa*. Journal of Natural Products 76, 2145−2149.

Meng, L.-H., Zhang, P., Li, X.-M., Wang, B.-G., 2015. Penicibrocazines A−E, five new sulfide diketopiperazines from the marine-derived endophytic fungus *Penicillium brocae*. Marine drugs 13, 276−287.

Nakamura, T., Suzuki, T., Rudianto Ariefta, N., Koseki, T., Aboshi, T., Murayama, T., et al., 2019. Meroterpenoids produced by Pseudocosmospora sp. Bm-1-1 isolated from *Acanthus ebracteatus* Vahl. Phytochemistry Letters 31, 85−91.

Nurunnabi, T.R., Nahar, L., Al-Majmaie, S., Rahman, S.M., Sohrab, M.H., Billah, M.M., et al., 2018. Anti-MRSA activity of oxysporone and xylitol from the endophytic fungus *Pestalotia* sp. growing on the Sundarbans mangrove plant *Heritiera fomes*. Phytotherapy Research 32, 348−354.

Palanichamy, P., Krishnamoorthy, G., Kannan, S., Marudhamuthu, M., 2018. Bioactive potential of secondary metabolites derived from medicinal plant endophytes. Egyptian Journal of Basic and Applied Sciences 5, 303−312.

Phyo, K.M.M., 2011. Isolation and identification of mangrove fungus from *Bruguiera sexangula* (Lour.) Poir. Universities Research Journal 273.

Prihanto, A., Firdaus, M., Nurdiani, R., 2011. Endophytic fungi isolated from mangrove (*Rhizophora mucronata*) and its antibacterial activity on *Staphylococcus aureus* and *Escherichia coli*. Journal of Food Science 1, 386.

Rahmawati, S., Izzati, F., Hapsari, Y., Septiana, E., Rachman, F., Simanjuntak, P., 2019. Endophytic microbes and antioxidant activities of secondary metabolites from mangroves *Avicennia marina* and *Xylocarpus granatum*. In: IOP Conference Series: Earth and Environmental Science. IOP Publishing, pp. 012065.

Ravindran, C., Naveenan, T., Varatharajan, G.R., Rajasabapathy, R., Meena, R.M., 2012. Antioxidants in mangrove plants and endophytic fungal associations. Botanica Marina 55, 269−279.

Sadeer, N.B., Fawzi, M.M., Gokhan, Z., Rajesh, J., Nadeem, N., Kannan, R.R.R., et al., 2019. Ethnopharmacology, phytochemistry, and global distribution of mangroves-a comprehensive review. Marine Drugs 17, 231.

Salini, G., 2014. Pharmaological profile of mangrove endophytes-a review. International Journal of Pharmacy and Pharmaceutical Sciences 7.

Saravanakumar, K., 2014. Antioxidant activity of the mangrove endophytic fungus (*Trichoderma* sp.). Journal of Coastal Life Medicine 2, 559−563.

Schulz, B., Boyle, C., Draeger, S., Römmert, A.-K., Krohn, K., 2002. Endophytic fungi: a source of novel biologically active secondary metabolites. In: Paper presented at the British Mycological Society symposium on Fungal Bioactive Compounds, the University of Wales Swansea, 22−27 April, 2001. Mycological Research 106, 996−1004.

Sharma, M., Kansal, R., Singh, D., 2018. Chapter 20—Endophytic microorganisms: their role in plant growth and crop improvement. In: Prasad, R., Gill, S.S., Tuteja, N. (Eds.), Crop Improvement through Microbial Biotechnology. Elsevier, pp. 391−413.

Shiono, Y., Sasaki, T., Shibuya, F., Yasuda, Y., Koseki, T., Supratman, U., 2013. Isolation of a phomoxanthone A derivative, a new metabolite of tetrahydroxanthone, from a *Phomopsis* sp. isolated from the mangrove, *Rhizhopora mucronata*. Natural Product Communications 8, 1735−1737.

Singh, B.P., 2019. Advances in Endophytic Fungal Research: Present Status and Future Challenges. Springer, Switzerland.

Strobel, G., Daisy, B., Castillo, U., Harper, J., 2004. Natural products from endophytic microorganisms. Journal of Natural Products 67, 257−268.

Sun, W., Wu, W., Liu, X., Zaleta-Pinet, D.A., Clark, B.R., 2019. Bioactive compounds isolated from marine-derived microbes in China: 2009−2018. Marine drugs 17, 339.

Tan, R.X., Zou, W.X., 2001. Endophytes: a rich source of functional metabolites. Natural Product Reports 18, 448–459.

Trewavas, A., 2005. Green plants as intelligent organisms. Trends in Plant Science 10, 413–419.

Venieraki, A., Dimou, M., Katinakis, P., 2017. Endophytic fungi residing in medicinal plants have the ability to produce the same or similar pharmacologically active secondary metabolites as their hosts. Hellenic Plant Protection Journal 10, 51–66.

Verma, V.C., Lobkovsky, E., Gange, A.C., Singh, S.K., Prakash, S., 2011. Piperine production by endophytic fungus *Periconia* sp. isolated from *Piper longum* L. The Journal of Antibiotics 64, 427–431.

Wang, J., Cox, D.G., Ding, W., Huang, G., Lin, Y., Li, C., 2014a. Three new resveratrol derivatives from the mangrove endophytic fungus *Alternaria* sp. Marine drugs 12, 2840–2850.

Wang, L., Han, X., Zhu, G., Wang, Y., Chairoungdua, A., Piyachaturawat, P., et al., 2018. Polyketides from the endophytic fungus *Cladosporium* sp. isolated from the mangrove plant *Excoecaria agallocha*. Frontiers in Chemistry 6, 344-344.

Wang, J.-F., Liang, R., Liao, S.-R., Yang, B., Tu, Z.-C., Lin, X.-P., et al., 2017. Vaccinols J–S, ten new salicyloid derivatives from the marine mangrove-derived endophytic fungus *Pestalotiopsis vaccinii*. Fitoterapia 120, 164–170.

Wang, J., Lu, Z., Liu, P., Wang, Y., Li, J., Hong, K., et al., 2012. Cytotoxic polyphenols from the fungus *Penicillium expansum* 091 006 endogenous with the mangrove plant *Excoecaria agallocha*. Planta Medica 78, 1861–1866.

Wang, K.-W., Wang, S.-W., Bin, W., Ji-Guang, W., 2014b. Bioactive natural compounds from the mangrove endophytic fungi. Mini-Reviews in Medicinal Chemistry 14, 370–391.

Wang, J., Wei, X., Qin, X., Chen, H., Lin, X., Zhang, T., et al., 2015. Two new prenylated phenols from endogenous fungus *Pestalotiopsis* vaccinii of mangrove plant *Kandelia candel* (L.) Druce. Phytochemistry Letters 12, 59–62.

Wang, S.-Y., Xu, Z.-L., She, Z.-G., Wang, H., Li, C.-R., Lin, Y.-C., 2008. Two new metabolites from the mangrove endophytic fungus no. 2106. Journal of Asian Natural Products Research 10, 622–626.

Wen, L., Wei, Q., Chen, G., Cai, J., She, Z., 2013. Chemical constituents from the mangrove endophytic fungus *Sporothrix* sp. Chemistry of Natural Compounds 49, 137–140.

Wu, Y.-Z., Qiao, F., Xu, G.-W., Zhao, J., Teng, J.-F., Li, C., et al., 2015. Neuroprotective metabolites from the endophytic fungus *Penicillium citrinum* of the mangrove *Bruguiera gymnorrhiza*. Phytochemistry Letters 12, 148–152.

Xiaoling, C., Xiaoli, L., Shining, Z., Junping, G., Shuiping, W., Xiaoming, L., et al., 2010. Cytotoxic and topoisomerase I inhibitory activities from extracts of endophytic fungi isolated from mangrove plants in Zhuhai, China. Journal of Ecology 2, 017–024.

Xia, X., Li, Q., Li, J., Shao, C., Zhang, J., Zhang, Y., et al., 2011. Two new derivatives of griseofulvin from the mangrove endophytic fungus *Nigrospora* sp. (strain No. 1403) from *Kandelia candel* (L.) Druce. Planta Medica 77, 1735–1738.

Xing, X., Guo, S., 2011. Fungal endophyte communities in four Rhizophoraceae mangrove species on the south coast of China. Ecological Research 26, 403–409.

Xu, J., Aly, A.H., Wray, V., Proksch, P., 2011. Polyketide derivatives of endophytic fungus *Pestalotiopsis* sp. isolated from the Chinese mangrove plant *Rhizophora mucronata*. Tetrahedron Letters 52, 21–25.

Xu, J., Kjer, J., Sendker, J., Wray, V., Guan, H., Edrada, R., et al., 2009. Cytosporones, coumarins, and an alkaloid from the endophytic fungus *Pestalotiopsis* sp. isolated from the Chinese mangrove plant *Rhizophora mucronata*. Bioorganic and Medicinal Chemistry 17, 7362–7367.

Xu, R., Li, X.-M., Wang, B.-G., 2016. Penicisimpins A–C, three new dihydroisocoumarins from *Penicillium simplicissimum* MA-332, a marine fungus derived from the rhizosphere of the mangrove plant *Bruguiera sexangula* var. rhynchopetala. Phytochemistry Letters 17, 114–118.

Yang, J., Huang, R., Qiu, S.X., She, Z., Lin, Y., 2013. A new isobenzofuranone from the mangrove endophytic fungus *Penicillium* sp. (ZH58). Natural Product Research 27, 1902–1905.

Yang, S.Q., Li, X.M., Xu, G.M., Li, X., An, C.Y., Wang, B.G., 2018. Antibacterial anthraquinone derivatives isolated from a mangrove-derived endophytic fungus *Aspergillus nidulans* by ethanol stress strategy. The Journal of Antibiotics (Tokyo) 71, 778–784.

Yu, H., Zhang, L., Li, L., Zheng, C., Guo, L., Li, W., et al., 2010. Recent developments and future prospects of antimicrobial metabolites produced by endophytes. Microbiological research 165, 437–449.

Zeng, Y.B., Gu, H.G., Zuo, W.J., Zhang, L.L., Bai, H.J., Guo, Z.K., et al., 2015. Two new sesquiterpenoids from endophytic fungus J3 isolated from mangrove plant *Ceriops tagal*. Arch Pharmaceutical Reseasrch 38, 673–676.

Zhang, M., Liu, J.-M., Zhao, J.-L., Li, N., Chen, R.-D., Xie, K.-B., et al., 2016. Two new diterpenoids from the endophytic fungus *Trichoderma* sp. Xy24 isolated from mangrove plant *Xylocarpus granatum*. Chinese Chemical Letters 27, 957–960.

Zhang, M., Li, N., Chen, R., Zou, J., Wang, C., 2014a. Two terpenoids and a polyketide from the endophytic fungus *Trichoderma* sp. Xy24 isolated from mangrove plant *Xylocarpus granatum*. Journal of Chinese Pharmaceutical Sciences 23, 421–424.

Zhang, P., Li, X.-M., Liu, H., Li, X., Wang, B.-G., 2015. Two new alkaloids from *Penicillium* oxalicum EN-201, an endophytic fungus derived from the marine mangrove plant *Rhizophora stylosa*. Phytochemistry Letters 13, 160–164.

Zhang, W., Xu, L., Yang, L., Huang, Y., Li, S., Shen, Y., 2014b. Phomopsidone A, a novel depsidone metabolite from the mangrove endophytic fungus *Phomopsis* sp. A123. Fitoterapia 96, 146–151.

Zheng, C., Chen, Y., Jiang, L.-L., Shi, X.-M., 2014. Antiproliferative metabolites from the endophytic fungus *Penicillium* sp. FJ-1 isolated from a mangrove *Avicennia marina*. Phytochemistry Letters 10, 272–275.

Zhou, J., Diao, X., Wang, T., Chen, G., Lin, Q., Yang, X., et al., 2018. Phylogenetic diversity and antioxidant activities of culturable fungal endophytes associated with the mangrove species *Rhizophora stylosa* and *R. mucronata* in the South China Sea. PLoS ONE 13, e0197359.

Zhou, X.-M., Zheng, C.-J., Chen, G.-Y., Song, X.-P., Han, C.-R., Li, G.-N., et al., 2014. Bioactive anthraquinone derivatives from the mangrove-derived fungus *Stemphylium* sp. 33231. Journal of Natural Products 77, 2021–2028.

Zhu, F., Chen, X., Yuan, Y., Huang, M., Sun, H., Xiang, W.-Z., 2009. The chemical investigations of the mangrove plant *Avicennia marina* and its endophytes. The Open Natural Products Journal 2, 24–32.

Zhu, F., Lin, Y., 2007. Three xanthones from a marine-derived mangrove endophytic fungus. Chemistry of Natural Compounds 43, 132–135.

Monographs of medicinally important mangrove plants

III

Acanthus ilicifolius L.

5

5.1 General description

5.1.1 Botanical nomenclature

Acanthus ilicifolius L. (Fig. 5.1)

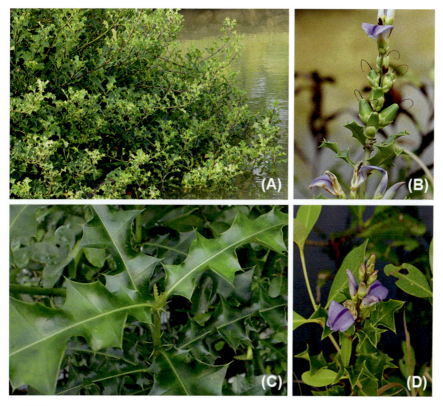

FIGURE 5.1

(A) Whole plant, (B) fruits, (C), and leaves (D) flowers of *Acanthus ilicifolius* (GBIF, 2020).

Mangroves with Therapeutic Potential for Human Health. DOI: https://doi.org/10.1016/B978-0-323-99332-6.00018-7

5.1.2 Botanical family

- Acanthaceae

5.1.3 Vernacular names

- Holy leaved acanthus, holy mangrove, sea holy (English)
- Harkukanta (Hindi)
- Jeruju, daruju (Indonesia)
- Daguari, diluariu (Philippines)
- Kaem mo, cha kreng, ngueak plaamo namngoen (Thailand)
- ô rô, nước, lão thử cân (Vietnam)
- Mulli (Tamil)
- Alchi, alisi (Telugu)

5.2 Geographical distribution

Acanthus ilicifolius is found in Bangladesh, India, Australia, Indonesia and South Thailand (Sadeer et al., 2019). It is a preserved specimen in Malaysia, Thailand and New Caledonia and is under human observation in Vanuatu, India, Sri Lanka, and Hong Kong. Fig. 5.2 illustrates the distribution of *A. ilicifolius* across the globe.

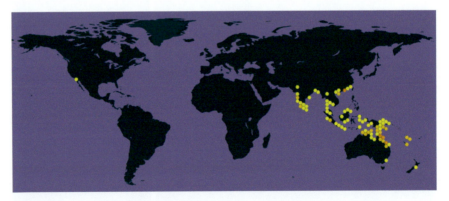

FIGURE 5.2

Distribution of *Acanthus ilicifolius* across the globe (GBIF, 2020).

5.3 Morphological characteristics

Acanthus ilicifolius is a small tree of height up to 2 m with stilt roots. It has simple, opposite, and sharp-edged leaves, with a narrow base. The petioles are short, 5–6 mm in length, slightly winged with two sharp spurs at the base, dark green in color. Flowers-sessile are 4 cm long, spike inflorescence, terminal and the corolla are light blue or violet. Fruits are 3 cm long, oblong, compressed, apiculate and brown in color (Bora et al., 2017). Fig. 5.1 illustrates the morphological characteristics of *A. ilicifolius*.

5.4 Ethnobotanical uses

In west Bengal and Bangladesh, the whole plant is traditionally used to manage a panoply of ailments, namely, rheumatism, relief for asthma, diabetes, diuretic, dyspepsia, leprosy, hepatitis, blood purifier, cure for cold, gangrenous wounds, skin allergies, snake bites, pain reliever, or as an aphrodisiac (Babu et al., 2001; Bandaranayake, 2002; Kumar et al., 2008). In India and Thailand, either the whole plant or the fruit is used against kidney stone, skin diseases, smallpox, leucorrhea, ulcer, paralysis or as an astringent (Islam et al., 2012; Rahmatullah et al., 2010; Ravindran et al., 2005).

5.5 Phytochemicals

This mangrove species contains a manifold of compounds from different phytochemical classes, including anthraquinones, alkaloids, flavonoids, steroids, tannins, saponins, terpenoids, glycosides, among others (Sadeer et al., 2019). Table 5.1 summarizes the different compounds identified from *A. ilicifolius*.

Table 5.1 Phytochemicals of *Acanthus ilicifolius*.

Plant part	Extract	Phytochemical class	Compounds	References
NI	NI	Aliphatic glycosides	Ilicifolioside B, ilicifolioside C	Saranya et al. (2015)
		Alkaloids	Acanthicifoline, trigonellin, 2-benzoxazolinone, benzoxazin-3-one, 5, 5'-bis-benzoxazoline-2,2'-dione, benzoxazinoid glucosides, 4-O-b-D-glucopyranosyl-benzoxazolin-2(3H)-one, (2R)-2-β-D-glucopyranosyloxy-2H-1,4-benzoxazine-3(4H)-one, (2R)-2-β-glucopyranosyloxy-4-hydroxy-1, 4-benzoxazine-3-one, 2-hydroxy-2H-1, 4-benzoxazin 3(4H) one	

(Continued)

Table 5.1 Phytochemicals of *Acanthus ilicifolius. Continued*

Plant part	Extract	Phytochemical class	Compounds	References
		Flavonoids	Quercetin, quercetin 3-O-β-D-glucopyranoside, apigenin 7-O-β-D-glucuronide, methylapigenin 7-O-β-D-glucopyranuronate, acacetin 7-O-β-L-rhamnopyranosyl-(1‴ 6")-O-β-D-glucopyranoside, vitexin	
		Lignan glycosides	(+)-Lyoniresinol 3a-[2-(3,5-dimethoxy-4-hydroxy)-benzoyl]-O-β-glucopyranoside, dihydroxymethyl-bis(3,5-dimethoxy-4-hydroxyphenyl) tetrahydrofuran-9(or9')-O-β-D-glucopyranosid, (8R,7'S,8'R)-5,5'-dimethoxylariciresinol-4-O-β-D-glucopyranoside, Acanfolioside, Alangilignoside C, (+)-syringaresinol-O-β-D-glucopyranoside (+) lyoniresinol3-O-β-D-glucopyranoside, (+)-lyoniresinol 2a-O-β-D-galactopyranosyl-3a-O-β-D-glucopyranoside, (+)-lyoniresinol 3a-O-β-D-galactopyranosyl-(1−6)-β-D-glucopyranoside, (-)-lyoniresinol 3-O-β-D-glucopyranoside	
		Phenylethanol glycosides	Phenylethyl-O-b-D-glucopyranosyl-(1/2)-O-b-D-glucopyranoside, phenylethyl-O-b-D-glucopyranoside, cistanoside F, isocistanoside F, cistanoside E, campneoside I, ilicifolioside A, ilicifolioside D, acteoside, isoacteoside	

(Continued)

Table 5.1 Phytochemicals of *Acanthus ilicifolius. Continued*

Plant part	Extract	Phytochemical class	Compounds	References
		Terpenoids	α-L-Arabinofuranosyl-(1/4)-β-D-glucuronopyranosyl-(1_3)-3-hydroxylup-20(29)-ene, pentacyclic triterpenes, β−amyrin, α−amyrin, lupeol, oleanolic acid, ursolic acid	
		Steroids	Cholesterol, campesterol, stigmasterol, β−sitosterol, stigmast-7-en-3-ol, stigmasteryl-D-glucopyanoside,28-isofucosterol, octacosyl alcohol, sitosterol-3-O-β-D-glucopyranoside, stigmasterol-3-O-β-D-glucopyranoside	
		Fatty acid derivatives	Palmitic acid, octadecanoic acid, stigmasterol octadecanoate, β-sitosterol octadecanoate, tetracosanol, octacosanol	
		Miscellaneous	(2R)-2-O-β-D-glucopyranosyl-4-hydroxy-*2H*-1,4-benzoxazin-3(4H)-one, 7-chloro-(2R)-2-O-β-D-glucopyranosyl-2H-1, 4-benzoxazin-3(4H)-one, betaine, vanillic acid, luteolin-7-O-b-D-glucuronide, uridine, uracil	
AP	EtOH	Alkaloids, steroids, terpenoids, saponins, tannins, phenolic compounds, glycosides and flavonoids	NI	Sardar et al. (2018)
NI	H, MeOH	Anthraquinones, alkaloids, flavonoids, glycosides, saponins, tannins, terpenoids	NI	Fabiyi (2015)
B, Fr, L, R	NI	Alkaloids, long-chain alcohols, steroids, sulfur, triterpenes, saponins	NI	Revathi et al. (2014)

(Continued)

Table 5.1 Phytochemicals of *Acanthus ilicifolius. Continued*

Plant part	Extract	Phytochemical class	Compounds	References
L	MeOH	Protein, resin, steroids, tannins, glycosides, reducing sugar, carbohydrates, saponins, sterols, terpenoids, acidic compounds, phenol, cardio glycosides, catechol	NI	Ganesh and Vennila (2011)
L	MeOH	Flavonoids, tannins, steroids, saponins, glycosides	NI	Islam et al. (2012)
R	EtOH	NI	Erigeside C	Lin et al. (2017)
R	EtOH	Terpenoids	NI	Singh and Aeri (2013)
L	Aq	NI	2-benzoxazolinone	
L	C	Terpenoids, sterols	NI	
L	MeOH	NI	Bisoxazolinone	
AP	MeOH	Lignan, cyclolignan glycosides	NI	
L	EtOH	NI	1β, 3β-dihydroxyrs-12-en-28-oic acid, 2α, 3β-dihyodroxyurs-12-en-28-oic acid, 3β, 19α, 23, 24-tetrahydroxyurs-12-en-28-oic acid, isotaraxenol, ursolic acid, decaffeoylactecoside, chrysosplenol C	Tan et al. (2016)
L, St	MeOH	Alkaloid	Acanthiline A	Cai et al. (2018)
F	MeOH	Terpenoids, alkaloids, saponins, flavonoids, tannins	NI	Firdaus et al. (2013)
L	Ac	Tannins	NI	Gong et al. (2019)
L	NI	NI	Blepharin, acteoside, isoverbascoside, daucosterol, 3-O-β-D-glucopyranosyl-stigmasterol	Chen et al. (2015b)

Ac, Acetone; *AP*, aerial part; *Aq*, Aqueous; *B*, bark; *C*, chloroform; *EtOH*, ethanol; *F*, Flower; *Fr*, fruit; *H*, hexane; *L*, leaf; *MeOH*, methanol; *N*, not indicatedl; *R*, root; *St*, stem.

5.6 Pharmacological activities

Acanthus ilicifolius possessed various important pharmacological properties including antioxidant, antinociceptive, antiinflammatory, cytotoxic, antiinfluenza and antimicrobial. There is an undeviating link between bioactive compounds and biological activities. For instance, the compounds blepharin, acteoside and isoverbascoside extracted from the leaves of *A. ilicifolius* exhibited antiinfluenza activities (Chen et al., 2015b). A study conducted by Gong et al. (2019) concluded that the condensed tannins derived from this mangrove species can be used as potential antioxidant and antityrosinase agents in the field of nutraceuticals, cosmetics, medicines and food preservations. The flower revealed to be the most potent and promising cytotoxic agent since its methanolic extract exhibited the highest anticancer activity (LC50 $= 22 \pm 40$ μg/mL) compared to acetone leaf extract (LC50 $= 1411 \pm 27$ μg/mL) (Firdaus et al., 2013). The in vivo test conducted on the methanolic leaf extract demonstrated potential peritoneal inflammation inhibition. Significant COX-1 and -2 and LOX inhibitions were also reported (Kumar et al., 2008). Table 5.2 summarizes further studies conducted on *A. ilicifolius*. From the table, it can be seen that the leaf of that plant has been well appraised in contrast to other plant parts and methanol was the preferred extraction solvent in most studies.

Table 5.2 Pharmacological activities of *Acanthus ilicifolius*.

Plant part (s)	Extract	Study	Results	References
L, R	MeOH	Antioxidant-DPPH	IC50 (mg/mL): L = 2501.53 ± 182.62, R = 1319.66 ± 150.76	Banerjee et al. (2008)
L, R	MeOH	Antioxidant-FRAP	AAE (mg/g): L = 1.10 ± 0.03, R = 1.62 ± 0.03	
L	MeOH	Antinociceptive-Acetic acid-induced writhing test	Control (10 mL/kg) number of writhing = 51.5 ± 4.1, at 250 and 500 mg/kg (extract), % inhibition = 33.0 and 51.1% respectively	Islam et al. (2012)
		Antinociceptive-Formalin test	At 250 and 500 mg/kg, % inhibition = 37.54 and 50.18 respectively for 5 min and 45.5% and 67.24% respectively for 30 min	
L	MeOH	Antiinflammatory-Carrageenan-induced paw edema	ED50 (mg/kg) = 146.2, 95% CI = 69.38−286.2 both at early and late phases. After 2 h, ED50 (mg/kg) = 194, 95% CI = 135.8-301.4. With BW755C (COX-LOX inhibitor) the paw edema decreased	Kumar et al. (2008)

(Continued)

Table 5.2 Pharmacological activities of *Acanthus ilicifolius. Continued*

Plant part(s)	Extract	Study	Results	References
			significantly. No significant inhibitory activity was shown with indomethacin	
		Antiinflammatory-Acetic acid-induced peritoneal inflammation	At 200 and 400 mg/kg, % inhibition = 48 and 77, respectively	
		Antioxidant-DPPH	IC50 (g/mL): extract = 8.40 ± 0.06, Quercetin = 5.28 ± 0.08, Vitamin C = 6.62 ± 0.05	
		Antioxidant-ABTS	IC50 (g/mL): extract = 10.34 ± 0.02, Quercetin = 3.60 ± 0.03, Vitamin C = 4.86 ± 0.03	
		Antioxidant-SO	IC50 (g/mL): extract = 78.12 ± 2.51, Quercetin = 30.19 ± 1.32, Vitamin C = 52.18 ± 3.14	
		Antioxidant-HO	IC50 (g/mL): extract = 24.60 ± 1.10, Quercetin = 14.32 ± 0.52, Vitamin C = 21.08 ± 0.34	
L	A	Antimicrobial	Zone of inhibition (mm) against BS = 20, SA = 18, PA = 18, CA = 22	Babu et al. (2001)
L	Bu		Zone of inhibition (mm) against BS = 16, SA = 8, PA = 10, CA = 15	
L	C		Zone of inhibition (mm) against BS = 22, SA = 21, PA = 20, CA = 26	
L	A	Antimicrobial-disk diffusion assay	Active against EC, AGT, STM, SA, AF and TR. Zone of inhibition (mm) = 7.5 ± 0.4, 8 ± 0.5, 7 ± 0.1, 8.2 ± 0.3, 8.0 ± 0.7 and 7.9 ± 0.3 respectively. MeOH and EA extracts are inactive against TR	Bakshi and Chaudhuri (2014)

A, Aqueous; *AAE*, ascorbic acid equivalent; *ABTS*, 2, 2-azino-bis-3-ethyl benzthiazoline-6-sulfonic acid; *AF*, Aspergillus flavus; *AGT*, Agrobacterium tumefaciens; *BS*, Bacillus subtilis; *Bu*, Butanol; *C*, Chloroform; *CA*, Candida albicans; *COX*, cyclooxigenase; *DPPH*, 2,2-diphenyl-1-picrylhydrazyl; *EA*, Ethyl acetate; *EC*, Escherichia coli; *ED50*, Effective dose; *FRAP*, Ferric reducing antioxidant power; *IC50*, Inhibitory concentration; *L*, Leaf; *LOX*, lipoxygenase; *MeOH*, Methanol; *PA*, Pseudomonas aeruginosa; *R*, Root; *SA*, Staphylococcus aureus; *STM*, Streptococcus mutans; *TR*, Tricophyton rubrum.

5.7 Associated fungal endophytes

Acanthus ilicifolius var. xiamenensis is one of the oldest mangrove plants on earth. However, the natural resource is in short supply due to overharvesting for urban development. Hence, to assess its biological properties in an ecological way, fungal endophytes hosted by the plant are isolated (Chi et al., 2019). In a recent study, 168 endophytic fungi were isolated from the leaves and stems of *A. ilicifolius var. xiamenensis* grown at Kinmen County in Taiwan. A total of 28 isolates successfully inhibited the growth of *Bacillus subtilis, Staphylococcus aureus, Escherichia coli, Candida albicans* and *Cryptococcus neoformans*. The isolates with high iNOS inhibition revealed to have low cell viability and those with low iNOS inhibition had high viability of cells (Chi et al., 2019). Two novel compounds were identified from the fungal endophyte, *Penicillium* sp. FJ-1, isolated from *A. ilicifolius*. The compound, (2R,3S)-pinobanksin-3-cinnamate, exhibited potent neuroprotective effects on corticosterone-damaged PC12 cells while the other compound, 15α-hydroxy-(22E,24R)-ergosta-3,5,8(14),22-tetraen-7-one, showed potent cytotoxic activity on glioma cell lines (Liu et al., 2014). Three new compounds, namely, aspergisocoumrins A-C and two known compounds, 8-dihydroxyisocoumarin-3-carboxylic acid and dichlorodiaportin were isolated from *Aspergillus* sp. HN15-5D. Aspergisocoumrin A and B displayed cytotoxic activity against MDA-MB-435 with IC50 values of 5.08 ± 0.88 and 4.98 ± 0.74 μM, respectively (Wu et al., 2019). A different research group isolated two novel indolic enamide diastereomers, terpeptin A and B, identified from the culture *Aspergillus* sp. (w-6). Both compounds demonstrated averaged cytotoxic activity against the cancerous human cell line, A-549 (Lin et al., 2008). The new nitro-phenyl glucoside isolated from the strain fungus B60 exhibited low antiglucosidase activity (IC50 = 160.5 μM) (Shao et al., 2007).

Table 5.3 summarizes further studies conducted on the fungal endophytes of *A. ilicifolius*. As shown by the mentioned studies, fungal endophytes isolated

Table 5.3 Pharmacological activities and phytochemicals identified from endophytic fungi isolated from *Acanthus ilicifolius*.

Plant part (s)	Endophytic fungi	Phytochemicals	Pharmacological activities	References
L	*Aspergillus flavipes* AIL8	Flavipesins A and B, phenyl dioxolanone	Flavipesins A exhibited low MIC against SA (IC50 = 8.0 μg/mL) and BS (IC50 = 0.25 μg/mL)	Bai et al. (2014)
L	*Aspergillus flavipes*	Guignardone J-M	All compounds were evaluated for antibacterial activity and cytotoxicity but none of them were active	Bai et al. (2015)

(Continued)

Table 5.3 Pharmacological activities and phytochemicals identified from endophytic fungi isolated from *Acanthus ilicifolius. Continued*

Plant part (s)	Endophytic fungi	Phytochemicals	Pharmacological activities	References
NI	*Aspergillus flavipes*	Cytochalasins Z_{16}–Z_{20}, rosellichalasin	Cytochalasin Z_{17} and rosellichalasin exhibited cytotoxic activities against A-549 cell lines with IC50 values of 5.6 and 7.9 μM, respectively	Lin et al. (2009)
L	*Phyllosticta, Cladosporium, Colletotrichum, Phomopsis, Xylaria* sp.	NI	*Xylaria* sp. inhibited the growth of BS, SA, EC and PA	Chaeprasert et al. (2010)
L	*Lasiodiplodia*	β-resorcylic acid derivative, (R, E)-ethyl 2,4-dihydroxy-6-(8-hydroxynon-1-en-1-yl) benzoate, (R)-lasicicol, lasicicol, lasiodiplodin, de-O-methyllasiodiplodin, (E)-9-ethenolasiodiplodin, 5R-hydroxylasiodiplodin, 5S-hydroxylasiodiplodin	The compounds β-resorcylic acid derivative, (R, E)-ethyl 2,4-dihydroxy-6-(8-hydroxynon-1-en-1-yl) benzoate, (R)-lasicicol, lasicicol, lasiodiplodin, de-O-methyllasiodiplodin and (E)-9-ethenolasiodiplodin exhibited anti-glucosidase activity better than acarbose	Chen et al. (2015a)
L	Taloromyces stipitatus SK-4	Tararomyones A and B	Tararomyone B inhibited the growth of BS with MIC value of 12.5 μg/mL	Cai et al. (2017)
NI	*Penicillium* sp., *Aspergillus flaviceps*	Penicinoline	NI	Salini (2015)
B	*Diaporthe phaseolorum*	Diaporphasines A-D, isoindolinones, meyeroguillines C and D, meyeroguilline A, 5-deoxybostrycoidin, fusaristatin A	5-deoxybostrycoidin displayed cytotoxicity against MDA-MB-435 and NCI-H460 human cancer cell lines with IC50 values of 5.32 and 6.57 μM, respectively.	Cui et al. (2017)

Table 5.3 Pharmacological activities and phytochemicals identified from endophytic fungi isolated from *Acanthus ilicifolius. Continued*

Plant part (s)	Endophytic fungi	Phytochemicals	Pharmacological activities	References
			Fusaristatin A showed growth-inhibitory activity against MDA-MB-435 human cancer cell line with IC50 value of 8.15 μM	
NI	*Cumulospora marina, Pestalotiopsis*	Flavonoids, terpenes steroids, triterpenoidal saponins (stigmasterol)	NI	Eldeen and Effendy (2013)

B, Branch; *BS, Bacillus subtilis; IC50,* inhibitory concentration; *L,* leaf; *MIC,* minimum inhibitory concentration; *NI,* not indicated; *PA, Pseudomonas aeruginosa; SA, Staphylococcus aureus.*

from the mangrove species, *A. ilicifolius*, are abounded with new compounds exhibiting promising pharmacological activities. However, the available studies conducted thus far on such plant are not enough which consequently fueled the need for more studies.

References

Babu, B.H., Shylesh, B.S., Padikkala, J., 2001. Antioxidant and hepatoprotective effect of *Acanthus ilicifolius*. Fitoterapia 72, 272−277.

Bai, Z.-Q., Lin, X., Wang, Y., Wang, J., Zhou, X., Yang, B., et al., 2014. New phenyl derivatives from endophytic fungus *Aspergillus flavipes* AIL8 derived of mangrove plant *Acanthus ilicifolius*. Fitoterapia 95, 194−202.

Bai, Z.-Q., Lin, X., Wang, J., Zhou, X., Liu, J., Yang, B., et al., 2015. New meroterpenoids from the endophytic fungus *Aspergillus flavipes* AIL8 derived from the mangrove plant *Acanthus ilicifolius*. Marine Drugs 13, 237−248.

Bakshi, M., Chaudhuri, P., 2014. Antimicrobial potential of leaf extracts of ten mangrove species from Indian Sundarban. International Journal of Pharma and Bio Sciences 5, 294−304.

Bandaranayake, W.M., 2002. Bioactivities, bioactive compounds and chemical constituents of mangrove plants. Wetlands Ecology and Management 10, 421−452.

Banerjee, D., Chakrabarti, S., Hazra, A.K., Banerjee, S., Ray, J., Mukherjee, B., 2008. Antioxidant activity and total phenolics of some mangroves in Sundarbans. African Journal of Biotechnology 7.

Bora, R., Adhikari, P.P., Das, A.K., Raaman, N., Sharma, G.D., 2017. Ethnomedicinal, phytochemical, and pharmacological aspects of genus Acanthus. International Journal of Pharmacy and Pharmaceutical Sciences 9, 8.

Cai, R., Chen, S., Long, Y., Li, C., Huang, X., She, Z., 2017. Depsidones from Talaromyces stipitatus SK-4, an endophytic fungus of the mangrove plant *Acanthus ilicifolius*. Phytochemistry Letters 20, 196–199.

Cai, Y.S., Sun, J.Z., Tang, Q.Q., Fan, F., Guo, Y.W., 2018. Acanthiline A, a pyrido[1,2-a] indole alkaloid from Chinese mangrove *Acanthus ilicifolius*. Journal of Asian Natural Products Research 20, 1088–1092.

Chaeprasert, S., Piapukiew, J., Whalley, A.J., Sihanonth, P., 2010. Endophytic fungi from mangrove plant species of Thailand: their antimicrobial and anticancer potentials. Botanica Marina 53, 555–564.

Chen, S., Liu, Z., Li, H., Xia, G., Lu, Y., He, L., et al., 2015a. β-Resorcylic acid derivatives with α-glucosidase inhibitory activity from *Lasiodiplodia* sp. ZJ-HQ1, an endophytic fungus in the medicinal plant *Acanthus ilicifolius*. Phytochemistry Letters 13, 141–146.

Chen, Y.P., Tan, D.P., Zeng, Q., Wang, Y., Yan, Q.X., Zeng, L.J., 2015b. Chemical constituents from leaves of *Acanthus ilicifolius* and their anti-influenza virus activities. Zhong Yao Cai = Zhongyaocai = Journal of Chinese Medicinal Materials 38, 527–530.

Chi, W.-C., Pang, K.-L., Chen, W.-L., Wang, G.-J., Lee, T.-H., 2019. Antimicrobial and iNOS inhibitory activities of the endophytic fungi isolated from the mangrove plant *Acanthus ilicifolius var. xiamenensis*. Botanical Studies 60, 4.

Cui, H., Yu, J., Chen, S., Ding, M., Huang, X., Yuan, J., et al., 2017. Alkaloids from the mangrove endophytic fungus *Diaporthe phaseolorum* SKS019. Bioorganic and Medicinal Chemistry Letters 27, 803–807.

Eldeen, M., Effendy, A.W.M., 2013. Antimicrobial agents from mangrove plants and their endophytes. In: Mendez-Vilas, A. (Ed.), Microbial Pathogens and Strategies for Combating them: Science, Technology and Education. Formatex, Badajoz, Spain.

Fabiyi, O.A., 2015. Toxicity of *Acanthus ilicifolius* (L) fractions against pratylechus spp. on maize (*Zea mays*). Albanian Journal of Agricultural Sciences 14.

Firdaus, M., Prihanto, A.A., Nurdiani, R., 2013. Antioxidant and cytotoxic activity of *Acanthus ilicifolius* flower. Asian Pacific Journal of Tropical Biomedicine 3, 17–21.

Ganesh, S., Vennila, J.J., 2011. Phytochemical analysis of *Acanthus ilicifolius* and *Avicennia officinalis* by GC-MS. Research Journal of Phytochemistry 5, 60–65.

GBIF, 2020. GBIF secretariat: GBIF backbone taxonomy. <https://www.gbif.org/> (accessed 06.11.20.).

Gong, C.F., Wang, Y.X., Wang, M.L., Su, W.C., Wang, Q., Chen, Q.X., et al., 2019. Evaluation of the structure and biological activities of condensed tannins from *Acanthus ilicifolius* Linn and their effect on fresh-cut Fuji apples. Applied Biochemistry and Biotechnology 189, 855–870.

Islam, M.A., Saifuzzaman, M., Ahmed, F., Rahman, M.M., Sultana, N.A., Naher, K., 2012. Antinociceptive activity of methanolic extract of *Acanthus ilicifolius* Linn leaves. Turkish. Journal of Pharmaceutical Sciences 9, 51–60.

Kumar, K.T.M.S., Gorain, B., Roy, D.K., Zothanpuia, Samanta, S.K., Pal, M., et al., 2008. Anti-inflammatory activity of *Acanthus ilicifolius*. Journal of Ethnopharmacology 120, 7–12.

Lin, N., Yi, B., Li, J., Zhang, W., Zhang, X., 2017. A new sugar ester from the roots of *Acanthus ilicifolius*. Records of Natural Products 11.

Lin, Z.J., Zhang, G.J., Zhu, T.J., Liu, R., Wei, H.J., Gu, Q.Q., 2009. Bioactive cytochalasins from *Aspergillus flavipes*, an endophytic fungus associated with the mangrove plant *Acanthus ilicifolius*. Helvetica Chimica Acta 92, 1538–1544.

Lin, Z., Zhu, T., Fang, Y., Gu, Q., 2008. 1H and 13C NMR assignments of two new indolic enamide diastereomers from a mangrove endophytic fungus *Aspergillus* sp. Magnetic Resonance in Chemistry 46, 1212–1216.

Liu, J.F., Chen, W.J., Xin, B.R., Lu, J., 2014. Metabolites of the endophytic fungus *Penicillium* sp. FJ-1 of *Acanthus ilicifolius*. Natural Product Communications 9, 799–801.

Rahmatullah, M., Sadeak, S., Bachar, S., Hossain, M.T., Abdullah al, M., Montaha, Jahan, N., et al., 2010. Brine shrimp toxicity study of different Bangladeshi medicinal plants. Advances in Natural and Applied Sciences .

Ravindran, K., Venkatesan, K., Balakrishnan, V., Chellappan, K., Balasubramanian, T., 2005. Ethnomedicinal studies of Pichavaram mangroves of East coast, Tamil Nadu. Indian Journal of Traditional Knowledge 4, 409–411.

Revathi, P., Senthinath, T.J., Thirumalaikolundusubramanian, P., Prabhu, N., 2014. An overview of antidiabetic profile of mangrove plants. International Journal of Pharmacy and Pharmaceutical Sciences 6, 1–5.

Sadeer, N.B., Fawzi, M.M., Gokhan, Z., Rajesh, J., Nadeem, N., R.R., R.K., et al., 2019. Ethnopharmacology, phytochemistry, and global distribution of mangroves—a comprehensive review. Marine Drugs 17, 231.

Salini, G., 2015. Pharmacological profile of mangrove endophytes-a review. Lipids 26.

Saranya, A., Ramanathan, T., Kesavanarayanan, K.S., Adam, A., 2015. Traditional medicinal uses, chemical constituents and biological activities of a mangrove plant, *Acanthus ilicifolius* linn. A brief review. American-Eurasian Journal of Agricultural and Environmental Sciences 15, 243–250.

Sardar, P.K., Dev, S., Bari, M.A.A., Paul, S., Yeasmin, M.S., Das, A., et al., 2018. Antiallergic, anthelmintic and cytotoxic potentials of dried aerial parts of *Acanthus ilicifolius* L. Clinical Phytoscience 4, 1–13.

Shao, C.L., Guo, Z.Y., Xia, X.K., Liu, Y., Huang, Z.J., She, Z.G., et al., 2007. Five nitrophenyl compounds from the South China Sea mangrove fungus. Journal of Asian Natural Products Research 9, 643–648.

Singh, D., Aeri, V., 2013. Phytochemical and pharmacological potential of *Acanthus ilicifolius*. Journal of Pharmacy and Bioallied Sciences 5, 17.

Tan, D., Jiang, C., Tao, Y., 2016. Chemical constituents of *Acanthus ilicifolius*. Chemistry of Natural Compounds 52, 951–952.

Wu, Y., Chen, S., Liu, H., Huang, X., Liu, Y., Tao, Y., et al., 2019. Cytotoxic isocoumarin derivatives from the mangrove endophytic fungus *Aspergillus* sp. HN15-5D. Archives of Pharmacal Research 42, 326–331.

Aegialitis rotundifolia Roxb.

6

6.1 General description

6.1.1 Botanical nomenclature

- *Aegialitis rotundifolia* Roxb. (Fig. 6.1)

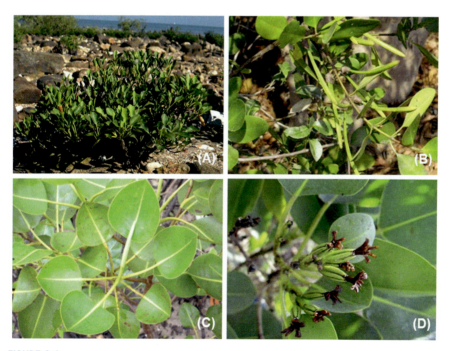

FIGURE 6.1

(A) Whole plant, (B) fruits, (C) leaves, and (D) flowers of *Aegialitis rotundifolia* (GBIF, 2020).

6.1.2 Botanical family

- Plumbaginaceae

Mangroves with Therapeutic Potential for Human Health. DOI: https://doi.org/10.1016/B978-0-323-99332-6.00012-6

6.1.3 Vernacular names

- Banrua (India)
- Nuniagach (Bengal)

6.2 Geographical distribution

Aegialitis rotundifolia is mainly found in Bangladesh. It is a preserved specimen in India, Thailand, Bangladesh, and Myanmar. Fig. 6.2 illustrates the distribution of *A. rotundifolia* across the globe.

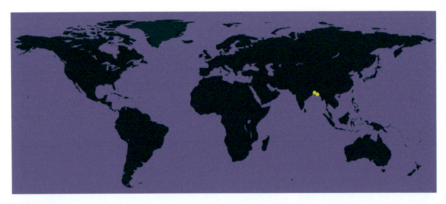

FIGURE 6.2

Distribution of *Aegialitis rotundifolia* across the globe (GBIF, 2020).

6.3 Morphological characteristics

Aegialitis rotundifolia is a small tree or shrub growing to a height of 2−3 m. The leaves are broad ovate, obtuse apex, 5−8.8 cm long, and 4.5−8.5 cm wide (Sadeer et al., 2019). The flowers are organized in terminal cymose racemous inflorescence forms, and the fruits are dehiscent and have a spongy mesocarp (Hasan et al., 2018). Fig. 6.1 illustrates the morphological characteristics of *A. rotundifolia*.

6.4 Ethnobotanical uses

The leaves can be used as a pain reliever and antiinflammatory and antiache agents (Ghosh et al., 2017; Raju et al., 2014; Ray, 2014). It can also act as an antidote against insect bites since this plant is pounded with oil. However, there is no scientific evidence yet to support this traditional use (Hasan et al., 2018).

6.5 Phytochemicals

There is a dearth of knowledge on the detailed characterization and identification of phytocompounds on this mangrove species. So far, only one report has been elucidated on its chemical composition. The work of Ghosh et al. (2017) revealed the presence of a wide spectrum of compounds in the methanolic leaf extract identified as benzene methanol, α-(chloromethyl)-, 2-[(tert-butyldimethylsilyl)oxy]-4,4-dimethyl-1,3-butan-diene, 2-[(benzo[1,3]dioxole-4-carbonyl)-amino]-3-hydroxy-propionic acid, methyl ester, 9-desoxo-9-x-acetoxy-3,8,12-tri-O-acetylingol, quercetin 7,3′,4′-trimethoxy, octadecane, 3-ethyl-5-(2-ethylbutyl)-, 1,1,3,3,5,5,7,7,9,9,11,11,13,13,15,15-hexadecamethyloctasiloxane, 17-pentatriacontene, 2-(benzylsulfanyl-fluoro-methylene)-malonic acid dimethyl ester, eicosamethylcyclodecasiloxane, 2-methoxy-5-trimethylstannylcyclohepta-2,4,6-trien-1-one, cyclodecasiloxane, eicosamethyl-, isochiapin B, heptasiloxane, hexadecamethyl-, 5-vinylsalicylaldoxime, 4-chlorobutyric acid, 4-methoxyphenyl ester, (−)-spiro[1-[(tert-Butyldimethylsiloxy)methyl]-3,5,8-trimethyl-bicyclo[4.3.0]non-2-en-5,7-diol-4,1′-cyclopropane], 1,3-dioxan-5-ol, 2-pentadecyl-, acetate, trans-, thiophene, tetrahydro-3-phenyl-, 1-oxide, emeguisin, stenophylline, tetramethyl ester and 5-methyl-dibenz(B,F)azapine.

6.6 Pharmacological activities

There is not much information available in the literature on the pharmacological activities of *A. rotundifolia* due to a lack of scientific attention given to this mangrove species. The few available studies report several biological activities. For instance, Raju et al. (2014) conducted a series of bioassays on the aqueous leaf extract to assess the antiinflammatory, analgesic, and antipyretic activities. Results were reported to be promising from this study. Reddy and Grace (2016) evaluated the aqueous leaf extract for cytotoxic effects against HepG2 cell line. At a dosage of 200 μg/mL, the IC50 was 97.77. Furthermore, Hasan et al. (2018) investigated on the in vitro thrombolytic, membrane stabilizing and antibacterial activities of the methanolic leaf extract of *A. rotundifolia*. Data reported 32.76% lysis of clot in the thrombolytic study, 38.40% and 27.04% inhibition of hemolysis and no antibacterial activity at a concentration of 10 mg/mL.

6.7 Associated fungal endophytes

Not available

References

GBIF, 2020. GBIF secretariat: GBIF backbone taxonomy. <https://www.gbif.org/> (accessed 06.11.20).

Ghosh, D., Mondal, S., Ramakrishna, K., 2017. Pharmacobotanical, physicochemical and phytochemical characterisation of a rare salt-secreting mangrove *Aegialitis rotundifolia Roxb.*, (Plumbaginaceae) leaves: a comprehensive pharmacognostical study. South African Journal of Botany 113, 212−229.

Hasan, I., Hussain, M.S., Millat, M.S., Sen, N., Rahman, M.A., Rahman, M.A., et al., 2018. Ascertainment of pharmacological activities of Allamanda neriifolia Hook and *Aegialitis rotundifolia* Roxb used in Bangladesh: an in vitro study. Journal of Traditional and Complementary Medicine 8, 107−112.

Raju, G.S., RahmanMoghal, M.M., Hossain, M.S., Hassan, M.M., Billah, M.M., Ahamed, S.K., et al., 2014. Assessment of pharmacological activities of two medicinal plant of Bangladesh: *Launaea sarmentosa* and *Aegialitis rotundifolia* roxb in the management of pain, pyrexia and inflammation. Biological Research 47, 1−11.

Ray, T., 2014. Customary use of mangrove tree as a folk medicine among the sundarban resource collectors. International Journal of Humanities, Arts and Literature 2, 43−48.

Reddy, A., Grace, J.R., 2016. Anticancer activity of methanolic extracts of selected mangrove plants. International Journal of Pharmaceutical Sciences and Research 7, 3852.

Sadeer, N.B., Fawzi, M.M., Gokhan, Z., Rajesh, J., Nadeem, N., Rengasamy Kannan, R.R., et al., 2019. Ethnopharmacology, phytochemistry, and global distribution of mangroves—a comprehensive review. Marine Drugs 17, 231.

Aegiceras corniculatum (L.) Blanco

7.1 General description

7.1.1 Botanical nomenclature

Aegiceras corniculatum (L.) Blanco (Fig. 7.1)

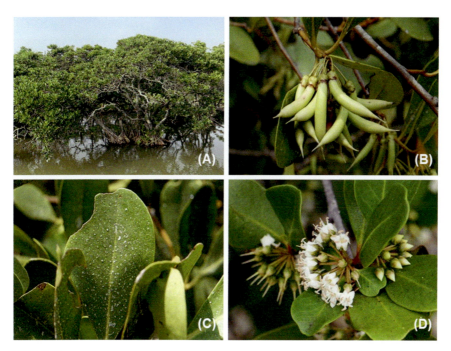

FIGURE 7.1

(A) Whole plant, (B) fruits, (C) leaves, and (D) flowers of *Aegiceras corniculatum* (GBIF, 2020).

Mangroves with Therapeutic Potential for Human Health. DOI: https://doi.org/10.1016/B978-0-323-99332-6.00025-4

7.1.2 Botanical family

- Primulaceae

7.1.3 Vernacular names

- Black mangrove, river mangrove, Goat's horn mangrove (English)
- খলশী khalsi (Bengali)
- हलसी halsi (Hindi)
- நரிக்கண்டல் narikandal (Tamil)
- 蜡烛果 La Zhu Guo (Chinese)

7.2 Geographical distribution

Aegiceras corniculatum is found in Bangladesh, India, Indonesia, South Thailand, and in many regions in Australia. It is a preserved specimen in Australia, India, Papua New Guinea, and Indonesia. Fig. 7.2 illustrates the distribution of *A. corniculatum* across the globe.

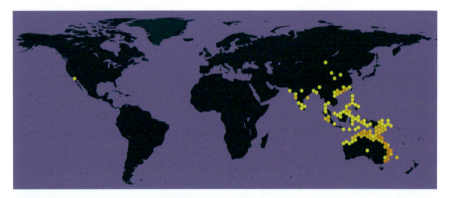

FIGURE 7.2

Distribution of *Aegiceras corniculatum* across the globe (GBIF, 2020).

7.3 Morphological characteristics

Aegiceras corniculatum is a mangrove species that grows up to 6 m. It has smooth and greyish bark, and the leaves are alternate, obovate, 3-to-10 cm long, and 1.5-to-5 cm wide. The color of the fruits ranged from light green to pink, curved cylinder, 2-to-7.5 cm long. Flowers are white, fragrant and form clusters of 10−30 (Web, 2019).

7.4 Ethnobotanical uses

In Pakistan, the stem is used to manage rheumatism, painful arthritis, and inflammation (Roome et al., 2008, 2011).

7.5 Phytochemicals

Different class of compounds have been identified from this plant including amino acids, benzoquinones, tannins, coumarins, flavonoids, saponins, polyphenols, triterpenoids, steroids, quinines, glycosides, sterols, and phenols (Janmanchi et al., 2017; Sadeer et al., 2019).

7.6 Pharmacological activities

Aegiceras corniculatum showed many potential pharmacological activities. For instance, the in vivo antinociceptive activity investigated by Roome et al. (2008, 2011) showed that ethyl acetate stem extracts at 50 mg/kg displayed an inhibition of $53 \pm 3.0\%$ while the hexane stem extract at the same concentration has an inhibition of $28 \pm 2.5\%$. Janmanchi et al. (2017) screened the plant for antibacterial activity. Results showed that the crude leaf extract inhibited the growth of *Bacillus subtilis* and *Escherichia coli*. The same extract exhibited antioxidant activity with DPPH assay with an IC50 value of 1.79 ± 0.0002 mg/mL. There is not much information available on the pharmacological activities of this mangrove species.

7.7 Associated fungal endophytes

The endophytic fungus *Trichoderma* sp. isolated from the leaves of this mangrove species revealed potent scavenging activity against DPPH and hydroxyl radicals (Saravanakumar, 2014). Phytochemical screening showed that the fungus *Emericella* sp. (HK-ZJ) produce six isoindolone derivatives termed emerimidine A and B and emeriphenolicins A and D, and six previously reported compounds, namely, aspernidine A and B, austin, austinol, dehydroaustin, and acetoxydehydroaustin, respectively (Zhang et al., 2011). Six novel tetramic acids derivatives, namely, penicillenols A (1), A (2), B (1), B (2), C (1), and C (2), together with citrinin, phenol A acid, phenol A, and dihydrocitrinin, were identified from *Penicillium* sp. GQ-7. Penicillenols A (1) and B (1) showed cytotoxicity activities against HL-60 cell line resulting in IC50 values of 0.76 and 3.20 μM, respectively (Lin et al., 2008). Ding et al. (2012) isolated a few alkaloids from *Fusarium incarnatum* (HKI0504), namely, N-2-methylpropyl-2-methylbutenamide, 2-acetyl-

1,2,3,4-tetrahydro-β-carboline, fusarine, fusamine, and 3-(1-aminoethylidene)-6-methyl-2H-pyran-2,4(3H)-dione. However, compound 2-acetyl-1,2,3,4-tetrahydro-β-carboline, fusamine and 3-(1-aminoethylidene)-6-methyl-2H-pyran-2,4(3H)-dione exhibited relatively weak antiproliferative and cytotoxicity activity against HUVEC, K562, and HeLa human cell lines, respectively. In a different study but from the same aforementioned fungus [*Fusarium incarnatum* (HKI0504)], Li et al. (2008) identified two new pyrrole alkaloids as N-[4-(2-formyl-5-hydroxymethyl-pyrrol-1-yl)-butyl]-acetamide and N-[5-(2-formyl-5-hydroxymethyl-pyrrol-1-yl)-pentyl]-acetamide and a new indole derivative as (3aR,8aR)-3a-acetoxy-1,2,3,3a,8,8a-hexahydropyrrolo-[2,3-b]indol. Five alkenyl phenol and benzaldehyde derivatives, pestalols A-E were isolated from *Pestalotiopsis* sp. AcBC2. These compounds showed interesting biological activity against 10 tumor cell lines (H1975, A549, MCF-7, SK-BR-3, BT474, DU145, BGC-823, K562, U937 and MOLT-4), influenza A, and Swine flu (H1N1) virus (Sun et al., 2014). Huang et al. (2011) discovered three new bianthraquinone derivatives, namely, alterporriol K, L and M from the endophytic fungus *Alternaria* sp. ZJ9−6B. Cytotoxicity assay showed that alterporriol K and L exhibited activity against MDA-MB-435 and MCF-7 cell lines with IC50 values ranging from 13.1 to 29.1 μM.

References

Ding, L., Dahse, H.M., Hertweck, C., 2012. Cytotoxic alkaloids from *Fusarium incarnatum* associated with the mangrove tree *Aegiceras corniculatum*. Journal of Natural Products 75, 617−621.

GBIF, 2020. GBIF secretariat: GBIF backbone taxonomy. <https://www.gbif.org/> (accessed 06.11.20).

Huang, C.H., Pan, J.H., Chen, B., Yu, M., Huang, H.B., Zhu, X., et al., 2011. Three bianthraquinone derivatives from the mangrove endophytic fungus *Alternaria* sp. ZJ9-6B from the South China Sea. Marine Drugs 9, 832−843.

Janmanchi, H., Raju, A., Degani, M., Ray, M., Rajan, M., 2017. Antituberculosis, antibacterial and antioxidant activities of *Aegiceras corniculatum*, a mangrove plant and effect of various extraction processes on its phytoconstituents and bioactivity. South African Journal of Botany 113, 421−427.

Li, L.Y., Ding, Y., Groth, I., Menzel, K.D., Peschel, G., Voigt, K., et al., 2008. Pyrrole and indole alkaloids from an endophytic *Fusarium incarnatum* (HKI00504) isolated from the mangrove plant *Aegiceras corniculatum*. Journal of Asian Natural Products Research 10, 775−780.

Lin, Z.J., Lu, Z.Y., Zhu, T.J., Fang, Y.C., Gu, Q.Q., Zhu, W.M., 2008. Penicillenols from *Penicillium* sp. GQ-7, an endophytic fungus associated with *Aegiceras corniculatum*. Chemical and Pharmaceutical Bulletin 56, 217−221.

Roome, T., Dar, A., Naqvi, S., Ali, S., Choudhary, M.I., 2008. *Aegiceras corniculatum* extract suppresses initial and late phases of inflammation in rat paw and attenuates the production of eicosanoids in rat neutrophils and human platelets. Journal of Ethnopharmacology 120, 248−254.

Roome, T., Dar, A., Naqvi, S., Choudhary, M.I., 2011. Evaluation of antinociceptive effect of *Aegiceras corniculatum* stems extracts and its possible mechanism of action in rodents. Journal of Ethnopharmacology 135, 351–358.

Sadeer, N.B., Fawzi, M.M., Gokhan, Z., Rajesh, J., Nadeem, N., Rengasamy Kannan, R.R., et al., 2019. Ethnopharmacology, phytochemistry, and global distribution of mangroves—a comprehensive review. Marine Drugs 17, 231.

Saravanakumar, K., 2014. Antioxidant activity of the mangrove endophytic fungus (*Trichoderma* sp.). Journal of Coastal Life Medicine 2, 559–563.

Sun, J.F., Lin, X., Zhou, X.F., Wan, J., Zhang, T., Yang, B., et al., 2014. Pestalols A-E, new alkenyl phenol and benzaldehyde derivatives from endophytic fungus *Pestalotiopsis* sp. AcBC2 isolated from the Chinese mangrove plant *Aegiceras corniculatum*. The Journal of Antibiotics 67, 451–457.

Web, F.A.F., 2019. Flora and fauna web. <https://florafaunaweb.nparks.gov.sg> (accessed 07.11.20).

Zhang, G., Sun, S., Zhu, T., Lin, Z., Gu, J., Li, D., et al., 2011. Antiviral isoindolone derivatives from an endophytic fungus *Emericella* sp. associated with *Aegiceras corniculatum*. Phytochemistry 72, 1436–1442.

Avicennia germinans (L.) L

8

8.1 General description

8.1.1 Botanical nomenclature

Avicennia germinans (L.) L (Fig. 8.1)

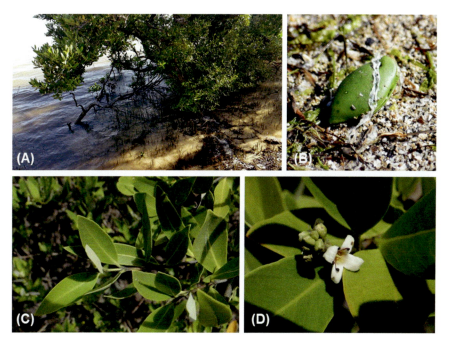

FIGURE 8.1

(A) Whole plant, (B) fruits, (C) leaves, and (D) flowers of *Avicennia germinans* (GBIF, 2020).

8.1.2 Botanical family

• Acanthaceae

Mangroves with Therapeutic Potential for Human Health. DOI: https://doi.org/10.1016/B978-0-323-99332-6.00008-4

8.1.3 Vernacular names

- Black mangrove, white mangrove, olive mangrove (English)
- Palétuvier blanc, mangle blanc, faux palétuvier (French)

8.2 Geographical distribution

Avicennia germinans is widely distributed along the coastlines of United States, Mexico, Central America, Colombia, Venezuela, Guyana, Cayenne, Brazil, and Ecuador. This species is also well distributed along the shores of the West regions of Africa including Senegal, Guinea, Côte d'Ivoire, and Cameroon as illustrated in Fig. 8.2. It is under human observation in Suriname, United States, Mexico, Costa Rica, Sint Maarten (Dutch part), Jamaica, and Brazil.

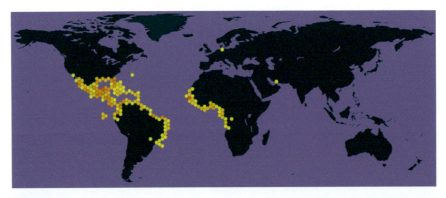

FIGURE 8.2

Distribution of *Avicennia germinans* across the globe (GBIF, 2020).

8.3 Morphological characteristics

Avicennia germinans is the tallest mangrove tree in its genus growing to a height of 30−50 m and has pneumatophore-type of roots. The bark is dark brown or black in color and has rough and irregular flattened scales. The leaves are opposite, elliptical, thick with glands on the upper surface, green on upper surface, gray on bottom surface, 3−15 cm long. Fruits are dark green, velvety pericarp beneath, 2−3 cm in diameter as illustrated in Fig. 8.1. Flowers are white, auxiliary clusters, 1−2 cm in diameter (Thatoi et al., 2016).

8.4 Ethnobotanical uses

The bark, leaf, and flower of *A. germinans* are used traditionally to treat malaria, hemorrhoids, rheumatism, swellings, throat pains, and hemorrhage. In the Bahamas, *A. germinans* is traditionally used to restore vitality and manage rheumatism. In Colombia, gargling the bark decoction helps to cure cancer of larynx and ulcers of the throat (Rajeshwari et al., 2013; Thatoi et al., 2016).

8.5 Phytochemical compounds

The compounds identified originate from the phytochemical class of glycosides, namely 20-cinnamoyl-mussaenosidic acid, 20-caffeoyl-mussaenosidic acid, and 20-CoUmamaheswarraoroyl-mussaenosidic acid (Fauvel et al., 1995; Fauvel et al., 1997; Thatoi et al., 2016). A dearth of knowledge is noticed in the phytocompounds present in this mangrove species.

8.6 Pharmacological activities

The methanolic extract of *A. germinans* exhibited significant antibacterial activity against *Escherichia coli*, *Klebsiella* sp., *Proteus* sp., *Staphylococcus aureus*, *Pseudomonas* sp., and *Salmonella* sp. This mangrove has been poorly explored in terms of their pharmacological activities (Sadeer et al., 2019).

8.7 Associated fungal endophytes

The fungus *Aspergillus* sp. isolated from the leaf, root, and stem can be a potential source of L-asparaginase enzyme (Prihanto et al., 2019).

References

Fauvel, M.-T., Bousquet-Melou, A., Moulis, C., Gleye, J., Jensen, S.R., 1995. Iridoid glucosides from *Avicennia germinans*. Phytochemistry 38, 893–894.

Fauvel, M.-T., Moulis, C., Bon, M., Fourasté, I., 1997. A new iridoid glucoside from African *Avicennia germinans*. Natural Product Letters 10, 139–142.

GBIF, 2020. GBIF secretariat: GBIF backbone taxonomy <https://www.gbif.org/> (accessed 06.11.20.).

Prihanto, A., Caisariyo, I., Pradarameswari, K., 2019. *Aspergillus* sp. as a potential producer for *L-Asparaginase* from mangrove (*Avicennia germinans*). IOP Conference Series: Earth and Environmental Science 230, 012101.

Rajeshwari, E., Gajendiran, Elamathy, S., 2013. Study of preliminary phytochemical analysis and antibacterial activity of selected medicinal plants (*Avicennia germinans*). International Journal 1, 952−954.

Sadeer, N.B., Fawzi, M.M., Gokhan, Z., Rajesh, J., Nadeem, N., Rengasamy Kannan, R.R., et al., 2019. Ethnopharmacology, phytochemistry, and global distribution of mangroves—a comprehensive review. Marine Drugs 17, 231.

Thatoi, H., Samantaray, D., Das, S.K., 2016. The genus *Avicennia*, a pioneer group of dominant mangrove plant species with potential medicinal values: a review. Frontiers in Life Science 9, 267−291.

Avicennia marina (Forssk.) Vierh.

9.1 General description

9.1.1 Botanical nomenclature

Avicennia marina (Forssk.) Vierh (Fig. 9.1).

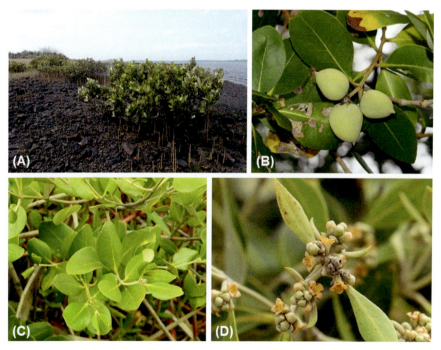

FIGURE 9.1

(A) Whole plant, (B) fruits, (C) leaves, and (D) flowers of *Avicennia marina* (GBIF, 2020).

Mangroves with Therapeutic Potential for Human Health. DOI: https://doi.org/10.1016/B978-0-323-99332-6.00023-0

9.1.2 Botanical family

- Acanthaceae

9.1.3 Vernacular names

- Gray mangrove, white mangrove, olive mangrove (English)
- Palétuvier blanc (French)
- Witseebasboom (African)
- Mangue branco, mangue nero, salgueiro (Portuguese)

9.2 Geographical distribution

Avicennia marina is mostly distributed in Australia, Indonesia, India, Madagascar, along the coastlines of Saudi Arabia and south-east of Africa and scarcely distributed in North America (Fig. 9.2). Fig. 9.2 illustrates the distribution of *A. marina* across the globe. It is a preserved specimen in South Africa and under human observation in Australia, New Zealand, United Arab Emirates, Hong Kong, and Egypt.

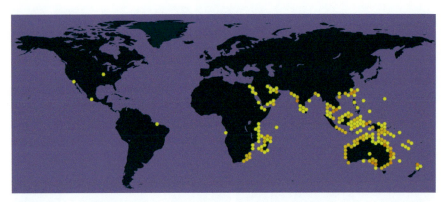

FIGURE 9.2

Distribution of *Avicennia marina* across the globe (GBIF, 2020).

9.3 Morphological characteristics

Avicennia marina is a mangrove plant growing up to a height of 14 m. It has pneumatophore roots that allow the plant to respire as shown in Fig. 9.1. It has smooth, light gray bark with thin, stiff, and brittle flakes. The leaves are thick, glossy on upper part and gray or silvery-white on the bottom, 5−8 cm long. The fruits are oval in shape, green, 20−25 mm in diameter. The flowers are white or golden-yellow forming clusters of 3−5 (Rippey and Rowland, 2004; Thatoi et al., 2016).

9.4 Ethnobotanical uses

The barks and leaves are used to treat smallpox, skin diseases, ulcers, and throat pains (Bandaranayake, 2002) and in Iran, the leaves are used to cure ulcers, burns and rheumatism (Khajehzadeh and Behbahani, 2016).

9.5 Phytochemicals

Avicennia marina is replete with promising biomolecules from different phytochemical classes namely alkaloids, tannins, terpenoids, fatty acids, to name a few. Various types of extracts have been prepared from extraction solvents of different polarities in order to extract and identify as many compounds as possible produced by this plant. Table 9.1 details the phytochemicals identified from different solvent extracts.

Table 9.1 Phytochemicals of *A. marina*.

Plant part	Extract	Phytochemical class	Compounds	References
St	NI	Phytoalexins, tannins, triterpenes, steroids	NI	Revathi et al. (2014)
L	MeOH, E, EE, EA, Aq	Alkaloids, glycosides, phenols, steroids, tannins, terpenoids	NI	Thatoi et al. (2016)
L	MeOH, EA	Saponins	NI	
L	MeOH, E, EE, EA, Aq	Flavonoids	Luteolin 7-O-methylether, Chrysoeriol 7-Oglucoside, Isorhamnetin 3-O-rutinoside, 5-hydroxy-4'; 7-dimethoxyflavone, Quercetin, Kaempferol, 4'5-dihydroxy-3'-5,7-diimethoxyflavone, 4',5-dihydroxy-3',7-trimethoxyflavone, 4',5,7-trihydroxyflavone, 3',4',5-trihydroxy-7-methoxyflavone, 2-[3'-3'-hydroxymethyloxiran-2'-yl-2' methoxy-4'-methoxymethylphenyl]-4H chromen-4-one	
L	MeOH, E, EE, EA, Aq	Naphthalene Derivatives	Naphtha[1,2-b]furan-4,5-dione, 3-hydroxy-naphtha[1,2-b]furan-4,5-dione, 2-[2'-2'-hydroxypropyl]-naphtha[1,2-b]furan-4,5-dione, Avicennone A, Avicenol A, Stenocarpoquinone B, 7'S, 8'R-4,4',9'-trihydroxy-3,3',5,5'-tetramethoxy-7,8-dehydro-9-al-2,7'-Cycloligan, Lyoniresinol	
L	MeOH, E, EE, EA, Aq	Tannins	Lapachol	
L	MeOH, E, EE, EA, Aq	Steroids	β-Sitosterol, Ergost-6,22-diene-5,8-epidioxy-3β-ol, Stigmasterol-3-O-β-D-galactopyranoside	
B, L, R	MeOH, E, EE, EA, Aq	Terpenoids	Lupeol, Taraxerol, Taraxerone, Betulinic acid, Betulin, Ursolic acid, 6Hα-11,12,16-trihydroxy-6,7-secoabieta-8,11,13-triene-6,7-dial11,6-hemiacetal, 6Hβ-11,12,16-trihydroxy-6,7-secoabieta-8,11,13-triene-6,7-dial11,6-hemiacetal	

L, R	MeOH, E, EE, EA, Aq	Fatty Acids	Oleic acid, Linolenic acid, Palmetic acid, Stearic acid, Lauric acid, Myristic acid
B, L	MeOH, E, EE, EA, Aq	Glycosides	Geniposidic acid, 2'-cinnamoyl-mussaenosidic acid, Mussaenoside, 2'-cinnamoyl-mussaenoside, 10-O-5-phenyl-2,4-pentadienoyl-geniposide, 7-O-5-phenyl-2,4-pentadienoyl-8-epiloganin, 10-O-[E-cinnamoyl]-geniposidic acid, 10-O-[E-p-coUmamaheswarraoroyl]-geniposidic acid, 10-O-[E-caffeoyl]-geniposidic acid, 2'-O-[E-cinnamoyl]mussaenosidic acid, 2'-O-[2E,4E-5-phenylpenta-2,4-dienoyl]mussaenosidic acid, 2'-O-4 mehtoxycinnamoylmussaenosidic acid, 2'-O-coUmamaheswarraoroylmussaenosidic acid, Marinoids A–E, Verbascoside, Isoverbascoside, Derhamnosylverbascosid, 11-hydroxy-8,11,13-abietatriene 12-O-β-xylopyranoside, Lyoniresinol 9'-O-β-D glucopyranoside
L	MeOH, E, EE, EA, Aq	Alkaloids, glycosides, phenols, steroids, tannins, terpenoids	NI
L	MeOH, EA	Saponins	NI
L	MeOH, E, EE, EA, Aq	Flavonoids	Luteolin 7-O-methylether, Chrysoeriol 7-Oglucoside, Isorhamnetin 3-O-rutinoside, 5-hydroxy-4'; 7-dimethoxyflavone, Quercetin, Kaempferol, 4'5-dihydroxy-3'-5,7-diimethoxyflavone, 4',5-dihydroxy-3',7-trimethoxyflavone, 4',5,7-trihydroxyflavone, 3',4',5-trihydroxy-7-methoxyflavone, 2-[3'-3'-hydroxymethyloxiran-2'-yl-2' methoxy-4'-methoxymethylphenyl]-4H chromen-4-one
L	MeOH, E, EE, EA, Aq	Naphthalene Derivatives	Naphtha[1,2-b]furan-4,5-dione, 3-hydroxy-naphtha[1,2-b]furan-4,5-dione, 2-[2'-2'-hydroxypropyl]-naphtha[1,2-b]furan-4,5-dione, Avicennone A, Avicenol A, Stenocarpoquinone B, 7'S, 8'R-4,4',9'-trihydroxy-3,3',5,5'-tetramethoxy-7,8-dehydro-9-al-2,7'-Cycloligan, Lyoniresinol

(Continued)

Table 9.1 Phytochemicals of *A. marina. Continued*

Plant part	Extract	Phytochemical class	Compounds	References
L	MeOH, E, EE, EA, Aq	Tannins	Lapachol	
L	MeOH, E, EE, EA, Aq	Steroids	β-Sitosterol, Ergost-6,22-diene-5,8-epidioxy-3β-ol, Stigmasterol-3-O-β-D-galactopyranoside	
B, L, R	MeOH, E, EE, EA, Aq	Terpenoids	Lupeol, Taraxerol, Taraxerone, Betulinic acid, Betulin, Ursolic acid, 6Hα-11,12,16-trihydroxy-6,7-secoabieta-8,11,13-triene-6,7-dial11,6-hemiacetal, 6Hβ-11,12,16-trihydroxy-6,7-secoabieta-8,11,13-triene-6,7-dial11,6-hemiacetal	
L, R	MeOH, E, EE, EA, Aq	Fatty Acids	Oleic acid, Linolenic acid, Palmetic acid, Stearic acid, Lauric acid, Myristic acid	
B, L	MeOH, E, EE, EA, Aq	Glycosides	Geniposidic acid, 2′-cinnamoyl-mussaenosidic acid, Mussaenoside, 2′-cinnamoyl-mussaenoside, 10-O-5-phenyl-2,4-pentadienoyl-geniposide, 7-O-5-phenyl-2,4-pentadienoyl-8-epiloganin, 10-O-[E-cinnamoyl]-geniposidic acid, 10-O-[E-p-coUmamaheswarraoroyl]-geniposidic acid, 10-O-[E-caffeoyl]-geniposidic acid, 2′-O-[E-cinnamoyl]mussaenosidic acid, 2′-O-[2E,4E-5-phenylpenta-2,4-dienoyl]mussaenosidic acid, 2′-O-4 mehtoxycinnamoylmussaenosidic acid, 2′-O-coUmamaheswarraoroylmussaenosidic acid, Marinoids A–E, Verbascoside, Isoverbascoside, Derhamnosylverbascosid, 11-hydroxy-8,11,13-abietatriene 12-O-β-xylopyranoside, Lyoniresinol 9-O-β-D glucopyranoside	
L	MeOH, E, EE, EA, Aq	Alkaloids, glycosides, phenols, steroids, tannins, terpenoids	NI	
L	MeOH, EA	Saponins	NI	

Part	Extract	Class	Compounds	Reference
L	MeOH, E, EE, EA, Aq	Flavonoids	Luteolin 7-O-methylether, Chrysoeriol 7-Oglucoside, Isorhamnetin 3-O-rutinoside, 5-hydroxy-4', 7-dimethoxyflavone, Quercetin, Kaempferol, 4'5-dihydroxy-3'-5,7-diimethoxyflavone, 4',5-dihydroxy-3',7-trimethoxyflavone, 4',5,7-trihydroxyflavone, 3',4',5-trihydroxy-7-methoxyflavone, 2-[3'-3'-hydroxymethyloxiran-2'-yl-2'-methoxy-4'-methoxymethylphenyl]-4H chromen-4-one	Shanmugapriya et al. (2012)
L	MeOH, E, EE, EA, Aq	Naphthalene Derivatives	Naphtha[1,2-b]furan-4,5-dione, 3-hydroxy-naphtha[1,2-b]furan-4,5-dione, 2-[2'-2'-hydroxypropyl]-naphtha[1,2-b]furan-4,5-dione, Avicennone A, Avicenol A, Stenocarpoquinone B, 7'S, 8'R-4,4',9-trihydroxy-3,3',5,5'-tetramethoxy-7,8-dehydro-9-al-2,7'-Cycloligan, Lyoniresinol	
L	MeOH, E, EE, EA, Aq	Tannins	Lapachol	
L	MeOH, E, EE, EA, Aq	Steroids	β-Sitosterol, Ergost-6,22-diene-5,8-epidioxy-3β-ol, Stigmasterol-3-O-β-D-galactopyranoside	
B, L, R	MeOH, E, EE, EA, Aq	Terpenoids	Lupeol, Taraxerol, Taraxerone, Betulinic acid, Betulin, Ursolic acid, 6Hα-11,12,16-trihydroxy-6,7-secoabieta-8,11,13-triene-6,7-dial11,6-hemiacetal, 6Hβ-11,12,16-trihydroxy-6,7-secoabieta-8,11,13-triene-6,7-dial11,6-hemiacetal	
L, R	MeOH, E, EE, EA, Aq	Fatty Acids	Oleic acid, Linolenic acid, Palmetic acid, Stearic acid, Lauric acid, Myristic acid	
B, L	MeOH, E, EE, EA, Aq	Glycosides	Geniposidic acid, 2'-cinnamoyl-mussaenosidic acid, Mussaenoside, 2'-cinnamoyl-mussaenoside, 10-O-5-phenyl-2,4-pentadienoyl-geniposide, 7-O-5-phenyl-2,4-pentadienoyl-8-epiloganin, 10-O-[E-cinnamoyl]-geniposidic acid, 10-O-[E-p-coUmamaheswarraoroyl]-geniposidic acid, 10-O-[E-caffeoyl]-geniposidic acid, 2'-O-[E-cinnamoyl]mussaenosidic acid, 2'-O-[2E,4E-5-phenylpenta-2,4-dienoyl]mussaenosidic acid, 2'-O-4 mehtoxycinnamoylmussaenosidic acid, 2'-O-coUmamaheswarraoroylmussaenosidic acid, Marinoids A–E, Verbascoside, Isoverbascoside, Derhamnosylverbascosid, 11-hydroxy-8,11,13-abietatriene 12-O-β-xylopyranoside, Lyoniresinol 9'-O-β-D glucopyranoside	
L	CE	Alkaloids, flavonoids, terpenoids, phenolics, saponins, amino acid	NI	

B, Bark; CE, crude extract; EA, ethyl acetate; EE, ethyl ether; L, leaf; MeOH, methanol; NI, not indicated; St, stem; R, root.

9.6 Pharmacological activities

The plant exhibits antimicrobial, anti-inflammatory, antiviral, antimutagenic, anti-cancer, and antioxidant properties. For instance, Ramanathan investigated the antimicrobial activity of the crude leaf extract using disk diffusion assay against *S. aureus, Klebsiella aerogenes, P. aeruginosa, Bacillus subtilis, E. coli, Enterobacter aerogenes, Proteus* sp, *Salmonella parathyphi, and Citrobacter* sp. The extracts showed activity against all tested microorganisms (Ramanathan, 2012). Shafie et al. (2013) conducted the anti-inflammatory activity on rat models, and it was observed that the inflammatory markers were reduced, and the joint lesions were also improved. The ethanolic leaf extracts were active against HIV (Human immunodeficiency virus), SFV (Semliki forest virus), EMVC (Encephalmyocarditis virus), and HBV (Hepatitis B virus) (Shafie et al., 2013). Table 9.2 summarized other studies conducted on *A. marina*.

Table 9.2 Pharmacological activities of *A. marina*.

Plant part (s)	Extract	Study	Results	References
L	A	Antimicrobial-Agar well diffusion	Active against BC, EF, SA, SM and AT	Thatoi et al. (2016)
L	E	Antimutagenic-MTT assay	Strong effect with inhibition rates of 68% and 71% with and without metabolic activation S9	Karami et al. (2012)
		Anticancer-MTT assay	Significant cytotoxic effect on HL-60 cells and induced apoptosis in HL-60 cell line	
NI	MeOH	Antioxidant-ABTS	Strong activity	Sharief and Umamaheswararao (2011)
L	NI	Antimicrobial	Zone of inhibition (mm) against EC, SA, BS, CA, and AN = 12, 6, 7, 9, and 10, respectively for 30 µL of extract	Al Maqtari Maher (2014)
L	Ac	Antimicrobial-Disk diffusion assay	Zone of inhibition (mm) against AGT, STM, SA, and TR are 6.8 ± 0.9, 7.5 ± 0.5, 9.1 ± 0.3, and 6.5 ± 0.35, respectively. Inactive against EC and TR	Bakshi and Chaudhuri (2014)

(Continued)

Table 9.2 Pharmacological activities of *A. marina. Continued*

Plant part (s)	Extract	Study	Results	References
L	CE	Antimicrobial-Disk diffusion assay	Zone of inhibition (mm) against SA, KP, PA, BS, EC, ENA, PS, SP, and CS = 18, 24, 26, 16, 27, 8, 12, 5, and 1, respectively	Ramanathan (2012)
		Antioxidant-DPPH (In vitro)	%radical scavenging = 88.93%	

A, Alcohol*; Ac,* acetone*; AT, Aspergillus tumefaciens; BC, Bacillus cereus; BS, Bacillus subtilis; CE,* crude extract*; CS, Citrobacter sp.; E,* ethanol*; EF, Enterococcus faecalis; ENA, Enterobacter aerogenes; L,* leaf*; SA, Staphylococcus aureus; NI,* not indicated*; PS: Proteus* sp.*; SP, Salmonella paratyphi; TR, Tricophyton rubrum.*

9.7 Associated fungal endophytes

A recent study identified a number of fungi as *Chaetomium madrasense, Chaetomium* sp., *Chaetomium globosum, Aspergillus hiratsukae, Aspergillus ochraceus, Alternaria tenuissima*, and *Curvularia lunata* isolated from 50 leaves of *A. marina* collected in Yanbu, Red sea coast, Saudi Arabia. Results from this work showed that the identified fungi displayed significant antioxidant properties and successfully inhibited the growth of *Candida albicans* and *Cryptococcus neoformans*. The extract of *Alternaria tenuissima* IE-9 displayed a strong activity against all Gram-negative and Gram-positive bacteria and yeasts with inhibition zones ranged between 12 and 20 mm (Khalil et al., 2021). Fungi isolated from the roots and stems of the mangrove collected in the mangrove forest in Serang, Indonesia possessed good radical scavenging activities with DPPH assay (Rahmawati et al., 2019). Table 9.3 summarizes further studies conducted on the fungal endophytes of *A. marina*.

Table 9.3 Pharmacological activities and phytochemicals identified from endophytic fungi isolated from *A. marina*.

Plant part (s)	Endophytic fungi	Phytochemicals	Pharmacological activities	References
NI	*Xylaria, Hypocrea lixii*	Alcohols, amino acids, carbohydrates, fatty acids, hydrocarbons, inorganic salts, minerals, phytoalexins, carboxylic acids, steroids, tannins, triterpenes, vitamins, n-hexadecanoic acid, cyclic peptides: xyloketals, xyloallenolides	Antimicrobial	Eldeen and Effendy (2013)
L	Unidentified	Farinomaleins C–E	NI	El Amrani et al. (2012)
NI	*Aspergillus niger* MA-132	Nigerapyrones A–H, asnipyrones A and B	Nigerapyrone B, D, E, asnipyrone A exhibited weak cytotoxicity activity against some tumor cell lines	Liu et al. (2011)
NI	*Dothiorella* sp. HTF3	Cytosporone B	Anticancer	Salini (2014)
L, Tw	*Phomopsis, Phomopsis azadirachtae, Leptosphaerulina chartarum, Phyllostica capitalensis, Pyronema, Fusarium equiseti, Hypoxylon investiens, Alternaria alternate, Cladosporium perangustum, Hortaea werneckii, Leptosphaeruline, Sordariomycetes*	NI	NI	Li et al. (2016)
S	*Xylaria*	Xyloketals A-I, Xyloallendide A and B, steroids, esters, lactones	NI	Zhu et al. (2009)
NI	*Penicillium brocae* MA-231	Brocazines A-F	NI	Meng et al. (2015)

NI	*Penicillium brocae* MA-231	Penicibrocazine A-E, epicoccin A, phomazine A, hexahydro-2-hydroxy-1-phenyl-1*H*-pyrrolizin-3-one, brocapyrrozins A	Brocapyrrozins A exhibited potent activity against SA with MIC value of 0.125 µg/mL	Meng et al. (2017)
L	*Aspergillus awamari, Aspergillus favipes, Aspergillus chevalieri, Aspergillus flavus, Aspergillus clavatus, Aspergillus fumigates, Penicillium candidum, Penicillium japonicum, Penicillium purpurogenum, Phomopsis*	NI	Methanolic extract of *Aspergillus flavus* demonstrated antibacterial activity with inhibition zones ranging from 10–14.7 mm	Bharathidasan and Panneerselvam (2015)
S	Endophytic fungus no. 2106	No. 2106A, cyclo-(N-MeVal-N-MeAla)	NI	Wang et al. (2008)
NI	*Penicillium citrinum*	(Z)-7,4′-dimethoxy-6-hydroxyaurone-4-O-β-glucopyranoside, (-)-4-O-(4-O-β-D glucopyranosylcaffeoyl) quinic acid	(-)-4-O-(4-O-β-D glucopyranosylcaffeoyl) quinic acid exhibited potent chemoreversal activity, mainly by inhibiting P-glycoprotein efflux pump function	Liu et al. (2015)
NI	*Penicillium* sp. FJ-1	4-(20,30-dihydroxy-30-methyl butanoxy)-phenethanol, 15-hydroxyl-6α,12-epoxy-7b,10aH,11bH-spiroax-4-ene-12-one	15-Hydroxyl-6α,12-epoxy-7b,10aH,11bH-spiroax-4-ene-12-one exhibited potent antitumoral activity on human osteosarcoma	Zheng et al. (2014)

L, Leaf; MIC, minimum inhibitory concentration; NI, not indicated; S, seed; SA, *Staphylococcus aureus*; Tw, twig.

References

Al Maqtari Maher, A., 2014. Screening of salt-stress, antioxidant enzyme, and antimicrobial activity of leave extracts of mangroves *Avicennia marina* L. from Hodaidah, Yemen. Journal of Stress Physiology and Biochemistry 10.

Bakshi, M., Chaudhuri, P., 2014. Antimicrobial potential of leaf extracts of ten mangrove species from Indian Sundarban. International Journal of Pharma and Bio Sciences 5, 294−304.

Bandaranayake, W.M., 2002. Bioactivities, bioactive compounds and chemical constituents of mangrove plants. Wetlands Ecology and Management 10, 421−452.

Bharathidasan, R., Panneerselvam, A., 2015. Antibacterial activity of endophytic fungi extracts from the mangrove plant *Avicennia marina* (Forsk) Vierh. International Journal of Advanced Research 2, 145−148.

El Amrani, M., Debbab, A., Aly, A.H., Wray, V., Dobretsov, S., Müller, W.E., et al., 2012. Farinomalein derivatives from an unidentified endophytic fungus isolated from the mangrove plant *Avicennia marina*. Tetrahedron Letters 53, 6721−6724.

Eldeen, M., Effendy, A.W.M., 2013. Antimicrobial agents from mangrove plants and their endophytes. In: Mendez-Vilas, A. (Ed.), Microbial Pathogens and Strategies for Combating Them: Science, Technology and Education. Formatex, Badajoz, Spain.

GBIF, 2020. GBIF secretariat: GBIF backbone taxonomy. <https://www.gbif.org/> (accessed 06.11.20).

Karami, L., Majd, A., Mehrabian, S., Nabiuni, M., Salehi, M., Irian, S., 2012. Antimutagenic and anticancer effects of *Avicennia marina* leaf extract on *Salmonella typhimurium* TA100 bacterium and human promyelocytic leukaemia HL-60 cells. ScienceAsia 38, 349−355.

Khajehzadeh, S., Behbahani, M., 2016. Activity of *Avicennia marina* methanol extracts on proliferation of lymphocytes and their mutagenicity using Ames test and in silico method. J. Mazandaran University of Medical Sciences 26, 32−42.

Khalil, A., Abdelaziz, A., Khaleil, M., Hashem, A., 2021. Fungal endophytes from leaves of *Avicennia marina* growing in semi-arid environment as a promising source for bioactive compounds. Letters in Applied Microbiology 72, 263−274.

Li, J.-L., Sun, X., Chen, L., Guo, L.-D., 2016. Community structure of endophytic fungi of four mangrove species in Southern China. Mycology 7, 180−190.

Liu, D., Li, X.-M., Meng, L., Li, C.-S., Gao, S.-S., Shang, Z., et al., 2011. Nigerapyrones A−H, α-pyrone derivatives from the marine mangrove-derived endophytic fungus *Aspergillus niger* MA-132. Journal of Natural Products 74, 1787−1791.

Liu, J., Xu, M., Zhu, M.-Y., Feng, Y., 2015. Chemoreversal metabolites from the endophytic fungus penicillium citrinum isolated from a mangrove avicennia marina. Natural Product Communications 10, 1934578X1501000717.

Meng, L.-H., Zhang, P., Li, X.-M., Wang, B.-G., 2015. Penicibrocazines A−E, five new sulfide diketopiperazines from the marine-derived endophytic fungus *Penicillium brocae*. Marine Drugs 13, 276−287.

Meng, L.-H., Li, X.-M., Liu, Y., Xu, G.-M., Wang, B.-G., 2017. Antimicrobial alkaloids produced by the mangrove endophyte *Penicillium brocae* MA-231 using the OSMAC approach. RSC Advances 7, 55026−55033.

Rahmawati, S., Izzati, F., Hapsari, Y., Septiana, E., Rachman, F., Simanjuntak, P., 2019. Endophytic microbes and antioxidant activities of secondary metabolites from mangroves *Avicennia marina* and *Xylocarpus granatum*. In: IOP Conference Series: Earth and Environmental Science. IOP Publishing, pp. 012065.

Ramanathan, T., 2012. Phytochemical characterization and antimicrobial efficiency of mangrove plants *Avicennia marina* and *Avicennia officinalis*. International Journal of Pharmaceutical and Biological Science Archive 3, 348–351.

Revathi, P., Senthinath, T.J., Thirumalaikolundusubramanian, P., Prabhu, N., 2014. An overview of antidiabetic profile of mangrove plants. International Journal of Pharmacy and Pharmaceutical Sciences 6, 1–5.

Rippey, E., Rowland, B., 2004. Coastal Plants: Perth and the South-West Region. UWA Publishing, Pimpri-Chinchwad, India.

Salini, G., 2014. Pharmacological profile of mangrove endophytes-a review. International Journal of Pharmacy and Pharmaceutical Sciences 7, 6–15.

Shafie, M., Forghani, A., Moshtaghiyan, J., 2013. Anti-inflammatory effects of hydro-alcoholic extracts of mangrove (*Avicennia marina*) and vitamin C on arthritic rats. Bulletin of Environment, Pharmacology and Life Sciences 2, 32–37.

Shanmugapriya, R., Ramanathan, T., Renugadevi, G., 2012. Phytochemical characterization and antimicrobial efficiency of mangrove plants Avicennia marina and *Avicennia officinalis*. International Journal of Pharmaceutical and Biological Science Archive 3, 348–351.

Sharief, M.N., Umamaheswararao, V., 2011. Antibacterial activity of stem and root extracts of *Avicennia officinalis L*. International Journal of Applied Pharmaceutics 2, 231–236.

Thatoi, H., Samantaray, D., Das, S.K., 2016. The genus Avicennia, a pioneer group of dominant mangrove plant species with potential medicinal values: a review. Frontiers in Life Science 9, 267–291.

Wang, S.-Y., Xu, Z.-L., She, Z.-G., Wang, H., Li, C.-R., Lin, Y.-C., 2008. Two new metabolites from the mangrove endophytic fungus no. 2106. Journal of Asian Natural Products Research 10, 622–626.

Zheng, C., Chen, Y., Jiang, L.-L., Shi, X.-M., 2014. Antiproliferative metabolites from the endophytic fungus Penicillium sp. FJ-1 isolated from a mangrove *Avicennia marina*. Phytochemistry Letters 10, 272–275.

Zhu, F., Chen, X., Yuan, Y., Huang, M., Sun, H., Xiang, W., 2009. The chemical investigations of the mangrove plant *Avicennia marina* and its endophytes. The Open Natural Products Journal 2, 24–32.

Avicennia officinalis L.

10.1 General description

10.1.1 Botanical nomenclature

- *Avicennia officinalis* L. (Fig. 10.1)

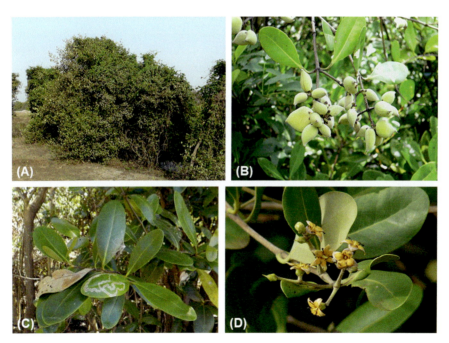

FIGURE 10.1

(A) Whole plant, (B) fruits, (C), and leaves (D) flowers of *Avicennia officinalis* (GBIF, 2020).

Mangroves with Therapeutic Potential for Human Health. DOI: https://doi.org/10.1016/B978-0-323-99332-6.00017-5

10.1.2 Botanical family

- Acanthaceae

10.1.3 Vernacular names

- White mangrove (English)
- ki balanak (Sundanese)
- api-api ludat (Peninsular)
- thame, theme-net (Myanmar)
- mắm-luói-dòng (Vietnam)

10.2 Geographical distribution

Avicennia officinalis is scarcely distributed across the globe as illustrated in Fig. 10.2. It is a preserved specimen in India, Australia, Africa, and Bangladesh.

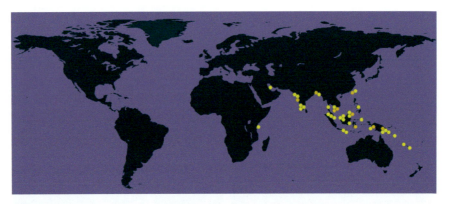

FIGURE 10.2

Distribution of *Avicennia officinalis* across the globe (GBIF, 2020).

10.3 Morphological characteristics

Avicennia officinalis is 30 m tall with pneumatophore roots system, smooth bark which is dirty green to dark gray, and is slightly fissured but does not flake compared to *A. germinans* (Sahoo et al., 2018). The leaves are shiny, green in color with round apex, 10 cm long, and 5 cm wide. The tree has pneumatophores similar to the other *Avicennia* species. The flower of *A. officinalis* is the largest of all the species in its genus and is orange-yellow to lemon-yellow as shown in Fig. 10.1. This species produced a heart-shaped propagule, green or brown (Sahoo et al., 2018; Thatoi et al., 2016).

10.4 Ethnobotanical uses

In Taiwan, the fruits are mixed with butter to form a paste to apply on smallpox to prevent them from bursting; in Indo-China, the bark is used to heal cutaneous affections, especially scabies; in Indonesia, the resin exuded from the bark is used as a contraceptive; in the Philippines, the resin from the sapwood is applied locally on snakebites (Perry, 1980). A decoction of the plant mixed with sugar candy and cumin is used against dyspepsia (Thirunavukkarasu et al., 2011).

10.5 Phytochemicals

Thatoi et al. (2016) identified 17 compounds from the terpenoid class as detailed in Table 10.1. The most studied part of this mangrove species is the leaves. Table 10.1 summarizes the different compounds identified from *A. officinalis*.

Table 10.1 Phytochemicals of *Avicennia officinalis*.

Plant part	Extract	Phytochemical class	Compounds	References
L	MeOH	Alkaloid, reducing sugar, tannins, gums, flavonoids, steroid	NI	Hossain et al. (2012)
L	CE	Alkaloid, flavonoid, terpenoids, phenolics, tannins, sterols, glycosides	NI	Ramanathan (2012)
L	MeOH	Pentacyclic triterpenoids	Lupeol, betulin, betulinaldehyde, betulinic acid, β-sitosterol	Sumithra et al. (2011)
		Glycosides, flavonoids, alkaloids, steroids, tannins, wax esters	NI	
L	NI	Flavonoid	Velutin	Thatoi et al. (2016)
		Naphthalene derivative	Avicenol	
		Tannins	Catechin, chlorogenic acid, gallic acid, ellagic acid	
		Steroids	β-sitosterol, stigmasterol, cholesterol, campesterol, stigmast-7-en-3β-ol	

(Continued)

Table 10.1 Phytochemicals of *Avicennia officinalis*. *Continued*

Plant part	Extract	Phytochemical class	Compounds	References
		Terpenoids	Taraxerol, saraxerone, setulinic acid, setulin, betulinaldehyde, β-amyrin, rhizophorins A-B, ent-13S-2,3-seco-14-labden-2,8-olide-3-oic acid, ribenone, ent-16-hydroxy-3-oxo-13-epi-manoyl oxide, ent-15-hydroxy-labda-8, 13E-dien-3-one, ent-3a,15-dihydroxylabda-8,13E-diene, excoecarin A, ent-beyerane	
		Glycosides	7-O-trans-cinnamoyl-4-epilogenin, geniposidic acid, 2'-cinnamoyl-mussaenosidic acid, 10-O-5-phenyl-2,4-pentadienoyl-geniposide, 7-O-cinnamoyl-8-epiloganic acid sodium salt, 8-O-cinnamoyl-mussaenosidic acid, officinosidic acid, loganin C	
L	E	Carbohydrate, reducing sugar, combined reducing sugar, glycosides, tannins, alkaloids, proteins, terpenoids and flavonoids	NI	Hossain (2016)

CE, Crude extract; *E*, ethanol; *L*, leaf; *MeOH*, methanol; *NI*, not indicated.

10.6 Pharmacological activities

Avicennia officinalis is largely studied for its pharmacological activities. For instance, the ethyl acetate leaf extract is analyzed for its antimicrobial activity against *Escherichia coli*, *Streptococcus mutans*, *Staphylococcus aureus*, *Aspergillus flavus*, and *Trichophyton rubrum*. The extract showed activity against *E. coli*, *S. mutans*, and *S. aureus* but found inactive for *A. flavus* and *T. rubrum*. Antiulcer activity was investigated on the ethanolic extract using indomethacin-induced gastric ulcer assay and it

Table 10.2 Pharmacological activities of *Avicennia officinalis*.

Plant part (s)	Extract	Study	Results	References
L	E	Antioxidant—DPPH	IC50 (control) = 65.12 ± 54, IC50 (extract) at 0.1 mg/mL = 40.77 ± 3.43	Thirunavukkarasu et al. (2011)
		Antioxidant—HO Antioxidant—NO	IC50 (control) = 64.35 ± 1.34, IC50 (extract) = 38.23 ± 3.84 At 0.1 mg/mL, IC50: control = 62.97 ± 8.64, extract = 39.87 ± 4.78	
		Antioxidant—ABTS	At 0.1 mg/mL, IC50: control = 61.84 ± 1.33, extract = 38.78 ± 9.62	
L	EA	Antimicrobial—disk diffusion assay	Zone of inhibition (mm) against EC, STM, and SA = 7.8 ± 0.7, 7 ± 0.1, and 7.7 ± 0.5, respectively, inactive against AF and TR	Bakshi and Chaudhuri (2014)
R	A, E, Me	Antimicrobial—agar well diffusion	For the three extracts activity observed with EC, SA, ENA, KP, PA, BS, LD, and SP	Sharief and Umamaheswararao (2011)
Nl	E	Antiulcer—indomethacine-induced gastric ulcer	Gastric ulcers observed to decrease when glutathione is reduced in the gastric mucosa	Sura et al. (2011)
L	MeOH	Antiinflammatory—carrageenan induced paw edema	Inhibition of prostaglandin effect more potent in chronic model than in acute model	Sumithra et al. (2011)
L	MeOH	Diuretic—lipschitz diuretic model	At dosage 200 and 400 mg/kg, volume of urine = 3.06 ± 0.18 and 3.89 ± 0.13 mL, respectively	Hossain et al. (2012)
L	MeOH	Neuropharmacological—pentobarbital-induced hypnosis test	At dosage 250 and 500 mg/kg, total sleeping time = 6.74 ± 2.83 and 82.07 ± 3.57 min, respectively while with control (0.1% Tween 80), time = 32.06 ± 1.20 min	Rege et al. (2010)

(Continued)

Table 10.2 Pharmacological activities of *Avicennia officinalis. Continued*

Plant part (s)	Extract	Study	Results	References
L	MeOH	Neuropharmacological—open field test	At dosage 250 mg/kg, number of movements before and after drug administration after 90 min = 110.50 ± 2.12 and 41.85 ± 3.35, respectively	Sharief and Umamaheswararao (2011)
			At dosage 500 mg/kg, number of movements before and after drug administration after 90 min = 107.99 ± 2.70 and 30.06 ± 2.64, respectively	
L	MeOH	Neuropharmacological—hole cross test	At dosage 250 mg/kg, number of holes crossed before and after drug administration after 90 min = 7.57 ± 0.18 and 5.30 ± 0.69, respectively	
			At dosage 500 mg/kg, number of movements before and after drug administration after 90 min = 6.61 ± 0.72 and 4.90 ± 0.67, respectively	
L	PE	Anti-HIV—reverse transcriptase inhibition assay	%inhibition: control = 71.04 ± 1.94, extract = 74.79 ± 3.47	Rege et al. (2010)
L	E	Antioxidant—ABTS	%inhibition: control (AZT) = 71.04 ± 1.94, extract = 82.00 ± 0.26	Sharief and Umamaheswararao (2011)
Fr	E		Activity highest with ABTS compared to DPPH and FRAP	
L	E	Toxicity	No significant change observed in the majority of the mice. Mortality rate was zero	Sura et al. (2011)
L	E	Antioxidant—DPPH	At dosage 10 and 100 µg/mL, %inhibition = 16.34% and 63.64%, respectively	Hossain (2016)
		Cytotoxic	LC50 (µg/mL) = 131.2	
		Antibacterial—disk diffusion	Active against EC and ST, MIC (µg/mL) against EC = 62.5, ST = 125	

ABTS, 2, 2-azino-bis-3-ethyl benzthiazoline-6-sulfonic acid; *AF*, *Aspergillus flavus*; *BS*, *Bacillus subtilis*; *DPPH*, 1-diphenyl-2-picryhydrazyl; *E*, ethanol; *EA*, ethyl acetate; *EC*, *Escherichia coli*; *ENA*, *Enterobacter aerogenes*; *Fr*, fruit; *HO*, hydroxyl; *KP*, *Klebsiella pneumonia*; *L*, leaf; *LD*, *Lactobacillus delbrueckii*; *MIC*, minimum inhibitory concentration; *NO*, nitric oxide; *PE*, petroleum ether; *SA*, *Staphylococcus aureus*; *SP*, *Salmonella paratyphi*; *ST*, *Salmonella typhi*; *STM*, *Streptococcus mutans*; *TR*, *Tricophyton rubrum*.

was observed that the gastric ulcers decreased when the amount of glutathione is reduced in the gastric mucosa (Sura et al., 2011). Hossain et al. (2012) investigated the diuretic and neuropharmacological properties of the methanolic leaf extracts. The Lipschitz diuretic model was used to test the diuretic activity of the sample. For the dosage of 200 and 400 mg/kg, the volume of urine excreted was 3.06 ± 0.18 mL and 3.89 ± 0.13 mL, respectively. It is reported that the amount of Na + ion excreted by the methanolic extract is higher compared to the excretion of K^+ ion and as a result the plant is classified as a good diuretic which causes less hyperkaliaemic side effects (Hossain et al., 2012). Table 10.2 summarized other studies conducted on A. officinalis.

10.7 Associated fungal endophytes

In a recent study, *Aspergillus, Penicillium, Acremonium, Curumlaria, Cladosporium, Phoma, Fusarium, Sterile mycelia, Candida* were isolated from the leaves and stems of *A. officinalis* collected at Ernakulam, Kerala, India (Job et al., 2015). Recently, a study concluded that the secondary metabolite, 2,4,6-triphenylaniline, identified from *Alternaria longipes* strain VITN14G can be an alternative to existing antidiabetic drugs (Ranganathan and Mahalingam, 2019a,b).

References

Bakshi, M., Chaudhuri, P., 2014. Antimicrobial potential of leaf extracts of ten mangrove species from Indian Sundarban. International Journal of Pharma and Bio Sciences 5, 294–304.

GBIF, 2020. GBIF secretariat: GBIF backbone taxonomy. <https://www.gbif.org/> (accessed 06.11.20).

Hossain, M.H., Howlader, M.S.I., Dey, S.K., Hira, A., Ahmed, A., 2012. Evaluation of diuretic and neuropharmacological properties of the methanolic extract of *Avicennia officinalis L.* leaves from Bangladesh. International Journal of Pharmaceutical and Phytopharmacological Research 2, 2–6.

Hossain, M.L., 2016. Medicinal activity of *Avicennia officinalis*: evaluation of phytochemical and pharmacological properties. Saudi Journal of Medical and Pharmaceutical Sciences 2, 250–255.

Job, N., Manomi, S., Philip, R., 2015. Isolation and characterisation of endophytic fungi from *Avicennia officinalis*. International Journal of Research in Biomedicine and Biotechnology 5, 4–8.

Perry, L.M., 1980. Medicinal Plants of East and Southeast Asia. MIT Press, Cambridge, United Kingdom.

Ramanathan, T., 2012. Phytochemical characterization and antimicrobial efficiency of mangrove plants *Avicennia marina* and *Avicennia officinalis*. International Journal of Pharmaceutical and Biological Science Archive 3, 348–351.

Ranganathan, N., Mahalingam, G., 2019a. 2,4,6-Triphenylaniline nanoemulsion formulation, optimization, and its application in type 2 diabetes mellitus. Journal of Cellular Physiology 234, 22505–22516.

Ranganathan, N., Mahalingam, G., 2019b. Secondary metabolite as therapeutic agent from endophytic fungi Alternaria longipes strain VITN14G of mangrove plant *Avicennia officinalis*. Journal of Cellular Biochemistry 120, 4021–4031.

Rege, A.A., Ambaye, R.Y., Deshmukh, R., 2010. In-vitro testing of anti-HIV activity of some medicinal plants. International Journal of Production Research 1, 193–199.

Sahoo, G., Ansari, Z., Shaikh, J.B., Varik, S.U., Gauns, M., 2018. Epibiotic communities (microalgae and meiofauna) on the pneumatophores of *Avicennia officinalis* (L.). Estuarine, Coastal and Shelf Science 207, 391–401.

Sharief, M.N., Umamaheswararao, V., 2011. Antibacterial activity of stem and root extracts of *Avicennia officinalis* L. International Journal of Applied Pharmaceutics 2, 231–236.

Sumithra, M., Anbu, J., Nithya, S., Ravichandiran, V., 2011. Anticancer activity of methanolic leaves extract of *Avicennia officinalis* on *Ehrlich ascitis* carcinoma cell lines in rodents. International Journal of Pharmtech Research 3, 1290–1292.

Sura, S., Anbu, J., Sultan, M., Uma, B., 2011. Antiulcer effect of ethanolic leaf extract of *Avicennia officinalis*. Pharmacologyonline 3, 12–19.

Thatoi, H., Samantaray, D., Das, S.K., 2016. The genus Avicennia, a pioneer group of dominant mangrove plant species with potential medicinal values: a review. Frontiers in Life Science 9, 267–291.

Thirunavukkarasu, P., Ramanathan, T., Ramkumar, L., Shanmugapriya, R., Renugadevi, G., 2011. The antioxidant and free radical scavenging effect of *Avicennia officinalis*. Journal of Medicinal Plants Research 5, 4754–4758.

Bruguiera cylindrica (L.) Blume

11.1 General description

11.1.1 Botanical nomenclature

- *Bruguiera cylindrica* (L.) Blume (Fig. 11.1)

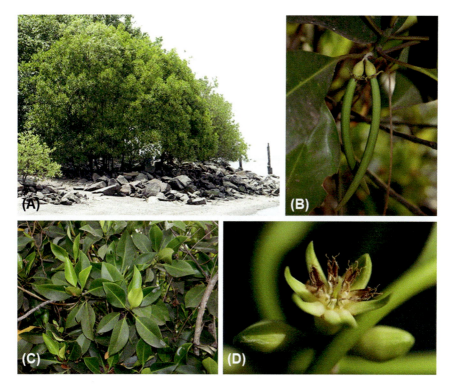

FIGURE 11.1

(A) Whole plant, (B) fruits, (C) leaves, and (D) flowers of *Bruguiera cylindrica* (GBIF, 2021).

Mangroves with Therapeutic Potential for Human Health. DOI: https://doi.org/10.1016/B978-0-323-99332-6.00020-5

11.1.2 Botanical family

• Rhizophoraceae

11.1.3 Vernacular names

• Black mangrove (English)
• Lindur (Madura), tanjang sukun (Java)
• Pototan lalaki (general), bakáuan (Tagalog), kalapínai (Ilokano)
• Byu, saung (Myanmar)
• thua-daeng (Chanthaburi), thua-khao (Ranong, Krabi), rui (Phetchaburi)
• vẹt trụ, vẹt khang (Vietnam)

11.2 Geographical distribution

Bruguiera cylindrica is scarcely distributed as illustrated in Fig. 11.2. It is a preserved specimen in Malaysia, Papua New Guinea, and the Philippines.

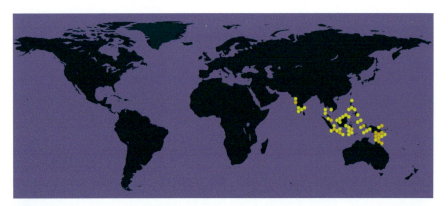

FIGURE 11.2

Distribution of *Bruguiera cylindrica* across the globe (GBIF, 2021).

11.3 Morphological characteristics

Bruguiera cylindrica coming from the Rhizophoraceae family, is 20 m tall with pneumatophore roots and has smooth bark, gray with corky-raised patches containing lenticels. The leaves are glossy in appearance and elliptical in shape with a pointed apex. The plant produces fruits of 15 cm long and has a curved/cylindrical shape. This species blooms greenish-white flowers in clusters of two to five (Fig. 11.1) (Putih, 2013).

11.4 Ethnobotanical uses

The bark is traditionally used to treat hemorrhages and ulcers by the local people of India (Krishnamoorthy et al., 2011).

11.5 Phytochemicals

Laphookhieo et al. (2004) conducted phytochemical screening on the fruit of *B. cylindrica* and the pentacyclic triterpenoids esters identified are E-feruloyltaraxerol, 3α-Z-feruloyltaraxerol, 3α-E-feruloyltaraxerol, 3α-Z-feruloyl-taraxerol, 3α-E-coumaroyltaraxerol, and 3α-Z-coumaroyltaraxenol. Gawali and Jadhav (2011) reported the presence of tannins, saponins, alkaloids, triterpenoids, anthraquinone, and flavonoids in the leaves of the plant.

11.6 Pharmacological activities

Results from DPPH assay revealed IC50 values for the methanolic leaf and stem extracts are 175 and 162.5 µg/mL, respectively (Gawali and Jadhav, 2011). Scavenging ability of the butanol, hexane, ethanol, and aqueous stem extract ranged from 18% to 77%, for superoxide anions (O^{2-}), 29% to 43% for hydroxyl radical (OH·), and 20% to 39% for microsomal lipid peroxidation (Lakshmi et al., 2012).

11.7 Associated fungal endophytes

Not available

References

Gawali, P., Jadhav, B.L., 2011. Antioxidant activity and antioxidant phytochemical analysis of mangrove species *Sonneratia alba* and *Bruguiera cylindrica*. Asian Journal of Microbiology, Biotechnology and Environmental Sciences 13, 257−261.

GBIF, 2021. GBIF secretariat: GBIF backbone taxonomy. <https://www.gbif.org/> (accessed 13.01.21).

Krishnamoorthy, M., Sasikumar, J., Shamna, R., Pandiarajan, C., Sofia, P., Nagarajan, B., 2011. Antioxidant activities of bark extract from mangroves, *Bruguiera cylindrica* (L.) Blume and Ceriops decandra Perr. Indian Journal of Pharmacology 43, 557.

Lakshmi, V., Sonkar, R., Khanna, A.K., 2012. Antihyperlipidemic and antioxidant activities of *Bruguiera cylindrinca* (L). Chronicles of Young Scientists 3.

Laphookhieo, S., Karalai, C., Ponglimanont, C., Chantrapromma, K., 2004. Pentacyclic tri-terpenoid esters from the fruits of *Bruguiera cylindrica*. Journal of Natural Products 67, 886–888.

Putih, B., 2013. *Bruguiera cylindrica*. <http://www.wildsingapore.com/wildfacts/plants/mangrove/bruguiera/cylindrica.htm> (accessed 13.01.21).

Bruguiera gymnorhiza (L.) Lam

12.1 General description

12.1.1 Botanical nomenclature

- *Bruguiera gymnorhiza* (L.) Lam (Fig. 12.1)

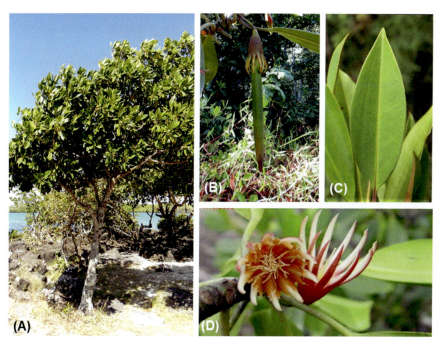

FIGURE 12.1

(A) Whole plant, (B) fruits, (C) leaves, and (D) flowers of *Bruguiera gymnorhiza* (GBIF, 2021).

Mangroves with Therapeutic Potential for Human Health. DOI: https://doi.org/10.1016/B978-0-323-99332-6.00016-3

12.1.2 Botanical family

- Rhizophoraceae

12.1.3 Vernacular names

- Large-leafed mangrove (English)
- Mangrove bean (Kavela; Papua New Guinea)
- オヒルギ (Japanese)
- പനേക്കണ്ടൽ (Malayalam)
- Manglier, Paletuvier (French)
- พังกาหัวสุมดอกแดง (Thai)

12.2 Geographical distribution

Bruguiera gymnorhiza is widely distributed in Malaysia, Indonesia, Thailand, East Australia, Papua New Guinea, and Madagascar (Fig. 12.2). It is a preserved specimen in South Africa, Mauritius, Japan, India, Namibia, and Mozambique and is under human observation in Seychelles and Australia.

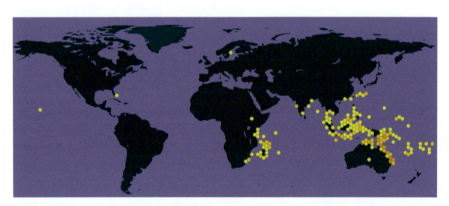

FIGURE 12.2

Distribution of *Bruguiera gymnorhiza* across the globe (GBIF, 2021).

12.3 Morphological characteristics

Bruguiera gymnorhiza is a common mangrove tree reaching a height of up to 15 m. Its bark is smooth and gray-brown in color. It has smooth and glossy leaves with pointed apex, 9.5−20 cm long and 3−7 cm wide. The propagules are green in color and have a cigar-shape which is 5−12 cm long and 1−2 cm wide. The flowers of the plant have pale yellow-green to pinkish orange sepals (Harvey, 2019).

12.4 Ethnobotanical uses

In India, the bark and root decoction are used to treat diabetes, fever, and diarrhea (Ahmed et al., 2007; Karimulla and Kumar, 2011). In Malaysia, the local people used its stem as a remedy for viral fever (Haq et al., 2011). In the Guangxi Province of China, the leaves and fruits are traditionally used to cure burns, intestinal worms, liver disorders, and diarrhea (Bandaranayake, 1998; Yi et al., 2015). The folk medicine practitioners in Indonesia uses the fruits to treat eye disease, malaria, and shingles, which is a viral infection that can occur anywhere on the body (Siemonsma and Piluek, 1993). In Comoros and Mauritius Islands, a decoction is prepared by boiling root (15 cm length) of *B. gymnorhiza* and five to seven leaves of *Piper borbonense* (Miq.) C. DC. in two cups of water. The decoction is taken to manage diabetes, hypertension, and hemorrhage (Gurib-Fakim and Brendler, 2004).

12.5 Phytochemicals

Phytochemicals present in the leaves, stems, flowers, roots, and fruits include flavonoids, saponins, reducing sugars, tannins, gums, dammarane triterpenes, aromatic compounds, sterols, diterpenoids, anthocyanins, and catechins, among others. Table 12.1 summarizes the different compounds identified from *B. gymnorhiza*.

Table 12.1 Phytochemicals of *Bruguiera gymnorhiza*.

Plant part	Extract	Phytochemical class	Compounds	References
L	MeOH	Flavonoids, saponins, reducing sugars, tannins, gums	NI	Ahmed et al. (2007)
F	NI	Dammarane triterpenes	Bruguierol A−C, bruguiesulfurol, brugierol, isobrugierol	Rahman et al. (2013)
St	NI	Pimaren diterpenes	ent-8(14)-pimarene-15R, 16-diol, ent-8(14)-pimarene-1alpha, 15 R,16-triol, isopimar-7-ene-15S,16-diol, (-)-1β,15(R)-ent-pimar-8(14)-en-1,15,16-triol	

(Continued)

Table 12.1 Phytochemicals of *Bruguiera gymnorhiza. Continued*

Plant part	Extract	Phytochemical class	Compounds	References
		Aromatic compounds	1-(3-hydroxyphenyl)-2,5-hexanediol, 3,4-dihydro-3-(3-hydroxybutyl)-1,1-dimethyl-1H-2-benzopyran-6,8-diol, (4α,8β,13β)-13-(hydroxymethyl)-16-oxo-17 norkauran-18-al, (4alpha,16alpha)-17-chloro-13,16-dihydroxy kauran-18-al, (4alpha)-13,16,17-trihydroxy-kaur-9(11)-en-18-oic acid, (4alpha)-16,17-dihydroxy-kaur-9(11)-en-18-al, ent-Kaurenol, ent-kaur-16-ene-13,19-diol, (-)-kauran-17,19-diol, (-)-17-hydroxy-16alpha-kauran-19-oic acid, (4α)-16,17-dihydroxy-Kauran-18-al, (-)-ent-kaur-16-en-13-hydroxy-19-al, 16,17-dihydroxy-9(11)-kauren-18-oic acid	
WP	NI	Gibberellin	Gymnorrhizol, gibberellin A3, A4, A7	
L	NI	Sterols	Cholesterol, campesterol, stigmasterol, 28-isofucosterol	
R	NI	Diterpenoids	Steviol, (-)-ent-kaur-16-en-13-hydroxy-19-al, 15(S)-isopimar-7-en-15,16-diol, ent-kaur-16-en-13,19-diol, methyl-ent-kaur-9(11)-en-13,17-epoxy-16-hydroxy-19-oate, apiculol (1-hydroxy-epimanoyl oxide)	
NI	NI	NI	Gymnorrhizol	Sun and Guo (2004)
R	MeOH	Gums, flavonoids, saponins, reducing sugar, tannins	NI	Rahman et al. (2011)
Fr	NI	Anthocyanins, catechins, diterpenes	NI	Revathi et al. (2014)

F, Flower; *L*, leaf; *MeOH*, methanol; *NI*, not indicated; *WP*, whole plant.

12.6 Pharmacological activities

The methanolic leaf extract has been studied for its antinociceptive activity using acetic acid—induced writhing in mice. At dosage 250 and 500 mg/kg, the %writhing inhibitions were 46% and 59%, respectively. The extract showed significant inhibition compared to the standard drug diclofenac sodium and confirmed the antinociceptive activity (Ahmed et al., 2007). Barik et al. (2016) investigated the anti-inflammatory activity on the crude leaf extract using COX (cyclooxygenase) inhibition assay. The %inhibitions at dosage 10 and 10 µg/mL were 9.7% ± 7.2% and 65.1% ± 5.8%, respectively. The ethanolic root extract was reported nontoxic with no significant change in behavior or neurological response up to 400 mg/kg body weight (Karimulla and Kumar, 2011). Methanolic leaf extract was found active against *Escherichia coli* (22 mm), while the hexane bark extract showed a broader spectrum of antimicrobial activity against *Klebsiella pneumonia* (23 mm), *Salmonella typhi* (22 mm), *Staphylococcus aureus* (19 mm), and *Shigella flexneri* (22 mm), respectively (Seepana et al., 2016). The plant was also reported to exhibit antioxidant, antihyperglycemic, antidiarrheal, and hepatoprotective activities (Table 12.2).

Table 12.2 Pharmacological activities of *Bruguiera gymnorhiza*.

Plant part (s)	Extract	Study	Results	References
L	MeOH	Antinociceptive—acetic acid—induced writhing in mice	At dosage 250 and 500 mg/kg, % writhing inhibition = 46% and 59%, respectively. Control (25 mg/kg) = 63%	Ahmed et al. (2007)
		Antidiarrheal	Latent period (h) for control (loperamide) and at dosage 500 mg = 1.71 ± 0.145 and 1.67 ± 0.163, respectively	
B	C, E, MeOH	Antioxidant—DPPH	IC50: C = 0.27 ± 0.017, E = 0.029 ± 0.004, Me = 0.038 ± 0.003	Haq et al. (2011)
L	MeOH	Antimicrobial	Zone of inhibition (mm) against BC, SA, EC, and PA are 12.67, 14.34, 8.87, and 7.85, respectively	
B	MeOH		Zone of inhibition (mm) against BC, SA, EC, and PA are 15.86, 17.85, 9.25, and 8.38, respectively	

(Continued)

Table 12.2 Pharmacological activities of *Bruguiera gymnorhiza*. *Continued*

Plant part (s)	Extract	Study	Results	References
R	E	Toxicity	Nontoxic, no significant change in behavior or neurological response up to 400 mg/kg body weight	Karimulla and Kumar (2011)
R	E	Antihyperglycemic— STZ-induced diabetic rats	Serum glucose levels of control and extract (400 mg/kg) at day 0 = 224.70 ± 15.52 and 237.0 ± 15.0 mg/mL, respectively	
			Serum glucose levels of control and extract (400 mg/kg) at day 7 = 214.5 ± 2.60 and 188.10 ± 3.14 mg/mL, respectively	
			Serum glucose levels of control and extract (400 mg/kg) at day 28 = 201 ± 16.32 and 89.04 ± 10.23 mg/mL, respectively. A significant decrease is observed in the blood glucose level compared to diabetic control rats	
L	MeOH	Antioxidant	IC50 (μg/mL) for FRAP, DPPH, NO, SO, HO and ABTS radical scavenging = 17.93 ± 0.161, 0.355 ± 0.005, 0.305 ± 0.004, 0.356 ± 0.007, 0.311 ± 0.004 and 0.056 ± 0.0003, respectively	Sur et al. (2016)
		Hepatoprotective— GalN-induced hepatic toxicity in rats	With sample GalN + extract (125 mg/kg), ALT, AST, AKP, and total protein was exhibited to be 76.6 ± 2.75, 79.3 ± 2.49, 121 ± 3.19, and 4.46 ± 0.12. With sample GalN + extract (250 mg/kg), ALT, AST, AKP, and total protein was exhibited to be 68.8 ± 2.27, 69.1 ± 1.66, 108.8 ± 3.43, and 5.01 ± 0.11	

(Continued)

Table 12.2 Pharmacological activities of *Bruguiera gymnorhiza. Continued*

Plant part (s)	Extract	Study	Results	References
L, Sb, R	MeOH	Antioxidant—FRAP	AAE (mg/g) for the 3 methanolic extracts of each plant parts = 1.25 ± 0.03, 2.85 ± 0.09, and 1.55 ± 0.16, respectively	
		Antioxidant—DPPH	IC50 (mg/g) for the 3 methanolic extracts of each plant parts = 2052.20 ± 172.01, 254.69 ± 21.26, and 1532.71 ± 46.32, respectively	
NI	MeOH	Cytotoxicity	IC50 > 2.5 mg/mL	
R	MeOH	Antioxidant—DPPH, CUPRAC; FRAP	492.62 ± 5.31, 961.46 ± 11.18, 552.49 ± 8.71 mg TE/g, respectively	Sadeer et al. (2020)

AAE, Ascorbic acid equivalent; *B*, bark; *C*, crude; *E*, ethanol; *L*, leaf; *MeOH*, methanol; *NI*, not indicated; *R*, root; *TE*, Trolox equivalent.

12.7 Associated fungal endophytes

Jiang et al. (2018a) collected the stems and barks of the mangrove plant in Fujian Province, China. The endophytic fungus *Penicillium* sp. GD6 isolated was found to produce one new sorbicillin derivatives and one new alkaloid namely 2-deoxy-sohirnone C and 5S-hydroxynorvaline-S-Ile, respectively and two other compounds, 3S-hydroxylcyclo(S-Pro-SPhe) and cyclo(S-Phe-S-Gln). The identified compounds were screened for their antibacterial activities. However, only 2-deoxy-sohirnone C moderately inhibited the growth of methicillin-resistant *S. aureus* (MRSA) with an MIC value of 80 mg/mL. Interestingly, Li et al. (2012) isolated the marine endophytic fungus *Aspergillus* sp. from leaves. Two new coumarins namely aspergillumarins A and B were identified from the fungus using 1H and 13C NMR techniques. The two compounds demonstrated weak antibacterial activity against *S. aureus* and *B. subtilis*. Later, Li et al. (2014) isolated a new naturally occurring 7-membered 2,5-dioxopiperazine alkaloid, (+)-cyclopenol, from the fungus *Penicillium sclerotiorum*. A novel pyrrolizidine alkaloid, penibruguieramine A, characterized by an unprecedented 1-alkenyl-2-methyl-8-hydroxymethylpyrrolizidin-3-one skeleton, was isolated from the endophytic fungus *Penicillium* sp. GD6 (Zhou et al., 2014). Jiang et al. (2018b) identified one new sorbicillin derivative, 2-deoxy-sohirnone C, one new diketopiperazine alkaloid, 5S-hydroxynorvaline-S-Ile, and two naturally occurring diketopiperazines, 3S-hydroxylcyclo(S-Pro-S-Phe) and cyclo(S-Phe-S-Gln) from the same type of fungus namely *Penicillium* sp. GD6.

References

Ahmed, F., Shahid, I., Gain, N., Reza, M., Sadhu, S., 2007. Antinociceptive and antidiarrhoeal activities of *Bruguiera gymnorrhiza*. Oriental Pharmacy and Experimental Medicine 7, 280–285.

Bandaranayake, W., 1998. Traditional and medicinal uses of mangroves. Mangroves and Salt Marshes 2, 133–148.

Barik, R., Sarkar, R., Biswas, P., Bera, R., Sharma, S., Nath, S., et al., 2016. 5, 7-dihydroxy-2-(3-hydroxy-4, 5-dimethoxy-phenyl)-chromen-4-one-a flavone from *Bruguiera gymnorrhiza* displaying anti-inflammatory properties. Indian Journal of Pharmacology 48, 304.

GBIF, 2021. GBIF secretariat: GBIF backbone taxonomy. <https://www.gbif.org/> (accessed 13.01.21).

Gurib-Fakim, A., Brendler, T., 2004. Medicinal and Aromatic Plants of Indian Ocean Islands: Madagascar, Comoros, Seychelles and Mascarenes. Medpharm GmbH Scientific Publishers, Stuttgart, Germany.

Haq, M., Sani, W., Hossain, A., Taha, R.M., Monneruzzaman, K., 2011. Total phenolic contents, antioxidant and antimicrobial activities of *Bruguiera gymnorrhiza*. Journal of Medicinal Plants Research 5, 4112–4118.

Harvey, P., 2019. Australian mangrove and saltmarsh resource: *Bruguiera sexangula*. <https://coastalresearch.csiro.au/?q = node/119> (accessed 19.01.21).

Jiang, C.-S., Zhen-Fang, Z., Xiao-Hong, Y., Le-Fu, L., Yu-Cheng, G., Bo-Ping, Y., et al., 2018a. Antibacterial sorbicillin and diketopiperazines from the endogenous fungus Penicillium sp. GD6 associated Chinese mangrove *Bruguiera gymnorrhiza*. Chinese Journal of Natural Medicines 16, 358–365.

Jiang, C.S., Zhou, Z.F., Yang, X.H., Lan, L.F., Gu, Y.C., Ye, B.P., et al., 2018b. Antibacterial sorbicillin and diketopiperazines from the endogenous fungus *Penicillium* sp. GD6 associated Chinese mangrove *Bruguiera gymnorrhiza*. Chinese Journal of Natural Medicines 16, 358–365.

Karimulla, S., Kumar, B.P., 2011. Antidiabetic and antihyperlipidemic activity of bark of *Bruguiera gymnorrhiza* on streptozotocin induced diabetic rats. Asian Journal of Pharmaceutical Science and Technology 1, 4–7.

Li, S., Wei, M., Chen, G., Lin, Y., 2012. Two new dihydroisocoumarins from the endophytic fungus *Aspergillus* sp. collected from the South China Sea. Chemistry of Natural Compounds 48, 371–373.

Li, J., Wang, J., Jiang, C.S., Li, G., Guo, Y.W., 2014. (+)-Cyclopenol, a new naturally occurring 7-membered 2,5-dioxopiperazine alkaloid from the fungus *Penicillium sclerotiorum* endogenous with the Chinese mangrove *Bruguiera gymnorrhiza*. Journal of Asian Natural Products Research 16, 542–548.

Rahman, M., Ahmed, A., Shahid, I., 2011. Phytochemical and pharmacological properties of *Bruguiera gymnorrhiza* roots extract. International Journal of Pharmaceutical Research 3, 63–67.

Rahman, S.M., Kabir, M.Z., Paul, P.K., Islam, M.R., Rahman, S., Jahan, R., et al., 2013. A review on a mangrove species from the Sunderbans, Bangladesh: *Bruguiera gymnorrhiza* (L.) Lam.(Rhizophoraceae). American-Eurasian. Journal of Sustainable Agriculture 7, 340–355.

Revathi, P., Senthinath, T.J., Thirumalaikolundusubramanian, P., Prabhu, N., 2014. An overview of antidiabetic profile of mangrove plants. International Journal of Pharmacy and Pharmaceutical Sciences 6, 1–5.

Sadeer, N.B., Sinan, K.I., Cziáky, Z., Jekő, J., Zengin, G., Jeewon, R., et al., 2020. Assessment of the pharmacological properties and phytochemical profile of *Bruguiera gymnorhiza* (L.) Lam using in vitro studies, in Silico docking, and multivariate analysis. Biomolecules 10, 731.

Seepana, R., Perumal, K., Kada, N.M., Chatragadda, R., Raju, M., Annamalai, V., 2016. Evaluation of antimicrobial properties from the mangrove *Rhizophora apiculata* and *Bruguiera gymnorrhiza* of Burmanallah coast, South Andaman, India. Journal of Coastal Life Medicine 4, 475–478.

Siemonsma, J., Piluek, K., 1993. Plant resources of south-east Asia. No. 8: vegetables. Wageningen Pudoc Publisher, Netherlands.

Sun, Y.-Q., Guo, Y.-W., 2004. Gymnorrhizol, an unusual macrocyclic polydisulfide from the Chinese mangrove *Bruguiera gymnorrhiza*. Tetrahedron Letters 45, 5533–5535.

Sur, T.K., Hazra, A., Hazra, A.K., Bhattacharyya, D., 2016. Antioxidant and hepatoprotective properties of Indian Sunderban mangrove *Bruguiera gymnorrhiza* L. leave. Journal of Basic and Clinical Pharmacy 7, 75.

Yi, X.-X., Deng, J.-G., Gao, C.-H., Hou, X.-T., Li, F., Wang, Z.-P., et al., 2015. Four new cyclohexylideneacetonitrile derivatives from the hypocotyl of mangrove (*Bruguiera gymnorrhiza*). Molecules 20, 14565–14575.

Zhou, Z.F., Kurtán, T., Yang, X.H., Mándi, A., Geng, M.Y., Ye, B.P., et al., 2014. Penibruguieramine A, a novel pyrrolizidine alkaloid from the endophytic fungus Penicillium sp. GD6 associated with Chinese mangrove *Bruguiera gymnorrhiza*. Organic Letters 16, 1390–1393.

Bruguiera parviflora (Roxb.) Wight & Arn. ex Griff.

13

13.1 General description

13.1.1 Botanical nomenclature

- *Bruguiera parviflora* (Roxb.) Wight & Arn. ex Griff. (Fig. 13.1)

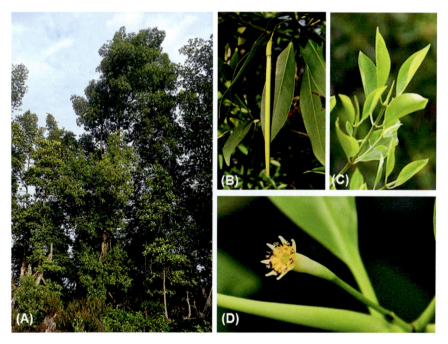

FIGURE 13.1

(A) Whole plant, (B) fruits, (C) leaves, and (D) flowers of *Bruguiera parviflora* (GBIF, 2021).

Mangroves with Therapeutic Potential for Human Health. DOI: https://doi.org/10.1016/B978-0-323-99332-6.00019-9

13.1.2 Botanical family

- Rhizophoraceae

13.1.3 Vernacular names

- Black mangrove (English)
- Vẹt tách. (Vietnam)
- Lang-kra-dai, rang ka thae, thua dam (Thailand)
- Berus lenggadai (Malaysia)

13.2 Geographical distribution

Bruguiera parviflora is mostly distributed in Malaysia, Indonesia, and Papua New Guinea (Fig. 13.2). It is a preserved specimen in Indonesia.

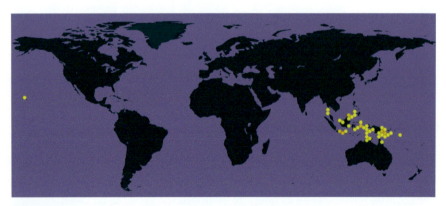

FIGURE 13.2

Distribution of *Bruguiera parviflora* across the globe (GBIF, 2021).

13.3 Morphological characteristics

It is a tree with brownish-gray trunk. It has a knee-roots system and elliptical and yellowish-green leaves (Suson et al., 2019), as illustrated in Fig. 13.1.

13.4 Ethnobotanical uses

In India, leaves decoction is prepared to cure constipation. The bark is used to regulate the blood glucose level (Rollet, 1981).

13.5 Phytochemicals

Arora et al. (2014) reported the presence of phenolic compounds in the bark while Revathi et al. (2014) reported the presence of tannins and triterpenes in the bark and leaves of the plant.

13.6 Pharmacological activities

The antioxidant activity was assessed using DPPH, lipid peroxidation, and the quinone reductase induction assay. Results showed that EC50 (μg/mL) was 105, IC50 (μg/mL) was 42.60, and IC50 (μg/mL) was > 20, respectively (Bunyapraphatsara et al., 2003).

13.7 Associated fungal endophytes

Not available

References

Arora, K., Nagpal, M., Jain, U., Jat, R., Jain, S., 2014. Mangroves: a novel gregarious phyto medicine for diabetes. International Journal of Research and Development in Pharmacy and Life Sciences 3, 1231–1244.

Bunyapraphatsara, N., Jutiviboonsuk, A., Sornlek, P., Therathanathorn, W., Aksornkaew, S., Fong, H.H., et al., 2003. Pharmacological studies of plants in the mangrove forest. Thai Journal of Pharmacology 10, 1–12.

GBIF, 2021. GBIF secretariat: GBIF backbone taxonomy. <https://www.gbif.org/> (accessed 19.01.21).

Revathi, P., Senthinath, T.J., Thirumalaikolundusubramanian, P., Prabhu, N., 2014. An overview of antidiabetic profile of mangrove plants. International Journal of Pharmacy and Pharmaceutical Sciences 6, 1–5.

Rollet, B., 1981. Bibliography on Mangrove Research 1600–1975. UNESCO, Paris.

Suson, P., Jondonero, M.A., Guihawan, J., Osing, P., Amparado, R., 2019. Species composition and diversity of natural and reforested mangrove forests in Panguil Bay, Mindanao, Philippines. Journal of Biodiversity and Environmental Sciences 15, 88–102.

Ceriops decandra (Griff.) W. Theob.

14

14.1 General description

14.1.1 Botanical nomenclature

- *Ceriops decandra* (Griff.) W. Theob. (Fig. 14.1)

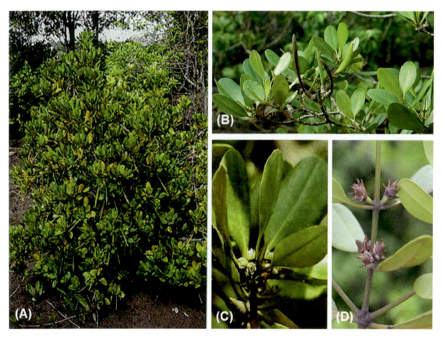

FIGURE 14.1

(A) Whole plant, (B) fruits, (C) leaves, and (D) flowers of *Ceriops decandra* (GBIF, 2021).

Mangroves with Therapeutic Potential for Human Health. DOI: https://doi.org/10.1016/B978-0-323-99332-6.00009-6

14.1.2 Botanical family

- Rhizophoraceae

14.1.3 Vernacular names

- Tengar (Brunei)
- Malatangal (Tagalog), tungung (Bisaya), tungug (Ibanag) (Philippines)
- Ka-pyaing (Burma)
- Smaè (Cambodia)
- Kapuulong (Phetchaburi), prong khaao (Samut Sakhon), samae manoh (Satun) (Thailand)
- Dzà (Vietnam)

14.2 Geographical distribution

Ceriops decandra is scarcely distributed across the globe as illustrated in Fig. 14.2. It is a preserved specimen in Bangladesh, Philippines, Papua New Guinea, Australia, and Indonesia and is under human observation in India.

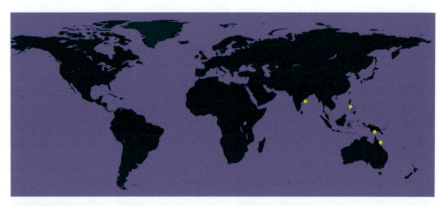

FIGURE 14.2

Distribution of *Ceriops decandra* across the globe (GBIF, 2021).

14.3 Morphological characteristics

The tree is straight, columnar, narrow crown, with short basal buttresses. Roots are superficial, with whitish or pale gray bark, branches jointed with swollen nodes, coriaceous leaves opposite clustered at the end of the twigs, flowers in head-like, deeply lobed calyx, white petals, stamens twice the number of calyx lobes, fruit as an ovoid-conical berry, persistent erect or ascending calyx lobes, seeds viviparous, hypocotyl club shaped, in tidal forest in high rainfall regions, mangrove swamp (Fig. 14.1) (Quattrochi, 2012).

14.4 Ethnobotanical uses

In Tamil Nadu, India, the leaves, fruits and barks are used by the local people to treat hepatitis, ulcers, viral infections, gastrointestinal disorders, liver disorders, diarrhea, and amebiasis (Premanathan et al., 1996). The whole plant is used to treat wounds, boils angina, diabetes, and diarrhea (Mahmud et al., 2018).

14.5 Phytochemicals

Different parts of the plant are rich with various phytoconstituents including diterpenoids (ceriopsin A-G), triterpenoids (lupeol, α-amyrin, oleanolic acid, ursolic acid), and phenolics (catechin, procyanidins) (Mahmud et al., 2018). Table 14.1 details the phytochemicals identified from *C. decandra*.

Table 14.1 Phytochemicals of *Ceriops decandra*.

Plant part	Extract	Phytochemical class	Compounds	References
B, Fr, L	NI	Polyphenols, tannins, triterpenes	NI	Revathi et al. (2014)
L	Bu, E	Protein, coumarin, phenols, flavonoids, saponins, glycosides, alkaloids, terpenoids, tannins	NI	Thirunavukkarasu et al. (2018), Thirunavukkarasu et al. (2011)
R	EA	Diterpenoids	Ceriopsin F, G	Anjaneyulu and Rao (2003)
		NI	ent-13-hydroxy-16-kauren-19-oic acid, methyl ent-16β,17-dihydroxy-9(11)-kauren-19-oat, ent-16β,17-dihydroxy-9(11)-kauren-19-oic acid, ent-16-oxobeyeran-19-oic acid (189), 8,15R-epoxypimaran-16-ol	

(Continued)

Table 14.1 Phytochemicals of *Ceriops decandra. Continued*

Plant part	Extract	Phytochemical class	Compounds	References
NI	NI	Alkaloids, flavonoids, phenols, saponins, steroids, tannins, terpenoids	NI	Poompozhil and Kumarasamy (2014)
L	H	Carbohydrates, free reducing sugars, tannins, steroids, cardiac glycosides, terpenoids, flavonoids	NI	Nagababu and Umamaheswara (2014)
	C	Carbohydrates, combined reducing sugars, steroids, cardiac glycosides, terpenoids	NI	
	Ac	Carbohydrates, monosaccharides, combined reducing sugars, tannins, free anthraquinones, flavonoids, soluble starch, alkaloids	NI	
	MeOH	Carbohydrates, monosaccharides, combined reducing sugars, tannins, free anthraquinones, flavonoids, soluble starch	NI	
R	NI	ent-abietanes	Decandrols A–I	Jiang et al. (2018)
Sb	EA	Diterpenes	Ceridecandrin A and B	Van Thanh et al. (2021)
B	EtOH	Diterpenes	Decandrins A–K	Wang et al. (2013)
		Abietanes	Podocarpanes	
W	NI	Diterpenoids	β, 13β-Dihydroxy-8-abietaen-7-one, 3β-Hydroxy-8,13-abietadien-7-one	Simlai et al. (2016)

Ac, Acetone; *B*, bark; *Bu*, butanol; *C*, chloroform; *EA*, ethyl acetate; *EtOH*, ethanol; *Fr*, fruit; *H*, hexane; *L*, leaf; *MeOH*, methanol; *NI*, not indicated; *Sb*, stem bark; *W*, wood.

14.6 Pharmacological activities

Black tea was extracted from *C. decandra*, which contains a large amount of flavoring agent theaflavin and theambrugin (neurostimulant). The black tea prevents oral cancer incidences and maintains the good health conditions of the animals. The tea showed no toxicity in mice and had better quality than commercial teas (Boopathy et al., 2011). Methanolic leaf, stem bark and root extracts were screened for their antioxidant activities using DPPH assay. The ascorbic acid equivalent of the extracts was 0.9, 13.04, and 9.81 mg/g, respectively (Banerjee et al., 2008). An in vivo study showed that the ethanolic bark extract (400 mg/kg) possessed anti-inflammatory activity with percentage inhibition of 67.72% while that of the control was 69.29% (Hossain et al., 2011). The zone of inhibition of ethyl acetate leaf extract against *Escherichia coli, Agrobacterium tumefaciens, Streptococcus mutans* and *Staphylococcus aureus* was 8.3, 9.0, 7.8 and 8.5 mm, respectively (Bakshi and Chaudhuri, 2014). Oral administration of ethanolic leaf extract (120 mg/kg) in alloxan-induced diabetic rats exhibited promising antidiabetic activity (Nabeel et al., 2010). Decandrols C and E identified from the root exhibited significant NF-κB inhibitory activity at the concentration of 100 μM (Jiang et al., 2018). Ceridecandrin A and B identified the stem bark exhibited weak cytotoxicity against three cancer cell lines (SK-LU-1, HepG2, and MCF7) with IC50 values in the range of 20.02 to 60.28 μg/mL (Van Thanh et al., 2021). The ethanolic extract of leaf and pneumatophore, at the oral doses of 250 and 500 mg/kg, showed a dose-dependent and significant inhibition of acetic acid-induced writhing in mice (Uddin et al., 2005). ABTS radical scavenging assay reported the EC50 of the methanolic stem bark extract as 13.5 μg/mL (Krishnamoorthy et al., 2011). Boopathy et al. (2011) reported that the black tea extracted from this mangrove plant prevented dimethyl benz[a]anthracene (DMBA)-induced buccal pouch carcinogenesis in hamsters.

14.7 Associated fungal endophytes

Not available.

References

Anjaneyulu, A.S., Rao, V.L., 2003. Ceriopsins F and G, diterpenoids from *Ceriops decandra*. Phytochemistry 62, 1207–1211.

Bakshi, M., Chaudhuri, P., 2014. Antimicrobial potential of leaf extracts of ten mangrove species from Indian Sundarban. International Journal of Pharma and Bio Sciences 5, 294–304.

Banerjee, D., Chakrabarti, S., Hazra, A.K., Banerjee, S., Ray, J., Mukherjee, B., 2008. Antioxidant activity and total phenolics of some mangroves in Sundarbans. African Journal of Biotechnology 7, 805–810.

Boopathy, N.S., Kandasamy, K., Subramanian, M., You-Jin, J., 2011. Effect of mangrove tea extract from *Ceriops decandra* (Griff.) Ding Hou. on salivary bacterial flora of DMBA induced Hamster buccal pouch carcinoma. Indian Journal of Microbiology 51, 338–344.

GBIF, 2021. GBIF secretariat: GBIF backbone taxonomy. <https://www.gbif.org/> (accessed 03.02.21.).

Hossain, H., Moniruzzaman, S., Nimmi, I., Kawsar, H., Hossain, A., Islam, A., et al., 2011. Anti-inflammatory and antioxidant activities of the ethanolic extract of *Ceriops decandra* (griff.) ding hou bark. Oriental Pharmacy and Experimental Medicine 11, 215–220.

Jiang, Z.P., Tian, L.W., Shen, L., Wu, J., 2018. Ent-abietanes from the Godavari mangrove, *Ceriops decandra*: absolute configuration and NF-κB inhibitory activity. Fitoterapia 130, 272–280.

Krishnamoorthy, M., Sasikumar, J.M., Shamna, R., Pandiarajan, C., Sofia, P., Nagarajan, B., 2011. Antioxidant activities of bark extract from mangroves, *Bruguiera cylindrica* (L.) Blume and *Ceriops decandra* Perr. Indian Journal of Pharmacology 43, 557–562.

Mahmud, I., Shahria, N., Yeasmin, S., Iqbal, A., Mukul, E.H., Gain, S., et al., 2018. Ethnomedicinal, phytochemical and pharmacological profile of a mangrove plant *Ceriops decandra* GriffDin Hou. Journal of Complementary and Integrative Medicine 16.

Nabeel, M.A., Kathiresan, K., Manivannan, S., 2010. Antidiabetic activity of the mangrove species *Ceriops decandra* in alloxan-induced diabetic rats. Journal of Diabetes 2, 97–103.

Nagababu, P., Umamaheswara, R., 2014. Phytochemical, antibacterial and antioxidant evaluation of *Ceriops decandra* (griff). Ding hou leaf extract. Journal of Chemical and Pharmaceutical Research 6, 428.

Poompozhil, S., Kumarasamy, D., 2014. Studies on phytochemical constituents of some selected mangroves. Journal of Academia and Industrial Research 2, 590–592.

Premanathan, M., Nokashima, H., Kathiresan, K., Rajendran, N., Yamamoto, N., 1996. In vitro anti human immunodeficiency virus activity of mangrove plants. Indian Journal of Medical Research 103, 278–281.

Quattrochi, U., 2012. CRC World of Dictionary of Medicinal and Poisonous Plants. CRC Press, Boca Raton, FL.

Revathi, P., Senthinath, T.J., Thirumalaikolundusubramanian, P., Prabhu, N., 2014. An overview of antidiabetic profile of mangrove plants. International Journal of Pharmacy and Pharmaceutical Sciences 6, 1–5.

Simlai, A., Mukherjee, K., Mandal, A., Bhattacharya, K., Samanta, A., Roy, A., 2016. Partial purification and characterization of an antimicrobial activity from the wood extract of mangrove plant *Ceriops decandra*. EXCLI Journal 15, 103–112.

Thirunavukkarasu, P., Asha, S., Reddy, R., Priya, D., Hari, R., Sudhakar, N., 2018. Phytochemical analysis of medicinal mangrove plant species *Ceriops decandra*. Global Journal of Pharmacology 12, 24–30.

Thirunavukkarasu, P., Ramanathan, T., Ramkumar, L., Shanmugapriya, R., Renugadevi, G., 2011. The antioxidant and free radical scavenging effect of *Avicennia officinalis*. Journal of Medicinal Plants Research 5, 4754–4758.

Uddin, S.J., Shilpi, J.A., Barua, J., Rouf, R., 2005. Antinociceptive activity of *Ceriops decandra* leaf and pneumatophore. Fitoterapia 76, 261–263.

Van Thanh, N., Linh, K.T.P., Binh, P.T., Thao, N.P., Cuong, N.T., Ha, T.T.B., et al., 2021. Structure elucidation of two new diterpenes from Vietnamese mangrove *Ceriops decandra*. Magnetic Resonance in Chemistry 59, 74–79.

Wang, H., Li, M.Y., Satyanandamurty, T., Wu, J., 2013. New diterpenes from a Godavari mangrove, *Ceriops decandra*. Planta Medica 79, 666–672.

Ceriops tagal (Perr.) C. B. Rob.

15

15.1 General description

15.1.1 Botanical nomenclature

- *Ceriops tagal* (Perr.) C. B. Rob. (Fig. 15.1)

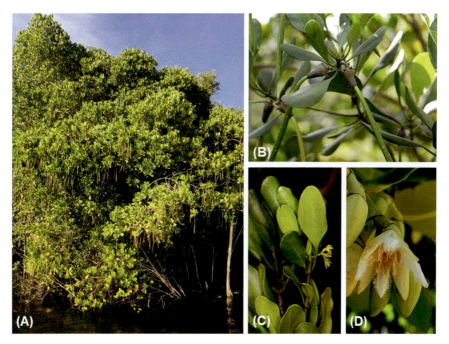

FIGURE 15.1

(A) Whole plant, (B) fruits, (C) leaves, (D) flowers of *Ceriops tagal* (GBIF, 2021).

Mangroves with Therapeutic Potential for Human Health. DOI: https://doi.org/10.1016/B978-0-323-99332-6.00022-9

233

15.1.2 Botanical family

- Rhizophoraceae

15.1.3 Vernacular names

- Indian mangrove, yellow mangrove (English)
- Indiese wortelboom (Afrikaans)
- Isinkaha (Zulu)

15.2 Geographical distribution

Ceriops tagal is largely distributed in North Australia, Indonesia, Malaysia, Madagascar, and East Africa (Fig. 15.2). It is under human observation in Mozambique, Australia, India, Kenya, Malaysia, and Madagascar.

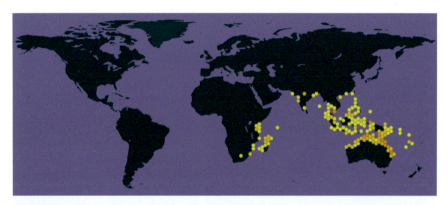

FIGURE 15.2

Distribution of *Ceriops tagal* across the globe (GBIF, 2021).

15.3 Morphological characteristics

Ceriops tagal grows to a height of 25 m. It has a buttress root system, smooth barks, and is silvery-gray to orangish-brown with lenticels on its surface. The leaves are obovate and yellowish-green on the bottom surface, and they are 6 cm long and 3 cm wide. The propagule is ovoid in shape, brown in color, and is generally 3 cm long. The flowers are creamy white. Cymes are on the terminal nodes of new shoots, and the deeply lobed calyx and stamens twice the number of calyx lobes, anthers much shorter than filaments (Quattrochi, 2012; Soepadmo and Wong, 1995).

15.4 Ethnobotanical uses

The bark has been used for the treatment of infected wounds in Thailand, obstetric and hemorrhagic conditions in the Philippines. The plant is also used to treat sores, hemorrhages, and malignant ulcers and malaria in China (Chan et al., 2015).

15.5 Phytochemicals

Chen et al. (2011) identified six compounds from the root extract as 8(14)-enyl-pimar-2′(3′)-en-4′(18′)-en-15′(16′)-endolabr-16,15,2′,3′-oxoan-16-one, tagalsin C, tagalsin I, lup-20(29)-ene-3_,28-diol, 3-oxolup-20(29)-en-28-oic acid, and 28-hydroxylup-20(29)-en-3-one, while Wang et al. (2011) identified 14 compounds from the ethanolic root extract as 3α-O-trans-feruloylbetulinic acid, 3α-O-trans-coumaroylbetulinic acid, 3α-O-cis-feruloylbetulin, 3α-O-cis-coumaroylbetulin, 3α-O-trans-coumaroylbetulin, 3α-O-trans-feruloylbetulin, 3α-O-trans-coumaroylbetulinic acid, 3α-O-cis-coumaroylbetulinic acid, lupeol, 3-epi-betulinic acid, betulin, 3-epi-betulin, and 28-hydroxylup-20(29)-en-3-one. Hu et al. (2010) also isolated phytochemicals such as dolabranes (tagalsins P, Q, R, S, T, U), pimarane, and abietane. The ethanolic aerial part was rich in terpenes namely ent-5α,3,15-dioxodolabr-1,4(18)-diene-2,16-diol, tagalsin S, tagalsin P, ent-5α,2,15 dioxodolabr-3-ene-3,16-diol, ent-8(14)-pimarene-15R,16-diol, 3a-lup-20(29)-ene-3,28-diol (Chen et al., 2016). Revathi et al. (2014) identified various types of phytochemicals in the bark extract such as inositols, steroids, polyphenols, and tannins. Two novel dolabrane diterpenes, tagalenes J and K (Ni et al., 2018), two new phenylpropanoids, tagalphenylpropanoidins A-B (Ni et al., 2018), four new diterpenes named tagalons A-D (Zhang et al., 2018), six new dolabrane-type diterpenes with the trivial names of tagalenes A-F (Yang et al., 2015) were identified from the mangrove.

15.6 Pharmacological activities

Tagalsin C exerted potent effects against a panel of drug-resistant human tumor cell lines, indicating it is a promising molecule for further evaluation as an antitumor lead compound (Yang et al., 2015). Antioxidant properties of gallic acid and quercetin isolated from the methanolic extract are found to be IC50 value of $0.77 \pm 0.41 \, \mu g/mL$ and $1.897 \pm 0.81 \, \mu g/mL$, respectively (Sachithanandam et al., 2020).

15.7 Associated fungal endophytes

Endophytic *Cytospora* sp., yielded a new bicyclic sesquiterpene seiricardine D, and eight known metabolites, xylariterpenoid A, xylariterpenoid B and regiolone, 4-hydroxyphenethyl alcohol, (22E, 24 R)5, 8-epidioxy-5α, 8α-ergosta-6,22E-dien-3ß-ol,

(22E, 24 R)5, 8-epidioxy-5α, 8α-ergosta-6,9(11), 22-trien-3 ß-ol, ß-sitosterol, and stigmast-4-en-3-one (Deng et al., 2020). Two new sesquiterpenoids, named 2α-hydroxyxylaranol B and 4β-hydroxyxylaranol B, together with a known diterpenoid 3,4-seco-sonderianol were isolated from the fermentation of endophytic fungus J3. The compound, 3,4-seco-sonderianol, exhibited cytotoxic activities against K562, SGC-7901, and BEL-7402 cell lines (Zeng et al., 2015). Four new xanthene derivatives, penicixanthenes A-D, were isolated from a marine mangrove endophytic fungus *Penicillium* sp. JY246 that was obtained from the stem of the plant. Penicixanthenes B and C showed growth inhibition activity against newly hatched larvae of *Helicoverpa armigera* Hubner with the IC50 values 100 and 200 µg/mL, respectively, and penicixanthenes A, C and D showed insecticidal activity against newly hatched larvae of *Culex quinquefasciatus* with LC50 values of 38.5 ± 1.16, 11.6 ± 0.58, and 20.5 ± 1 µg/mL, respectively (Bai et al., 2019). Compounds such as 7-hydroxydeoxytalaroflavone and deoxytalaroflavone were isolated and identified from the endophytic fungus *Penicillium* sp. FJ-1. The isolated compounds showed weak activity against *Staphylococcus aureus* and methicillin-resistant *Staphylococcus aureus* (Jin et al., 2013).

References

Bai, M., Zheng, C.J., Nong, X.H., Zhou, X.M., Luo, Y.P., Chen, G.Y., 2019. Four new insecticidal xanthene derivatives from the mangrove-derived fungus *Penicillium* sp. JY246. Marine Drugs 17.

Chan, E., Tangah, J., Kezuka, M., Hoan, H., Binh, C., 2015. Botany, uses, chemistry and bioactivities of mangrove plants II: *Ceriops tagal*. ISME/GLOMIS Electronic Journal 13, 39–43.

Chen, J.-D., Yi, R.-Z., Lin, Y.-M., Feng, D.-Q., Zhou, H.-C., Wang, Z.-C., 2011. Characterization of terpenoids from the root of *Ceriops tagal* with antifouling activity. International Journal of Molecular Sciences 12, 6517–6528.

Chen, Y., Wang, W.-J., Wu, J., 2016. Two new dolabranes from the Chinese mangrove *Ceriops tagal*. Journal of Asian Natural Products Research 18, 41–45.

Deng, Q., Li, G., Sun, M., Yang, X., Xu, J., 2020. A new antimicrobial sesquiterpene isolated from endophytic fungus *Cytospora* sp. from the Chinese mangrove plant *Ceriops tagal*. Natural Product Research 34, 1404–1408.

GBIF, 2021. GBIF secretariat: GBIF backbone taxonomy. <https://www.gbif.org/> (accessed 13.02.21.).

Hu, W.-M., Li, M.-Y., Li, J., Xiao, Q., Feng, G., Wu, J., 2010. Dolabranes from the Chinese mangrove, *Ceriops tagal*. Journal of Natural Products 73, 1701–1705.

Jin, P.F., Zuo, W.J., Guo, Z.K., Mei, W.L., Dai, H.F., 2013. Metabolites from the endophytic fungus *Penicillium* sp. FJ-1 of *Ceriops tagal*. Yao Xue Xue Bao 48, 1688–1691.

Ni, S.J., Li, J., Li, M.Y., 2018. Two new dolabrane diterpenes from the Chinese mangrove *Ceriops tagal*. Chemistry and Biodiversity 15, e1700563.

Quattrochi, U., 2012. CRC World of Dictionary of Medicinal and Poisonous Plants. CRC Press, Boca Raton, FL.

Revathi, P., Senthinath, T.J., Thirumalaikolundusubramanian, P., Prabhu, N., 2014. An overview of antidiabetic profile of mangrove plants. International Journal of Pharmacy and Pharmaceutical Sciences 6, 1−5.

Sachithanandam, V., Parthiban, A., Lalitha, P., Muthukumaran, J., Jain, M., Elumalai, D., et al., 2020. Biological evaluation of gallic acid and quercetin derived from *Ceriops tagal*: insights from extensive in vitro and in silico studies. Journal of Biomolecular Structure and Dynamics 1−13.

Soepadmo, E., Wong, K.M., 1995. Tree Flora of Sabah and Sarawak. Forest Research Institute Malaysia, Kuala Lumpur, Malaysia.

Wang, L., Mu, M., Li, X., Lin, P., Wang, W., 2011. Differentiation between true mangroves and mangrove associates based on leaf traits and salt contents. Journal of Plant Ecology 4, 292−301.

Yang, Y., Zhang, Y., Liu, D., Li-Weber, M., Shao, B., Lin, W., 2015. Dolabrane-type diterpenes from the mangrove plant *Ceriops tagal* with antitumor activities. Fitoterapia 103, 277−282.

Zeng, Y.B., Gu, H.G., Zuo, W.J., Zhang, L.L., Bai, H.J., Guo, Z.K., et al., 2015. Two new sesquiterpenoids from endophytic fungus J3 isolated from mangrove plant *Ceriops tagal*. Archives of Pharmacal Research 38, 673−676.

Zhang, X., Li, W., Shen, L., Wu, J., 2018. Four new diterpenes from the mangrove *Ceriops tagal* and structure revision of four dolabranes with a 4,18-epoxy group. Fitoterapia 124, 1−7.

Excoecaria agallocha L.

16.1 General description

16.1.1 Botanical nomenclature

Excoecaria agallocha L. (Fig. 16.1)

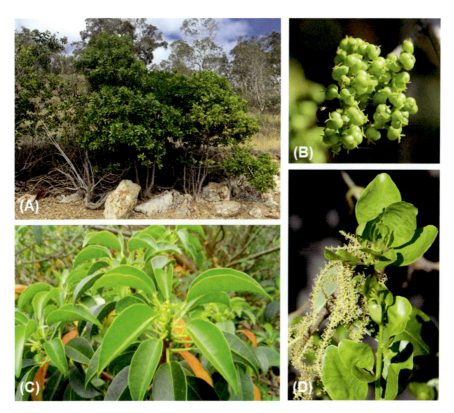

FIGURE 16.1

(A) Whole plant, (B) fruits, (C) leaves, and (D) flowers of *Excoecaria agallocha* (GBIF, 2021).

Mangroves with Therapeutic Potential for Human Health. DOI: https://doi.org/10.1016/B978-0-323-99332-6.00003-5

16.1.2 Botanical family

- Euphorbiaceae

16.1.3 Vernacular names

- Blind-your-eye mangrove, blinding tree, buta tree, milky mangrove, poison fish tree, and river poison tree (English)
- தில்லை tillai, அகதி akati, ஆக்கொல்லி akkolli, அம்பலவிருட்சம் ampala-virutcam, அம்பலத்தி ampalatti, ஆடியகூத்தன் atiya-kuttan, கொக்குமேனி kokkumeni, பருவி paruvi, வரிவனம் vari-vanam (Tamil)
- తెల్ల tella (Telegu)
- Thelakiriya, thela (Singhalese)
- Gewa (Bengali)
- Gangiva (Hindi)
- Tejbala (Kannada)
- കോമട്ടി koomatti (Marathi)

16.2 Geographical distribution

Excoecaria agallocha is distributed in Australia, Indonesia, Malaysia, Papua New Guinea, Philippines, Thailand, and India (Fig. 16.2). It is a preserved specimen in Austria, Australia, and New Zealand.

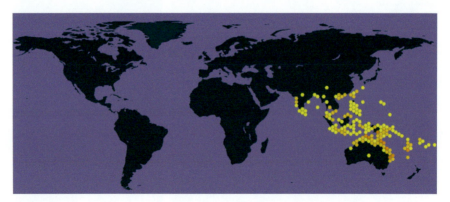

FIGURE 16.2

Distribution of *Excoecaria agallocha* across the globe (GBIF, 2021).

16.3 Morphological characteristics

Excoecaria agallocha is 15 m tall. Its root system is described as elbow-shaped pegs. The leaves are alternating and elliptical, with an acuminate apex and narrow base. They are 3−8 cm long and 1.5−3 cm wide. The fruits are small triangular capsules (Mondal et al., 2016).

16.4 Ethnobotanical uses

This tree is known to produce a latex that has therapeutic effects. The plant is traditionally used to treat rheumatism, epilepsy, leprosy, ulcers, and paralysis. This species is widely distributed in India, Africa, and northwest Australia. The local people of India, New Caledonia, and Malaysia traditionally use the latex and leaves to cure dart and fish poisoning. In Pakistan, besides using it for ulcers, paralysis, rheumatism, and leprosy, the latex is used as an abortifacient (Li et al., 2010). In Tamil Nadu, the latex is also used to alleviate a painful toothache (Ravindran et al., 2005). Another source reported that the plant is traditionally used against epilepsy, ulcers, leprosy, rheumatism, paralysis (Mondal et al., 2016).

16.5 Phytochemicals

A wide array of phytoconstituents were isolated. The main constituents identified were flavonoids, terpenoids, diterpenes, alkaloids, and tannins as shown in Table 16.1.

Table 16.1 Phytochemicals of *Excoecaria agallocha*.

Plant part	Extract	Phytochemical class	Compounds	References
St, Tw	NI	ent-kaurane diterpenoids	Agallochaol K, L, M, N, O, P	Li et al. (2010)
		Atisane-type diterpenoid	Agallochaol Q	
		Diterpenoids	NI	
B	NI	Ent-isopimarane-type diterpenoid	NI	Ponnapalli et al. (2013)
NI	NI	Diterpenoids	Excoecarins D, E, K	Konishi et al. (2000)
WP	NI	Alkaloids, tannins, phorbol esters, polyphenols	NI	Revathi et al. (2014)

(Continued)

Table 16.1 Phytochemicals of *Excoecaria agallocha. Continued*

Plant part	Extract	Phytochemical class	Compounds	References
NI	NI	Diterpenoids	3-oxo-ent-13-epi-8 (13)-epoxy-15-chloro-14-hydroxylabdane, ent-15-chloro-13,14-dihydroxylabd-8 (9)-en-3-one, ent-15-chloro-labd-8 (9) ene-3α,13,14-triol, 8,13-epoxy-3-nor-2,3-seco-14-epilabden-2,4-olide, ent-3β-hydroxy-13-epi-manoyl oxide (ribenol), (13 R,14 S)-ent-8α,13;14,15-diepoxy-13-epi-labda-3-one (excoecarin B)	Mondal et al. (2016)
		Triterpenoids	3β-(2E,4E)-5-oxo-decadienoyloxy-olean-12-ene, β-amyrin acetate, taraxerone, 3-epitaraxerol, taraxerol, 3-epilupeol, acetylaleuritolic acid	
		Flavonoids	2′,4′,6′,4-tetramethoxychalcone, 3,5,7,3′,5′-pentahydroxy-2R,3R-flavanonol 3-O-α-l-rhamnopyranoside	
		Alkaloid	2,4-dimethoxy-3-, -dimethylallyl-trans-cinnamoylpiperidine	
		Sterols	β-Sitostenone, (24 R)-24-ethylcholesta-4,22-dien-3-one	
		Tannin	3,4,5-trimethoxyphenol 1-O-D-(6-galloyl)-glucopyranoside	

B, *Bark;* NI, *not indicated;* St, *stem;* Tw, *twig;* WP, *whole plant.*

16.6 Pharmacological activities

This mangrove species possesses many pharmacological activities namely antioxidant, antiinflammatory, analgesic, anticancer, antifilarial, and antimicrobial activities. Mondal et al. (2016) investigated the antiinflammatory activity on the stem extract using two different methods, namely the carrageenan-induced paw edema test and pellet-induced granuloma test. The ethanolic and aqueous (3:1) extract of the plant showed a significant inhibition of 62.29% in carrageenan-induced paw edema model while the pellet-induced granuloma test showed an inhibition of 57.03% with the stem extract. Analgesic activity was tested using acetic acid-induced writhing test in mice. At dosage 500 mg/kg, the ethanolic and aqueous (3:1) bark extract showed the highest activity with a reduction of 53.87%. The antimicrobial properties of *E. agallocha* were tested by Bakshi and Chaudhuri

(2014) using disk-diffusion assay and the results showed the extract was active against *Escherichia coli, Agrobacterium tumefaciens, Streptococcus mutans,* and *Staphylococcus aureus* but inactive against *Aspergillus flavus* and *Trichophyton rubrum.*

16.7 Associated fungal endophytes

Expansols A and B were isolated from *Penicillium expansum* (salini). In Guangxi province, China, 3-arylisoindolinone enantiomers: (+)-asperglactam A, (-)-asperglactam A, nor-bisabolane enantiomers: (+)-1-hydroxyboivinianic acid, (-)-1-hydroxyboivinianic acid were identified from *Aspergillus versicolor* SYSU-SKS025 isolated from bark (cui). Another study isolated phomopsin A, B and C, cytosporone B and C, 5-hydroxy-6,8-dimethoxy-2-benzyl-4H-naphtho[2,3-b]-pyran-4-one, 5,7-dihydroxy-2-methylbenzopyran-4-one, 3,5-dihydroxy-2,7-dimethylbenzopyran-4-one, cyclo(Tyr-Tyr) from the fungus *Phomopsis* sp. ZSU-H76 hosted by the stem of the plant. Phomopsin A, B and C had no significant antibiotic activities, but cytosporone B and C inhibited two fungi, *Candida albicans* and *Fusarium oxysporum,* with an MIC ranging from 32 to 64 μg/mL (Huang et al., 2008). Compounds (R)-ethyl 35-dihydroxy-7-(8-hydroxynonyl) benzoate, ethyl-2,4-dihydroxy-6-(8-oxononyl) benzoate, (R)-Zearalane, 2,4-dihydroxy-6-nonylbenzoate, (R)-de-O-methyllasiodiplodin were identified from *Lasiodiplodia* sp. 318. However, compound ethyl-2,4-dihydroxy-6-(8-oxononyl) benzoate was the most potent, with IC50 values of 5.29 μM against MMQ, 13.05 μM against GH3 (Huang et al., 2017). Wang et al. (2012) identified expansols C-F and 3-O-methyldiorcinol from the fungal endophyte *Penicillium expansum* 091006.

References

Bakshi, M., Chaudhuri, P., 2014. Antimicrobial potential of leaf extracts of ten mangrove species from Indian Sundarban. International Journal of Pharma and Bio Sciences 5, 294−304.

GBIF, 2021. GBIF secretariat: GBIF backbone taxonomy. <https://www.gbif.org/> (accessed 13.02.21).

Huang, Z., Cai, X., Shao, C., She, Z., Xia, X., Chen, Y., et al., 2008. Chemistry and weak antimicrobial activities of phomopsins produced by mangrove endophytic fungus *Phomopsis* sp. ZSU-H76. Phytochemistry 69, 1604−1608.

Huang, J., Xu, J., Wang, Z., Khan, D., Niaz, S.I., Zhu, Y., et al., 2017. New lasiodiplodins from mangrove endophytic fungus *Lasiodiplodia* sp. 318#. Natural Product Research 31, 326−332.

Konishi, T., Konoshima, T., Fujiwara, Y., Kiyosawa, S., 2000. Excoecarins D, E, and K, from *Excoecaria agallocha*. Journal of Natural Products 63, 344−346.

Li, Y., Liu, J., Yu, S., Proksch, P., Gu, J., Lin, W., 2010. TNF-α inhibitory diterpenoids from the Chinese mangrove plant *Excoecaria agallocha* L. Phytochemistry 71, 2124−2131.

Mondal, S., Ghosh, D., Ramakrishna, K., 2016. A complete profile on blind-your-eye mangrove *Excoecaria agallocha* L. (Euphorbiaceae): ethnobotany, phytochemistry, and pharmacological aspects. Pharmacognosy Reviews 10, 123.

Ponnapalli, M.G., Ankireddy, M., Annam, S.C.V.R., Ravirala, S., Sukki, S., Tuniki, V.R., 2013. Unusual ent-isopimarane-type diterpenoids from the wood of *Excoecaria agallocha*. Tetrahedron Letters 54, 2942−2945.

Ravindran, K., Venkatesan, K., Balakrishnan, V., Chellappan, K., Balasubramanian, T., 2005. Ethnomedicinal studies of Pichavaram mangroves of East coast, Tamil Nadu. Indian Journal of Traditional Knowledge 4, 409−411.

Revathi, P., Senthinath, T.J., Thirumalaikolundusubramanian, P., Prabhu, N., 2014. An overview of antidiabetic profile of mangrove plants. International Journal of Pharmacy and Pharmaceutical Sciences 6, 1−5.

Wang, J., Lu, Z., Liu, P., Wang, Y., Li, J., Hong, K., et al., 2012. Cytotoxic polyphenols from the fungus *Penicillium expansum* 091 006 endogenous with the mangrove plant *Excoecaria agallocha*. Planta Medica 78, 1861−1866.

Heritiera fomes Buch.-Ham. 17

17.1 General description

17.1.1 Botanical nomenclature

- *Heritiera fomes* Buch.-Ham. (Fig. 17.1)

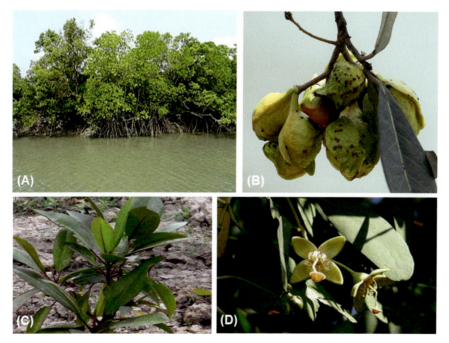

FIGURE 17.1

(A) Whole plant, (B) fruits, (C) leaves, and (D) flowers of *Heritiera fomes* (GBIF, 2021).

Mangroves with Therapeutic Potential for Human Health. DOI: https://doi.org/10.1016/B978-0-323-99332-6.00006-0

17.1.2 Botanical family

- Sterculiaceae

17.1.3 Vernacular names

- Sundari, sunder, jekanazo and pinlekanazo (Hindi)

17.2 Geographical distribution

Heritiera fomes is scarcely distributed across the globe as illustrated in Fig. 17.2. It is a preserved specimen in India, and Myanmar.

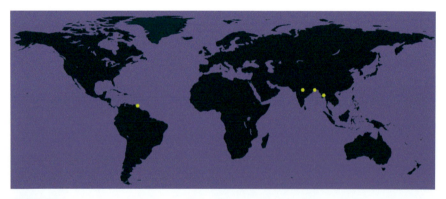

FIGURE 17.2

Distribution of *Heritiera fomes* across the globe (GBIF, 2021).

17.3 Morphological characteristics

Heritiera fomes is a tall mangrove tree which can attain a height of 15−25 m. It has pneumatophore roots, elliptical leaves, and blooms bell-shaped flowers pink to orange in color about 5 mm across, calyx cup shaped, solitary seeds can float on the tidal water, fruit does not possess vivipary germination (Mahmud et al., 2014).

17.4 Ethnobotanical uses

In Bhitarkanika and Sunderbans, India, the leaves, roots, and stems are traditionally used to treat cardiovascular diseases, gastrointestinal disorders (diarrhea, dyspepsia, stomach ache, dysentery, constipation), and skin diseases (rash, eczema, boils, itch, sores) (Hossain et al., 2013; Mahmud et al., 2014; Patra and Thatoi, 2013; Thatoi et al., 2016). Ali et al. (2011) and Rahmatullah et al. (2010) also reported that the whole plant or twig could be used against bloating, diabetes, heart disease, hepatic disorders, goiter, toothache, and oral infection.

17.5 Phytochemicals

The ethanolic leaf extract, bark extract, and the acetone and aqueous stem extracts were screened for the phytochemical compositions, and the constituents include alkaloids, cardiac glycosides, tannins, steroids, saponins, gums, carbohydrates, proteins, amino acids, terpenoids, anthraquinone glycoside, proanthocyanidins (Hossain et al., 2013; Mahmud et al., 2014; Patra and Thatoi, 2013).

17.6 Pharmacological activities

Heritiera fomes showed antihyperglycemic, antidiabetic, and antinociceptive activities in the methanolic bark extract. Ali et al. (2011) showed that the methanolic bark extract of the plant exhibited good antihyperglycemic and anti-nociceptive activities, validating the folk medicinal uses of the plant in treating diabetes and alleviating pain. Hossain et al. (2013) conducted antioxidant, anti-nociceptive, and antimicrobial assays on the ethanolic leaf extract. Results from DPPH radical scavenging assay showed that the IC50 was 26.30 μg/mL. The toxicity test on the leaf extract and the % writhing inhibitions at dosage 250 and 500 mg/kg was 34.83% and 59.20%, respectively. The extract also showed excellent antimicrobial activity against *Escherichia coli, Salmonella typhi, Salmonella paratyphi*, and *Staphylococcus aureus* with zone of inhibition of 3.92, 7.63, 5.21, and 6.41 mm, respectively. After 60 min of glucose loading at dosage 250 mg/kg, serum glucose level was 49.2. After 120 min, serum glucose level of extracts (250 and 500 mg/kg) and standard drug (glibenclamide) were reduced by 35.6, 44.7, and 30.1, respectively (Mahmud et al., 2014). The LC50 from toxicity test conducted on crude leaf and methanolic bark extracts were 234.77 and 47.081 mg/mL, respectively (Rahmatullah et al., 2010). A recent study suggested that the two phytocompounds extracted from the plant: a ses-quiterpene lactone and a flavone glycoside can act as candidate inhibitors of multiple catalytic checkpoints of the inflammatory network (Salekeen et al., 2020). The ethanolic stem bark extract showed high DPPH activity resulting in EC50 of 19.4 μg/mL. The extract also showed antibacterial activities against *Kocuria rhizophila, S. aureus, Bacillus subtilis*, and *Pseudomonas aeruginosa* (Wangensteen et al., 2009).

17.7 Associated fungal endophytes

The anti-MRSA potential of the isolated compounds present in the fungus *Pestalotia* sp. were determined against various MRSA strains, that is, ATCC 25923, SA-1199B, RN4220, XU212, EMRSA-15, and EMRSA-16, with minimum inhibitory concentration values ranging from 32 to 128 μg/mL (Nurunnabi et al., 2018).

References

Ali, M., Nahar, K., Sintaha, M., Khaleque, H.N., Jahan, F.I., Biswas, K.R., et al., 2011. An evaluation of antihyperglycemic and antinociceptive effects of methanol extract of *Heritiera fomes* Buch.-Ham.(Sterculiaceae) barks in Swiss albino mice. Advances in Natural and Applied Sciences 5, 116−121.

GBIF, 2021. GBIF secretariat: GBIF backbone taxonomy. <https://www.gbif.org/> (accessed 17.02.21.).

Hossain, M.A., Panthi, S., Asadujjaman, M., Khan, S.A., Ferdous, F., Sadhu, S.K., 2013. Phytochemical and pharmacological assessment of the ethanol leaves extract of *Heritiera fomes* Buch. Ham.(Family-Sterculiaceae). Journal of Porphyrins and Phthalocyanines 2, 95−101.

Mahmud, I., Islam, M.K., Saha, S., Barman, A.K., Rahman, M.M., Anisuzzman, M., et al., 2014. Pharmacological and ethnomedicinal overview of *Heritiera fomes*: future prospects. International Scholarly Research Notices 2014.

Nurunnabi, T.R., Nahar, L., Al-Majmaie, S., Rahman, S.M.M., Sohrab, M.H., Billah, M.M., et al., 2018. Anti-MRSA activity of oxysporone and xylitol from the endophytic fungus Pestalotia sp. growing on the Sundarbans mangrove plant *Heritiera fomes*. Phytotherapy Research 32, 348−354.

Patra, J.K., Thatoi, H., 2013. Anticancer activity and chromatography characterization of methanol extract of *Heritiera fomes* Buch. Ham., a mangrove plant from Bhitarkanika, India. Oriental Pharmacy and Experimental Medicine 13, 133−142.

Rahmatullah, M., Sadeak, I., Bachar, S.C., Hossain, T., Jahan, N., Chowdhury, M.H., et al., 2010. Brine shrimp toxicity study of different Bangladeshi medicinal plants. Advances in Natural Sciences 4, 163−174.

Salekeen, R., Mou, S.N., Islam, M.E., Ahmed, A., Billah, M.M., Rahman, S.M.M., et al., 2020. Predicting multi-enzyme inhibition in the arachidonic acid metabolic network by *Heritiera fomes* extracts. Journal of Biomolecular Structure and Dynamics 1−14.

Thatoi, H., Samantaray, D., Das, S.K., 2016. The genus Avicennia, a pioneer group of dominant mangrove plant species with potential medicinal values: a review. Frontiers in Life Science 9, 267−291.

Wangensteen, H., Dang, H.C., Uddin, S.J., Alamgir, M., Malterud, K.E., 2009. Antioxidant and antimicrobial effects of the mangrove tree *Heritiera fomes*. Natural Product Communications 4, 371−376.

Heritiera littoralis Aiton

18

18.1 General description

18.1.1 Botanical nomenclature

- *Heritiera littoralis* Aiton (Fig. 18.1)

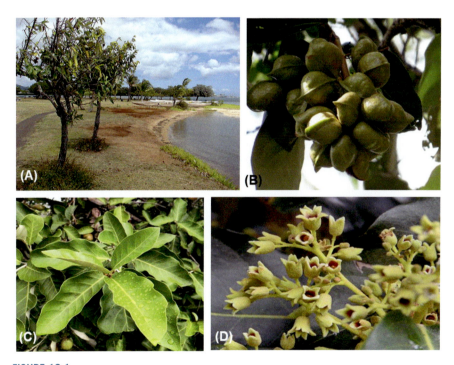

FIGURE 18.1

(A) Whole plant, (B) fruits, (C) leaves, and (D) flowers of *Heritiera littoralis* (GBIF, 2021).

18.1.2 Botanical family

- Sterculiaceae

Mangroves with Therapeutic Potential for Human Health. DOI: https://doi.org/10.1016/B978-0-323-99332-6.00021-7

18.1.3 Vernacular names

- Looking glass mangrove, looking glass tree, beach tulip-oak (English)
- Dhala sundari, kamreout, kannadi yele, sundri (Hindi)
- Sakishima-suho-no-ki (Japanese)
- Bengkulang, dungun, mengkulang (Malay)
- Barit (Philippines language)
- Moukoumafi, mouroumouny (Comoros language)
- Moromony, msikundazi, rogniny, rogno, tsilaintsango, voandrongo (Malagasy)

18.2 Geographical distribution

Heritiera littoralis is distributed along the East coasts of Australia, Papua New Guinea, Indonesia, Malaysia, and Madagascar as illustrated in Fig. 18.2.

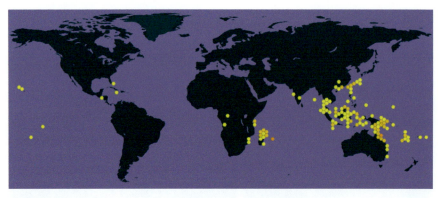

FIGURE 18.2

Distribution of *Heritiera littoralis* across the globe (GBIF, 2021).

18.3 Morphological characteristics

Heritiera littoralis reaches a height of 25 m. Shrubby, slow-growing tree, strong horizontal roots, dark green shiny simple leaves with acute apex which are generally 10−23 cm long and 4−10 cm wide, inflorescences axillary, white scented very small flowers, in habitats of low salinity, high tide line, along beach, infructescence pendulous, fruits ovoid with flattened base and winged keel as illustrated in Fig. 18.1 (Mahmud et al., 2014; Quattrochi, 2012).

18.4 Ethnobotanical uses

In the Philippines, the sap is traditionally used to counteract fish, arrowhead, and spearhead poisoning and the seed is used to treat diarrhea, dysentery, and hematuria (Ge et al., 2016).

18.5 Phytochemicals

Ge et al. (2016) conducted phytochemical screening and isolated four compounds namely 3,5,7-trihydroxychromone-3-O-α-l-rhamnopyranoside, quercetin-3-O-α-l-rhamnopyranoside, (2R,3R)-dihydroquercetin-3-O-α-l-rhamnopyranoside, and kaempferol-3-O-α-l-rhamnopyranoside from the ethanolic leaf extract and Revathi et al. (2014) reported the presence of alkaloids, tannins, polyphenols, and saponins in the stem, bark, fruit, and leaf extracts.

18.6 Pharmacological activities

Wang et al. (2014) studied the antioxidant activities on the leaves and roots using three different assays, namely DPPH, HO and SO. The IC50 value for the leaf extracts for all the three methods are 0.028, 0.600, and 0.606 mg/mL, respectively. Fruit extract has protective effects against DSS-induced colitis by keeping the balance of the gut microbiota and suppressing the NF-κB pathway (Lin et al., 2020). Ergosterol peroxide identified in bark extract was found to down regulate mRNA expressions of iNOS and COX-2 in dose-dependent manners (Tewtrakul et al., 2010). Ethanolic leaf extract exhibited antimycobacterial activity against the non-pathogenic Mycobacterium species *Mycobacterium madagascariense* and *Mycobacterium indicus pranii*, with a MIC of 5.0 mg/mL (Christopher et al., 2014).

18.7 Associated fungal endophytes

Compounds, namely, TMC-264 and penicilliumolide B were identified from the fungus *Penicillium chermesinum* hosted by the root of the plant (Darsih et al., 2015).

References

Christopher, R., Nyandoro, S.S., Chacha, M., de Koning, C.B., 2014. A new cinnamoylglycoflavonoid, antimycobacterial and antioxidant constituents from *Heritiera littoralis* leaf extracts. Natural Product Research 28, 351−358.

Darsih, C., Prachyawarakorn, V., Wiyakrutta, S., Mahidol, C., Ruchirawat, S., Kittakoop, P., 2015. Cytotoxic metabolites from the endophytic fungus *Penicillium chermesinum*: discovery of a cysteine-targeted Michael acceptor as a pharmacophore for fragment-based drug discovery, bioconjugation and click reactions. RSC Advances 5, 70595−70603.

GBIF, 2021. GBIF secretariat: GBIF backbone taxonomy. <https://www.gbif.org/> (accessed 21.02.21).

Ge, L., Li, Y., Yang, K., Pan, Z., 2016. Chemical constituents of the leaves of *Heritiera littoralis*. Chemistry of Natural Compounds 52, 702−703.

Lin, G., Li, M., Xu, N., Wu, X., Liu, J., Wu, Y., et al., 2020. Anti-inflammatory effects of *Heritiera littoralis* fruits on dextran sulfate sodium- (DSS-) induced ulcerative colitis in mice by regulating gut microbiota and suppressing NF-κB pathway. BioMed Research International 2020, 8893621.

Mahmud, I., Islam, M.K., Saha, S., Barman, A.K., Rahman, M.M., Anisuzzman, M., et al., 2014. Pharmacological and ethnomedicinal overview of *Heritiera fomes*: future prospects. International Scholarly Research Notices 2014.

Quattrochi, U., 2012. CRC World of Dictionary of Medicinal and Poisonous Plants. CRC Press, Boca Raton, FL.

Revathi, P., Senthinath, T.J., Thirumalaikolundusubramanian, P., Prabhu, N., 2014. An overview of antidiabetic profile of mangrove plants. International Journal of Pharmacy and Pharmaceutical Sciences 6, 1−5.

Tewtrakul, S., Tansakul, P., Daengrot, C., Ponglimanont, C., Karalai, C., 2010. Anti-inflammatory principles from *Heritiera littoralis* bark. Phytomedicine 17, 851−855.

Wang, Y., Zhu, H., Tam, N.F.Y., 2014. Polyphenols, tannins and antioxidant activities of eight true mangrove plant species in South China. Plant and Soil 374, 549−563.

Kandelia candel (L.) Druce 19

19.1 General description

19.1.1 Botanical nomenclature

- *Kandelia candel* (L.) Druce. (Fig. 19.1)

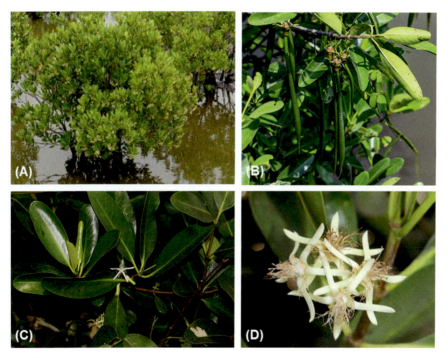

FIGURE 19.1

(A) Whole plant, (B) fruits, (C) leaves, and (D) flowers of *Kandelia candel* (GBIF, 2021).

19.1.2 Botanical family

- Rhizophoraceae

Mangroves with Therapeutic Potential for Human Health. DOI: https://doi.org/10.1016/B978-0-323-99332-6.00001-1

19.1.3 Vernacular names

- Sindhuguan, sinduka, tsjeru kandel (tsjeru = small) (Hindi)
- Matsafushi, me-hirugi, Ryukyu-kogai (Japanese)
- Aleh-aleh, beras-beras, berus-berus, pisangpisang laut, pulut-pulut (Malay)

19.2 Geographical distribution

Kandelia candel is scarcely distributed across the globe as illustrated in Fig. 19.2.

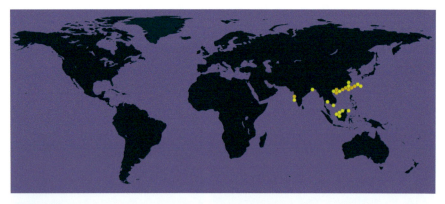

FIGURE 19.2

Distribution of *Kandelia candel* across the globe (GBIF, 2021).

19.3 Morphological characteristics

Kandelia candel grows to a height of up to 10 m. It has flaky barks with lenticels on its surface and is reddish-brown. The plant produces oval-shaped fruits, 25-cm long and blooms white flowers (Soepadmo, 1995).

19.4 Ethnobotanical uses

Bark mixed with dried ginger or long pepper said to be useful in diabetes and to reduce blood pressure. The plant is traditionally used to treat cardiovascular diseases, cancer, and neurodegenerative disorders (Sadeer et al., 2019).

19.5 Phytochemicals

The plant possessed a variety of compounds originating from different phytochemical classes namely alkaloids, tannins, saponins, polyphenols, carbohydrate, protein, amino acid, and glycoside (Jasna et al., 2017; Revathi et al., 2014).

19.6 Pharmacological activities

The ethyl acetate hypocotyl extract has an IC50 value of $124.19 \pm 3.02\,\mu g/mL$ with DPPH assay and an AAE value of $4.39 \pm 3.17\,mmol/g$ with FRAP assay (Wei et al., 2010).

19.7 Associated fungal endophytes

A variety of different species of fungal endophytes have been isolated such as *Sporothrix* sp., *Pestalotiopsis* sp., *Botryosphaeria* sp., *Phomopsis* sp., *Penicillium* sp. Table 19.1 summarizes studies conducted on the fungal endophytes of *K. candel*.

Table 19.1 Pharmacological activities and phytochemicals identified from endophytic fungi isolated from *K. candel*.

Plant part (s)	Endophytic fungi	Phytochemicals	Pharmacological activities	References
NI	*Talaromyces*	7-epiaustdiol, 8-O-methylepiaustdiol stemphyperylenol, secalonic acid A	NI	Salini (2014)
L	Endophytic fungus 1962	Two new cyclic depsipeptides, 1962A and 1962B. Cyclic depsipeptides: cyclo-(Leu-Tyr), cyclo-(Phe-Gly), cyclo-(Leu-Leu)	1962A showed activity against human breast cancer MCF-7 cells with an IC50 value of 100 μg/mL	Huang et al. (2007)
B	*Sporothrix* sp. KAC-1985	Sporothrin A, B and C, 3-methoxy-6-methyl-1,2-benzenediol (182), 5-hydroxy-2-methyl-4 chromanone, 5-carboxymellein, diaporthin, 7-chloro-2′,5,6-trimethoxy-6′-methylspiro [benzofuran-2(3 H),1′-(2) cyclohexene] 3,4′-dione, 7-methylbenzofuran-2 carboxylate, cerevisterol, peroxyergosterol, 1,8-dihydroxy-4 methylanthraquinone, cytochalasin IV, 3,5 dimethylphenol, 1,8-dimethoxynaphthalene, 1-hydroxy-8 methoxynaphthalene, 1,8-dihydroxy-5-methoxy-3-methyl-9H-xanthen-9-one, ergosterol, cyclo(L-Leu-L-Pro), cyclo-L-phenylalanyl-L-alanine, 2,4-dihydroxypyrimidine	NI	Wen et al. (2013)
B	*Pestalotiopsis vaccinii* cgmcc3.9199	Vaccinols J-S	Vaccinol J exhibited in vitro anti-EV71 with IC50 value of 30.7 μM (IC50 177.0 μM for the positive control ribavirin)	Wang et al. (2017)
Fr	*Botryosphaeria* sp. SCSIO KcF6	Botryosphaerin A and B, botryoisocoumarin A	Botryoisocoumarin A exhibited significant COX-2 inhibitory activity with an IC50 value of 6.51 μM, whereas none of the compounds exhibited cytotoxicity on the tested cancer cell lines (IC50 > 100 μM)	Ju et al. (2015)
R	*Nigrospora* sp. strain No. 1403	Methyl 3-chloro-6-hydroxy-2-(4-hydroxy-2-methoxy-6-methylphenoxy)-4-methoxybenzoate, (2 S,50 R, E)-7-hydroxy-4,6-dimethoxy-2-(1-methoxy-3-oxo5-methylhex-1-enyl)-benzofuran-3(2 H)-one, griseofulvin, dechlorogriseofulvin, bostrycin, deoxybostrycin	Bostrycin, and deoxybostrycin showed moderate antitumor and moderate antimicrobial activity	Xia et al. (2011)

L	Endophytic fungus ZZF13, Guignardia sp. 4382	(+)- and (−)-ascomindone D, ascomfurans C, ascomarugosin A	(+) and (−) exhibited potential antinflammatory effects by inhibiting against the production of nitric oxide (NO) in lipopolysaccharide (LPS)-induced RAW 246.7 mouse macrophages with the IC50 values of 17.0 and 17.1 μM, respectively	Liu et al. (2018)
L	Phomopsis sp. A123	Phomopsidone A	Compound possessed cytotoxic, antioxidant, and antifungal activities	Zhang et al. (2014)
NI	Diaporthe phaseolorum var. sojae	Lactones: 1893A, 1893B	NI	Cheng et al. (2008)
St	Streptomyces griseus subsp.	7-(4-aminophenyl)-2,4-dimethyl-7-oxo-hept-5-enoic acid, 9-(4-aminophenyl)-7-hydroxy-2,4,6-trimethyl-9-oxo-non-2-enoic acid, 12-(4-aminophenyl)-10-hydroxy-6-(1-hydroxyethyl)-7,9-dimethyl-12-oxo-dodeca-2,4-dienoic acid	NI	Guan et al. (2005)
L	Penicillium sp. sk5GW1L	Arigsugacin I, arigsugacin F, territrem B	NI	Huang et al. (2013)
L	Penicillium sp. ZH58	4-(methoxymethyl)-7-methoxy-6-methyl-1(3 H)-isobenzofuranone, lumichrome, curvulari, 5,50-oxy-dimethylene-bis(2-furaldehyde), chromone, harman(1-methyl-b-carboline), N9-methyl-1-methyl-b-carboline	4-(methoxymethyl)-7-methoxy-6-methyl-1 (3 H)-isobenzofuranone exhibited cytotoxicity against KB and KBV200 cells with IC50 values of 6 and 10 μg/mL, respectively.	Yang et al. (2013)
NI	Colletotrichum salsolae SCSIO 41021	Collacyclumines A–D	No cytotoxic effects reported	Lin et al. (2020)

B, Bark; Fr, fruit; L, leaf; NI, not indicated; R, root; St, stem.

References

Cheng, Z.-s, Tang, W.-c, Xu, S.-l, Sun, S.-f, Huang, B.-Y., Yan, X., et al., 2008. First report of an endophyte (*Diaporthe phaseolorum var. sojae*) from *Kandelia candel*. Journal of Forestry Research 19, 277—282.

GBIF, 2021. GBIF secretariat: GBIF backbone taxonomy. <https://www.gbif.org/> (accessed 21.02.21.).

Guan, S.-H., Sattler, I., Lin, W.-H., Guo, D.-A., Grabley, S., 2005. p-Aminoacetophenonic acids produced by a mangrove endophyte: *Streptomyces griseus* subsp. Journal of Natural Products 68, 1198—1200.

Huang, H., She, Z., Lin, Y., Vrijmoed, L.L.P., Lin, W., 2007. Cyclic peptides from an endophytic fungus obtained from a mangrove leaf (*Kandelia candel*). Journal of Natural Products 70, 1696—1699.

Huang, X., Sun, X., Ding, B., Lin, M., Liu, L., Huang, H., et al., 2013. A new anti-acetylcholinesterase α-pyrone meroterpene, arigsugacin I, from mangrove endophytic fungus *Penicillium* sp. sk5GW1L of *Kandelia candel*. Planta medica 79, 1572—1575.

Jasna, T., Chandra, P.R., Khaleel, K., 2017. Preliminary phytochemical screening and gc ms analysis of chloroform extract of *Kandelia candel* (l.) Druce. International Journal of Pharmaceutical Sciences and Research (IJPSR) 8, 3530—3533.

Ju, Z., Lin, X., Lu, X., Tu, Z., Wang, J., Kaliyaperumal, K., et al., 2015. Botryoisocoumarin A, a new COX-2 inhibitor from the mangrove *Kandelia candel* endophytic fungus *Botryosphaeria* sp. KcF6. The Journal of Antibiotics 68, 653—656.

Lin, X., Ai, W., Li, M., Zhou, X., Liao, S., Wang, J., et al., 2020. Collacyclumines A—D from the endophytic fungus *Colletotrichum salsolae* SCSIO 41021 isolated from the mangrove *Kandelia candel*. Phytochemistry 171, 112237.

Liu, Z., Qiu, P., Li, J., Chen, G., Chen, Y., Liu, H., et al., 2018. Anti-inflammatory polyketides from the mangrove-derived fungus *Ascomycota* sp. SK2YWS-L. Tetrahedron 74, 746—751.

Revathi, P., Senthinath, T.J., Thirumalaikolundusubramanian, P., Prabhu, N., 2014. An overview of antidiabetic profile of mangrove plants. International Journal of Pharmacy and Pharmaceutical Sciences 6, 1—5.

Sadeer, N.B., Fawzi, M.M., Gokhan, Z., Rajesh, J., Nadeem, N., Kannan, R.R.R., et al., 2019. Ethnopharmacology, phytochemistry, and global distribution of mangroves-a comprehensive review. Marine Drugs 17, 231.

Salini, G., 2014. Pharmaological profile of mangrove endophytes-a review. International Journal of Pharmacy and Pharmaceutical Sciences 7, 6—15.

Soepadmo, E.W., 1995. Tree Flora of Sabah and Sarawak. Forest Research Institute Malaysia, Kuala Lumpur, Malaysia.

Wang, J.-F., Liang, R., Liao, S.-R., Yang, B., Tu, Z.-C., Lin, X.-P., et al., 2017. Vaccinols J—S, ten new salicyloid derivatives from the marine mangrove-derived endophytic fungus *Pestalotiopsis vaccinii*, Fitoterapia, 120. pp. 164—170.

Wei, S.-D., Zhou, H.-C., Lin, Y.-M., 2010. Antioxidant activities of extract and fractions from the hypocotyls of the mangrove plant *Kandelia candel*, International journal of molecular sciences, 11. pp. 4080—4093.

Wen, L., Wei, Q., Chen, G., Cai, J., She, Z., 2013. Chemical constituents from the mangrove endophytic fungus *Sporothrix* sp, Chemistry of Natural Compounds, 49. pp. 137—140.

Xia, X., Li, Q., Li, J., Shao, C., Zhang, J., Zhang, Y., et al., 2011. Two new derivatives of griseofulvin from the mangrove endophytic fungus *Nigrospora* sp.(strain No. 1403) from *Kandelia candel* (L.) Druce. Planta medica 77, 1735−1738.

Yang, J., Huang, R., Qiu, S.X., She, Z., Lin, Y., 2013. A new isobenzofuranone from the mangrove endophytic fungus *Penicillium* sp. (ZH58). Natural Product Research 27, 1902−1905.

Zhang, W., Xu, L., Yang, L., Huang, Y., Li, S., Shen, Y., 2014. Phomopsidone A, a novel depsidone metabolite from the mangrove endophytic fungus *Phomopsis* sp. A123. Fitoterapia 96, 146−151.

Lumnitzera racemosa Willd. 20

20.1 General description

20.1.1 Botanical nomenclature

- *Lumnitzera racemosa* Willd. (Fig. 20.1)

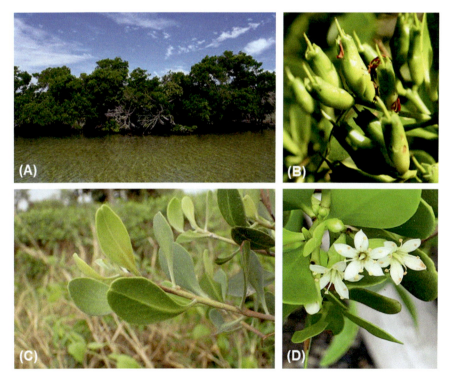

FIGURE 20.1

(A) Whole plant, (B) fruits, (C) leaves, and (D) flowers of *Lumnitzera racemosa* (GBIF, 2021).

20.1.2 Botanical family

- Combretaceae

20.1.3 Vernacular names

- Black mangrove, Kosi mangrove, Tonga mangrove, white-flowered black mangrove (English)
- Kikandaa, mkandaa-mwitu, mkandaa-dume (Swahili)
- Lovinjo, lovizo, rongo, rono, tanga, vahona, votishonko (Malagasy)
- Tongawortelboom (Afrikaans); isiKhahaesibomvu (Zulu)
- Mteda (Swahili)
- lan li (Chinese)
- Hirugi-modoki, matsafushi (Japanese)
- Sesup, teruntum, teruntum bunga puteh, white teruntum (Malaya)
- Kulasi (Philippines language)
- Beriya, tipparuthin (Sinhala: Sri Lanka)

20.2 Geographical distribution

Lumnitzera racemosa is widely distributed in Madagascar, Australia, Papua New Guinea, Indonesia, Malaysia, the Philippines, Thailand, India as illustrated in Fig. 20.2. It is a preserved specimen in Austria, New Zealand, Australia.

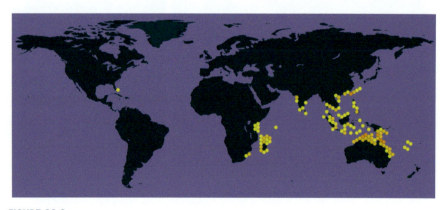

FIGURE 20.2

Distribution of *Lumnitzera racemosa* across the globe (GBIF, 2021).

20.3 Morphological characteristics

Shrub to small tree, evergreen, bushy, brittle branches, leaves slightly fleshy to leathery, white flowers, greenish yellow fruits turning black when ripe, in habitats with low salinity, on sandy soils, fruits eaten by birds, inner wood red when cut (Quattrochi, 2012).

20.4 Ethnobotanical uses

Latex from the stem is used for itch, boils, herpes while the fruits are used to treat skin disorders. In India, the plant is used against snake bites, rheumatism, skin allergies, blood purifier, asthma, diabetes, and to treat infertility (Pattanaik et al., 2008).

20.5 Phytochemicals

The aqueous leaf, methanolic twig, and dichloromethane: methanol stem extracts were screened for phytochemicals and most constituents present were alkaloids, phenols, flavonoids, terpenoids, tannins, sterols, carbohydrates, quinines, saponins, quercetin, and aromatic ester (Anjaneyulu and Rao, 2003; DeSouza and Wahidullah, 2010; Paul and Ramasubbu, 2017). Racelactone A was isolated from the methanolic extract of the leaves and twigs of the plant (Yu et al., 2018). Phytochemical investigation of the n-BuOH fraction of the mangrove plant led to the isolation of one new flavonoid glycoside; myricetin 3-O-methyl glucuronate, one new phenolic glycoside; lumniracemoside and one new aliphatic alcohol glycoside; n-hexanol 1-O-rutinoside (Darwish et al., 2016).

20.6 Pharmacological activities

Lumnitzera racemosa showed antioxidant, cytotoxicity, and anticoagulant properties. Cytotoxicity test was conducted on the aqueous leaf extract against Hep G2 cancer cell line using MTT assay. The resulting IC50 value was 26.05 μg/mL, and the extract was reported to exhibit potent cytotoxicity activity on the Hep G2 cell lines (Paul and Ramasubbu, 2017). Racelactone A showed significant anti-inflammatory effects with IC50 value of 4.95 ± 0.89 μM (Yu et al., 2018). Leaf extract treated rats showed maximum reduction of serum glutamic oxaloacetic transaminase [(210.36 ± 19.63) IU/L], serum glutamic pyruvic transaminase [(82.37 ± 13.87) IU/L], alkaline phosphatase [(197.63 ± 23.43) IU/L], bilirubin [(2.15 ± 0.84) mg/dL], cholesterol [(163.83 ± 15.63) mg/dL], sugar [(93.00 ± 7.65) mg/dL] and LDH [(1134.00 ± 285.00) IU/L] were observed with the high dose (300 mg/kg bw) of leaf extract treated rats (Ravikumar and Gnanadesigan, 2011).

20.7 Associated fungal endophytes

Sumalarins A, B, C were isolated from *Penicillium sumatrense* MA-92 (Meng et al., 2013).

References

Anjaneyulu, A.S.R., Rao, V.L., 2003. Ceriopsins F and G, diterpenoids from *Ceriops decandra*. Phytochemistry 62, 1207–1211.

Darwish, A.G., Samy, M.N., Sugimoto, S., Otsuka, H., Abdel-Salam, H., Matsunami, K., 2016. Effects of hepatoprotective compounds from the leaves of *Lumnitzera racemosa* on acetaminophen-induced liver damage in vitro. Chemical and Pharmaceutical Bulletin 64, 360–365.

DeSouza, L., Wahidullah, S., 2010. Antibacterial phenolics from the mangrove *Lumnitzera racemosa*. Indian Journal of Marine Sciences 39, 294–298.

GBIF, 2021. GBIF secretariat: GBIF backbone taxonomy. <https://www.gbif.org/> (accessed 22.02.21.).

Meng, L.H., Li, X.M., Lv, C.T., Li, C.S., Xu, G.M., Huang, C.G., et al., 2013. Sulfur-containing cytotoxic curvularin macrolides from *Penicillium sumatrense* MA-92, a fungus obtained from the rhizosphere of the mangrove *Lumnitzera racemosa*. Journal of Natural Products 76, 2145–2149.

Pattanaik, C., Reddy, C., Dhal, N., Das, R., 2008. Utilisation of mangrove forests in Bhitarkanika wildlife sanctuary, Orissa. Indian Journal of Traditional Knowledge 7, 598–603.

Paul, T., Ramasubbu, S., 2017. The antioxidant, anticancer and anticoagulant activities of *Acanthus ilicifolius* L. roots and *Lumnitzera racemosa* Willd. leaves, from southeast coast of India. Journal of Applied Pharmaceutical Science 7, 81–87.

Quattrochi, U., 2012. CRC World of Dictionary of Medicinal and Poisonous Plants. CRC Press, Boca Raton, FL.

Ravikumar, S., Gnanadesigan, M., 2011. Hepatoprotective and antioxidant activity of a mangrove plant *Lumnitzera racemosa*. Asian Pacific Journal of Tropical Biomedicine 1, 348–352.

Yu, S.Y., Wang, S.W., Hwang, T.L., Wei, B.L., Su, C.J., Chang, F.R., et al., 2018. Components from the leaves and twigs of mangrove *Lumnitzera racemosa* with anti-angiogenic and anti-inflammatory effects. Marine Drugs 16.

Nypa fruticans Wurmb

21

21.1 General description

21.1.1 Botanical nomenclature

- *Nypa fruticans* Wurmb (Fig. 21.1)

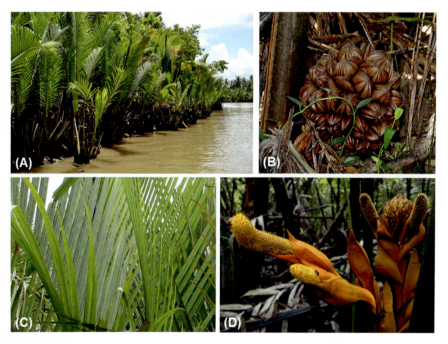

FIGURE 21.1

(A) Whole plant, (B) fruits, (C) leaves, and (D) flowers of *Nypa fruticans* (GBIF, 2021).

Mangroves with Therapeutic Potential for Human Health. DOI: https://doi.org/10.1016/B978-0-323-99332-6.00004-7

21.1.2 Botanical family

- Arecaceae

21.1.3 Vernacular names

- Mangrove palm, nipa palm, nypa palm, water coconut, water palm (English)
- Palmeira do mangue, palmeira ripa (Portuguese)
- Dane (Myanmar)
- Cha:k (Cambodia)
- Phudo, railoi (Hindi)
- Bobo, buyuk, nipah (Indonesian)
- Nippa-yashi (Japanese)
- Nipah (Malay)
- Biri-biri (Papua New Guinea language)
- Anipa, lasa, nipa, pawid, pinog, pinok, saga, sasa, tata (Philippines language)
- Gin-pol (Sinhala)
- Atta, chak (Thailand)
- D[uwf]a n[uw][ows]c, d[uwf]a l[as] (Vietnamese)

21.2 Geographical distribution

Nypa fruticans is found in Northern Australia, Papua New Guinea, Indonesia, Malaysia, the Philippines (Fig. 21.2).

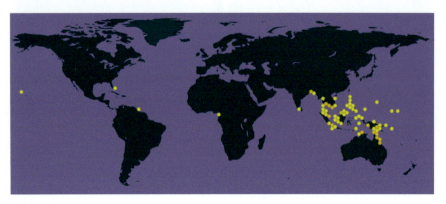

FIGURE 21.2

Distribution of *Nypa fruticans* across the globe (GBIF, 2021).

21.3 Morphological characteristics

Palm, creeping, unarmed, pleonanthic, monecious, prostrate or subterranean (rhizome), leaves erect, inflorescence solitary erect branched, globose head of female flowers, solitary male flowers, fruiting head subglobose, fruit eaten, young seeds and buds edible, sub humid to humid, sap used as beverage, swamp soils, tidal mud as illustrated in Fig. 21.1 (Quattrochi, 2012).

21.4 Ethnobotanical uses

Leaves decoction applied to snake and centipede bites. Juice prepared from young shoots is used against herpes. A decoction prepared from leaves is taken as a remedy for bloody diarrhea; ashes against toothache and headache. In Malaysia, the local inhabitants used the plant to manage diabetes (Yusoff et al., 2015) and in the Philippines, the flowers and leaves are traditionally used to treat diabetes and snake bites (Rollet, 1981).

21.5 Phytochemicals

Acetic acid, 2,3-butanediol, 1-(2-butoxyethoxy)-ethanol, 5-bromo-2-hydroxybenzaldehyde, (4-aminophenyl)-phenylmethanone have been identified from the plant (Yusoff et al., 2015). Prasad et al. (2013) identified gallic acid, protocatechuic acid, 4-hydroxybenzoic acid, chlorogenic acid, rutin, cinnamic acid, quercetin, kaempferol from the aqueous fruit extract. Compounds from different phytochemical classes alkaloids, cardiac glycosides, anthranoids, polyphenols, flavonoids, phlobatannins, and saponins were identified (Ebana et al., 2015).

21.6 Pharmacological activities

The methanolic leaf extract showed antimicrobial activity against *Escherichia coli, Agrobacterium tumefaciens, Streptococcus mutans*, and *Staphylococcus aureus* while the extract was inactive against *Aspergillus flavus* and *Trichophyton rubrum* (Bakshi and Chaudhuri, 2014). The antioxidant activity of ethyl acetate extract was investigated for its antioxidant activity using DPPH assay, and the result showed an IC50 value of 2.770 $\pm$ 0.012 mg/mL (Yusoff et al., 2015).

21.7 Associated fungal endophytes

Not available

References

Bakshi, M., Chaudhuri, P., 2014. Antimicrobial potential of leaf extracts of ten mangrove species from Indian Sundarban. International Journal of Pharma and Bio Sciences 5, P294–P304.

Ebana, R., Etok, C., Edet, U., 2015. Phytochemical screening and antimicrobial activity of *Nypa fruticans* harvested from Oporo River in the Niger Delta region of Nigeria. International Journal of Innovation and Applied Studies 10, 1120–1124.

GBIF, 2021. GBIF secretariat: GBIF backbone taxonomy. <https://www.gbif.org/> (accessed 22.02.21.).

Prasad, N., Yang, B., Kong, K.W., Khoo, H.E., Sun, J., Azlan, A., et al., 2013. Phytochemicals and antioxidant capacity from *Nypa fruticans* Wurmb. fruit. Evidence-Based Complementary and Alternative Medicine 2013, 154606.

Quattrochi, U., 2012. CRC World of Dictionary of Medicinal and Poisonous Plants. CRC Press, Boca Raton, Florida.

Rollet, B., 1981. Bibliography on Mangrove Research 1600–1975. UNESCO, Paris, France.

Yusoff, N.A., Yam, M.F., Beh, H.K., Abdul Razak, K.N., Widyawati, T., Mahmud, R., et al., 2015. Antidiabetic and antioxidant activities of *Nypa fruticans* Wurmb. vinegar sample from Malaysia. Asian Pacific Journal of Tropical Medicine 8, 595–605.

Pelliciera rhizophorae Planch. & Triana

22

22.1 General description

22.1.1 Botanical nomenclature

- *Pelliciera rhizophorae* Planch. & Triana (Fig. 22.1)

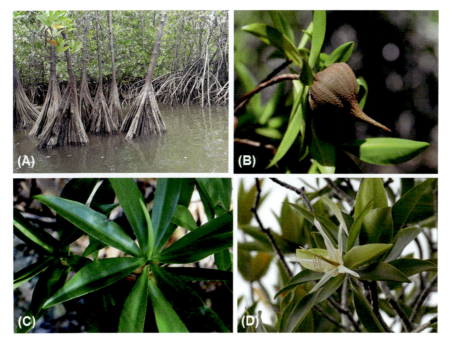

FIGURE 22.1

(A) Whole plant, (B) fruits, (C) leaves, and (D) flowers of *Pelliciera rhizophorae* (GBIF, 2021).

22.1.2 Botanical family

- Tetrameristaceae

22.1.3 Vernacular names

- Tea mangrove (English)

22.2 Geographical distribution

Pelliciera rhizophorae is scarcely distributed across the globe as illustrated in Fig. 22.2. It is a preserved specimen in Costa Rica, Honduras and is under human observation in Colombia, Panama, and Nicaragua.

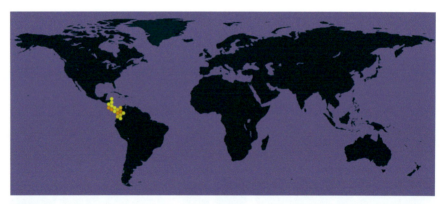

FIGURE 22.2

Distribution of *Pelliciera rhizophorae* across the globe (GBIF, 2021).

22.3 Morphological characteristics

Pelliciera rhizophorae attains a height of up to 20 m, has a buttress root system that spread themselves around the trunk, and dark-green, elongated, pointed leaves which are 20-cm long and 5-cm wide. Develops 5 rayed symmetric white flowers are which often also colored white and red and can reach up to 13 cm in diameter. The single flowers grow at the end of branches between the cluster-like leaves. The ripped brown fruit is about 10 cm in diameter. Sometimes the fruits reach sizes up to 14 cm. The fruit contains exactly one viviparous seed (Fig. 22.1) (Mangroves, 2021).

22.4 Ethnobotanical uses

Not available

22.5 Phytochemicals

α-Amyrin, β-amyrin, ursolic acid, oleanolic acid, betulinic acid, brugierol, iso-brugierol, kaempferol, and quercetin was identified in the leaf crude extract (López et al., 2015).

22.6 Pharmacological activities

Oleanolic acid, kaempferol, and quercetin showed antiparasitic activity against *Leishmania donovani*, and their respective IC50 values were 5.3, 22.9, and 3.4 μM while α-amyrin and betulinic acid exhibited activity against *Trypanosoma cruzi* and *Plasmodium falciparum* with the corresponding IC50 values of 19.0 and 18.0 μM (López et al., 2015).

22.7 Associated fungal endophytes

Not available

References

GBIF, 2021. GBIF secretariat: GBIF backbone taxonomy. <https://www.gbif.org/> (accessed 07.03.21.).

López, D., Cherigo, L., Spadafora, C., Loza-Mejía, M.A., Martínez-Luis, S., 2015. Phytochemical composition, antiparasitic and α-glucosidase inhibition activities from *Pelliciera rhizophorae*. Chemistry Central Journal 9, 53.

Mangroves, 2021. *Pelliciera rhizophorae*. <http://www.mangrove.at/pelliciera-rhizophorae_tea-mangrove.html> (accessed 07.03.21).

Rhizophora apiculata Blume

23

23.1 General description

23.1.1 Botanical nomenclature

- *Rhizophora apiculata* Blume (Fig. 23.1)

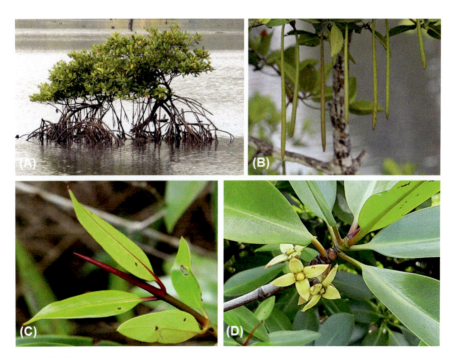

FIGURE 23.1

(A) Whole plant, (B) fruits, (C) leaves, and (D) flowers of *Rhizophora apiculata* (GBIF, 2021).

Mangroves with Therapeutic Potential for Human Health. DOI: https://doi.org/10.1016/B978-0-323-99332-6.00010-2

23.1.2 Botanical family

- Rhizophoraceae

23.1.3 Vernacular names

- Mangrove (English)
- Hong shu (Chinese)
- Char, cirugandal, daboja, kaaki ponna, kaandla, kandal, kantal, pee-kandel, ponna, rai, turu, uppu ponna (Hindi)

23.2 Geographical distribution

Rhizophora apiculata is distributed in Papua New Guinea, Indonesia, Malaysia, India as illustrated in Fig. 23.2. It is a preserved specimen in India and Thailand and is under human observation in Jamaica.

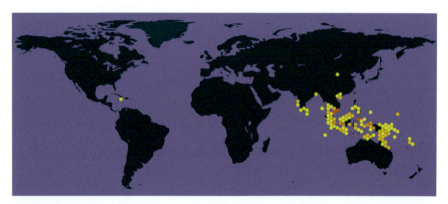

FIGURE 23.2

Distribution of *Rhizophora apiculata* across the globe (GBIF, 2021).

23.3 Morphological characteristics

Rhizophora apiculata is 30-m tall, has stilt roots, and almost smooth bark. The leaves are decussate, have the acute apex and reddish petiole, are 1.5−3 cm long, and bloom yellow, bisexual, 4-lobed calyx flowers, brown, ovoid or inversely pear-shaped berry, rough, 2−3.5 cm long fruits (Fig. 23.1) (Use, 2016).

23.4 Ethnobotanical uses

In Sidha, respiratory roots are chewed and applied to treat fish bite. Bark decoction is given to manage dysentery and stomach pain. In Tamil Nadu, the whole plant is used to treat colitis, inflammatory and bowel disease and in Pichavaram, the bark is traditionally used to manage amebiasis, diarrhea, nausea, and vomiting (Prabhu and Guruvayoorappan, 2014; Premanathan et al., 1999; Ravindran et al., 2005).

23.5 Phytochemicals

Compounds from different phytochemical classes such as aliphatic alcohols, hydrolysable tannins, steroids, triterpenoids, phenolic compounds are identified (Revathi et al., 2014). Lyoniresinol-3α-O-β-arabinopyranoside, lyoniresinol-3α-O-β-rhamnoside, afzelechin-3-rahmnoside were identified from the twig, leaf and bark extracts (Gao and Xiao, 2012). Alcohols, ketones, furan and pyran derivatives, guaiacol and derivatives, phenol and derivatives, syringol and derivatives, pyrocatechol, alkyl aryl ether, nitrogenated compounds, are carbohydrate derivatives, were identified in the dichloromethane extract of the plant (Loo et al., 2008).

23.6 Pharmacological activities

Rhizophora apiculata possessed many pharmacological properties namely antioxidant, antimicrobial and anti-HIV activities. The butanol, ethanolic, ethyl acetate, and water stem extracts were tested for the antioxidant activity using DPPH, ABTS, and HO assays (Gao and Xiao, 2012). Lim et al. (2006) investigated the antimicrobial activity of the crude bark extract using disk diffusion assay. The extract was found active against 11 microorganisms such as *Proteus mirabilis, Acinetobacter calcoaceticus, Staphylococcus epidermidis, Yersinia enterocolitica, Staphylococcus aureus, Pseudomonas aeruginosa, Bacillus cereus, Escherichia coli, Bacillus subtilis, Candida albicans*, and *Cryptococcus neoformans*. However, no fungal activity was reported. Varahalarao and Naidu (2009) investigated the antimicrobial activity on the crude extract using agarwell diffusion and the extract was active against seven bacterial pathogens namely *Acremonium strictum* (7 mm), *Aspergillus flavus* (8 mm), *Candida albicans* (11 mm), *Streptococcus mutans* (15 mm), *Streptococcus salivarius* (19 mm), *Staphylococcus aureus* (11 mm), and *Lactobacillus acidophilus* (22 mm), respectively. Activity was highest against *Lactobacillus acidophilus*. Table 23.1 summarized other studies conducted on *R. apiculata*.

Table 23.1 Pharmacological activities of *Rhizophora apiculata*.

Plant part (s)	Extract	Study	Results	References
St	Bu, E, EE, Aq	Antioxidant-DPPH	IC50 (µg/mL): Bu = 9.68 ± 1.86, E = 19.31 ± 1.56, EE = 13.56 ± 1.79, Aq = 23.72 ± 1.94, control (BHT) = 52.20 ± 1.57	Gao and Xiao (2012)
		Antioxidant-ABTS	IC50 (µg/mL): Bu = 1.26 ± 0.05, E = 3.01 ± 0.75, EE = 1.71 ± 0.39, Aq = 4.32 ± 0.96, control (BHT) = 9.63 ± 0.15	
		Antioxidant-HO	IC50 (µg/mL): Bu = 9.07 ± 0.99, E = 17.93 ± 1.51, EE = 13.57 ± 1.59, Aq = 33.59 ± 1.66, control (BHT) = 45.58 ± 2.14	
B	CE	Antimicrobial-disk diffusion	Activity tested with MT. Complete inhibition with PM, AC, SE, YE, SA, PA, and BC. Partial inhibition with EC, BS, CA, and CN. No fungal activity reported	Lim et al. (2006)
B	MeOH	Antimicrobial-disk diffusion	Activity tested with MT. Complete inhibition with PM, AC, SE, YE, SA, PA, and BC. Partial inhibition with EC, BS, CA, and CN. No fungal activity reported	
			MIC (mg/mL): 1.56 against AC, 3.12 against BC, 6.25 against PA, 6.25 against SA, 3.13 against SS	
NI	NI	Antioxidant-DPPH	Most potent radical scavengers: catechol, methoxycatechol, syringol.	Loo et al. (2008)
			Their respective EC50 (mg/mL): 0.1239 ± 0.0004, 0.2001 ± 0.0005, 0.2218 ± 0.0009. EC50 (mg/mL) Ascorbic acid (control) = 0.2562 ± 0.0023	
L	NI	Anti-HIV-MTT assay	CC50 (µg/mL) = 998.21 ± 81.57, EC50 (µg/mL) = 108.55 ± 16.24, SI = 9.19	Premanathan et al. (1996)

(Continued)

Table 23.1 Pharmacological activities of *Rhizophora apiculata. Continued*

Plant part (s)	Extract	Study	Results	References
B	NI	Antioxidant-FRAP	Reducing power increased as concentration of mangrove tannins increased from 20 to 60 µg/mL	Rahim et al. (2008), Sulaiman et al. (2011)
		Antioxidant-DPPH	Scavenging activity increased as concentration of tannins increased.	
			Maximum scavenging activity ($>90\%$) exhibited at 30 µg/mL	
NI	NI	Antimicrobial-disk diffusion	Zone of inhibition (mm) against BC = 14, SS = 9. For bacteria, AC, KP, BS, SA, BL, SE, BC, SM, PA, MIC (mg/mL) ranged from 3.13 to 386.25	

AC, Acinetobacter calcoaceticus; Aq, aqueous; B, bark; BC, Bacillus cereus; BL, Bacillus licheniformis; BS, Bacillus subtilis; Bu, butanol; CA, Candida albicans; CE, crude extract; CN, Cryptococcus neoformans; E, ethanol; EC, Escherichia coli; EE, ethyl ether; KP, Klebsiella pneumonia; L, leaf; MeOH, methanol; MT, mixed tannin; NI, not indicated; PA, Pseudomonas aeruginosa; PM, Proteus mirabilis; SA, Staphylococcus aureus; SE, Staphylococcus epidermidis; SI, selective index (CC50/EC50); St, stem; SM, Serratia marcescens; SS, Staphylococcus saprophyticus; YE, Yersinia enterocolitica.

23.7 Associated fungal endophytes

Not available

References

Gao, M., Xiao, H., 2012. Activity-guided isolation of antioxidant compounds from *Rhizophora apiculata*. Molecules 17, 10675–10682.

GBIF, 2021. GBIF secretariat: GBIF backbone taxonomy. <https://www.gbif.org/> (accessed 24.02.21).

Lim, S.H., Darah, I., Jain, K., 2006. Antimicrobial activities of tannins extracted from *Rhizophora apiculata* barks. Journal of Tropical Forest Science 18, 59–65.

Loo, A.Y., Jain, K., Darah, I., 2008. Antioxidant activity of compounds isolated from the pyroligneous acid, *Rhizophora apiculata*. Food Chemistry 107, 1151–1160.

Prabhu, V., Guruvayoorappan, C., 2014. Protective effect of marine mangrove *Rhizophora apiculata* on acetic acid induced experimental colitis by regulating anti-oxidant enzymes, inflammatory mediators and nuclear factor-kappa B subunits. International Immunopharmacology 18, 124—134.

Premanathan, M., Arakaki, R., Izumi, H., Kathiresan, K., Nakano, M., Yamamoto, N., et al., 1999. Antiviral properties of a mangrove plant, *Rhizophora apiculata* Blume, against human immunodeficiency virus. Antiviral Research 44, 113—122.

Premanathan, M., Nakashima, H., Kathiresan, K., Rajendran, N., Yamamoto, N., 1996. In vitro anti human immunodeficiency virus activity of mangrove plants. Indian Journal of Medical Research 103, 278—281.

Rahim, A.A., Rocca, E., Steinmetz, J., Jain Kassim, M., Sani Ibrahim, M., Osman, H., 2008. Antioxidant activities of mangrove *Rhizophora apiculata* bark extracts. Food Chemistry 107, 200—207.

Ravindran, Venkatesan, K., Balakrishnan, V., Balasubramanian, K.P., 2005. Ethnomedicinal studies of Pichavaram mangroves of East coast, Tamil Nadu. Indian Journal of Traditional Knowledge 4, 409—411.

Revathi, P., Senthinath, T.J., Thirumalaikolundusubramanian, P., Prabhu, 2014. An overview of antidiabetic profile of mangrove plants. International Journal of Pharmacy and Pharmaceutical Sciences 6, 1—5.

Sulaiman, S., Ibrahim, D., Kassim, J., Lim, S.-H., 2011. Antimicrobial and antioxidant activities of condensed tannin from *Rhizophora apiculata* barks. Journal of Chemical and Pharmaceutical Research 3, 436—444.

Use, P., 2016. *Rhizophora apiculata* (prosea). <https://uses.plantnet-project.org/en/Rhizophora_apiculata_(PROSEA)> (accessed 24.02.21).

Varahalarao, V., Naidu, K.C., 2009. In vitro bioefficiency of marine mangrove plant activity of *Rhizophora conjugata*. International Journal of PharmTech Research 1, 1598—1600.

Rhizophora mucronata **Lam.** 24

24.1 General description

24.1.1 Botanical nomenclature

- *Rhizophora mucronata* Lam. (Fig. 24.1)

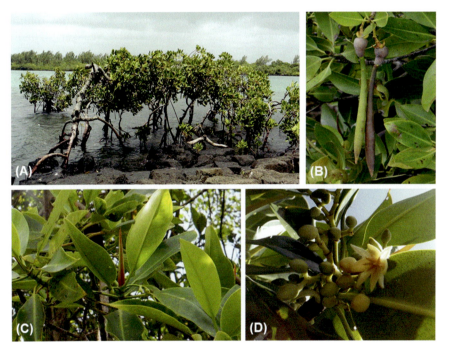

FIGURE 24.1

(A) Whole plant, (B) fruits, (C) leaves, and (D) flowers of *Rhizophora mucronata* (GBIF, 2021).

Mangroves with Therapeutic Potential for Human Health. DOI: https://doi.org/10.1016/B978-0-323-99332-6.00028-X

24.1.2 Botanical family

- Rhizophoraceae

24.1.3 Vernacular names

- Four-petaled mangrove, loop-root mangrove, long-fruited red mangrove, red mangrove, true mangrove (English)
- Mkaka, mkoko (East Africa)
- Beebasboom, rooiwortelboom; umNgombamkhonto, umHlume, umHluma (Zulu); umHluma (Xhosa)
- Hong qie dong (Chinese)
- Adavi ponna, adaviponna, bairada, bhara, bhora, coripunnai, jumuda, kaandla, kamdlam, kamdli, kamo, kandaale, kandal, kandale, kandia, kandla, kandlaa, kandle, kantal, kattuppunnai, manciponna, manjiponna, nija kaandla, olle kaandla, panachikandal, panaccikantal, paniccha kandal, panicchakandal, peecandel, peykkandal, peykkantal, pikandal, pikantal, ponna, pyu, rai, rohi, sorapinnai, upooponna, uppu ponna, uppuponna, venkandal, venkantal (Hindi)
- Funiki, oba-hirugi, pushiki, Yaeyama-hirugi (Japanese)
- Bakau belukap, bakau jangkar, bakau kurap, belukap, lenggayong (Malayam)

24.2 Geographical distribution

Rhizophora mucronata is widely distributed across the globe and is present in various countries, namely, North America, East Africa, Madagascar, Mauritius, India, Malaysia, Indonesia, Papua New Guinea, Solomons Island as illustrated in Fig. 24.2. It is a preserved specimen in Madagascar, Mauritius, India, Japan, Vietnam and is under

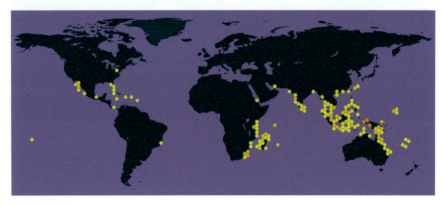

FIGURE 24.2

Distribution of *Rhizophora mucronata* across the globe (GBIF, 2021).

human observation in Indonesia, Kenya, India, Mozambique, Seychelles, Iran, Singapore, South Africa, Sri Lanka, Mayotte, Thailand, and Australia.

24.3 Morphological characteristics

Rhizophora mucronata is a 20−25 m tall mangrove tree and has stilt roots buttressing the trunk. It has dark green thick leaves with a distinct mucronate tip and covered with minute black spots on the inferior surface. The mangrove tree produces green fruits with a cigar shape. The flowers are creamy white in color (Fig. 24.1) (Sadeer et al., 2019).

24.4 Ethnobotanical uses

Folk medicinal practitioners in Tamil Nadu used the whole plant to prevent colitis and inflammatory bowel disease (Prabhu and Guruvayoorappan, 2014) and in Pichavaram region in India, the bark is used to treat amebiasis, diarrhea, nausea, and vomiting (Ravindran et al., 2005). In Mauritius, a decoction of the leaves or roots are used to manage diabetes, fever, hypertension, astringent and as an antidote against toxic fish stings (Sadeer et al., 2019). In Porong, Indonesia, the whole plant is used for elephantiasis, hematoma, hepatitis, ulcer, febrifuge (Nurdiani et al., 2012; Rollet, 1981). In Malaysia, the leaf and root are used for childbirth and hemorrhage (Suganthy and Devi, 2016). In Papua New Guinea, the stem is used to control constipation, cure fertility, and menstruation disorders (Liebezeit and Rau, 2006). In Thailand, the bark is used to treat diarrhea, dysentery, and leprosy (Miles et al., 1999).

24.5 Phytochemicals

The different plant parts contain a wide variety of phytochemicals, namely, condensed tannins, polyphenols, lipids, inositol, gibberellins, alkaloids, tannins, and proteins, among others. Table 24.1 summarizes the different compounds identified from *R. mucronata*.

Table 24.1 Phytochemicals of *Rhizophora mucronata*.

Plant part	Extract	Phytochemical class	Compounds	References
B, Fr, F, R	NI	Alkaloids, tannins, gibberellins, inositol saponins, lipids	NI	Revathi et al. (2014)

(Continued)

Table 24.1 Phytochemicals of *Rhizophora mucronata. Continued*

Plant part	Extract	Phytochemical class	Compounds	References
NI	NI	Proteins, minerals, carotenoids, hydrolysable tannins, lipids, polysaccharides, steroids, triterpenes, condensed tannins, procyanidins, anthocyanidins, alkaloids, carbohydrates, chlorophyll, gibberellins, flavonoids, inositols, polyphenols, saponins	NI	Balasubramanian et al. (2015)
L	C	Oleanenes	olean-18(19)-en-3β-yl-(3,6-dimethyl-3E,6Z-dienoate), (13α)-27-frido-olean-14(15)-en-(17α)-furanyl-3β-ol	Chakraborty and Raola (2017)
L, B, Fr, F	MeOH	Alkaloid, tannin, saponin, phenolic, flavonoid, terpenoid, steroid, glycosides	NI	Nurdiani et al. (2012)
R	MeOH	Alkaloid, tannin, saponin, steroids, Glycosides	NI	
R	EA	Diterpenoids	Rhizophorin A, rhizophorin B, rhizophorin C-E	Anjaneyulu and Lakshmana (2003)
B	NI	Lupeol, quercetin, caffeic acid	NI	Rohini and Das (2010)
L, F	H	Tannin, saponin, terpenoid, alkaloid, flavonoid	NI	Wahyuni et al. (2015)
AP	CE	Ethanone	1-(2-hydroxy-5-methylphenyl)	Manilal et al. (2015)
L, R, Tw, Fr	MeOH, EA, Aq	Phenolic acids, flavonols, flavones, anthocyanins, tyrosols, lignans, alkyl phenols, stilbenes	Pelargonidin 3,5-O-diglucoside, 8-prenylnaringenin, nepetin, nobiletin, (+)-catechin, trachelogenin, 4-vinylphenol	Sadeer et al. (2019)

AP, Aerial part; *B*, bark; *C*, chloroform; *CE*, crude extract; *EA*, ethyl acetate; *F*, flower; *Fr*, fruit; *H*, hexane; *L*, leaf; *NI*, not indicated; *MeOH*, methanol; *R*, root.

24.6 Pharmacological activities

Rhizophora mucronata possesses many pharmacological properties, namely, antioxidant, antiinflammatory, antibacterial, antimicrobial, antidiabetic, analgesic, anti-HIV, and anticholinesterase properties. Chakraborty and Raola (2017) conducted the antioxidant study on the crude chloroform leaf extract using DPPH assay and the resulting IC50 value was 1.38 ± 0.03 mg/mL, while Suganthy and Devi (2016) conducted the same assay to obtain an IC50 value of 47.39 ± 0.43 μg/mL. Interestingly, a study conducted by Hardoko et al. (2015) reported that the ripe flour of the fruit contained 7.50% soluble dietary fiber and 38.60% insoluble dietary flour. Additionally, the antidiabetic in vivo study conducted showed a decline in the blood glucose level, which, as a result, makes the ripe flour of *R. mucronata* a good functional food for diabetic patients. Pimpliskar et al. (2012) investigated the antimicrobial activity on the ethanolic stem extract. However, to the best of the knowledge of the authors, no other studies were conducted on ripe flour to support or confirm these results obtained by Hardoko et al. (2015). Alikunhi et al. (2012) added that the antidiabetic properties of *R. mucronata* were due to the presence of the insulin-like protein present in the leaves. Table 24.2 summarized other studies conducted on *R. mucronata*.

Table 24.2 Pharmacological activities of *Rhizophora mucronata*.

Plant part (s)	Extract	Study	Results	References
L, Sb, R	MeOH	Antioxidant-FRAP	AAE (mg/g) for the 3 methanolic extracts of each plant parts = 2.89 ± 0.23, 3.62 ± 0.16, and 1.40 ± 0.00, respectively	Banerjee et al. (2008)
		Antioxidant-DPPH	IC50 (mg/g) for the 3 methanolic extracts of each plant parts = 365.37 ± 23.95, 193.82 ± 11.14, and 1377.45 ± 50.62, respectively	
L	C	Antioxidant-DPPH	IC50 (mg/mL) = 1.38 ± 0.03	Chakraborty and Raola (2017)
		Antiinflammatory-COX-1 inhibition	IC50 (mg/mL) = 1.42 ± 0.01	
L	EA	Antibacterial-agar well diffusion	With 50 μL of extract, zone of inhibition(mm) against EC, SA, KP, PV, PA, PSF, ST, and BS = 15, 18, 9, 11, 13, 9, 13, and 6, respectively	Joel and Bhimba (2010)
R	H	Antimicrobial-disk diffusion	Zone of inhibition (mm) against BS, SA, PA, PV, CA, AFM, and AN = 20, 16, 19, 17, 16, 17, and 18, respectively	Kusuma et al. (2012)

(Continued)

Table 24.2 Pharmacological activities of *Rhizophora mucronata. Continued*

Plant part (s)	Extract	Study	Results	References
L	MeOH	Antidiabetic-STZ induced diabetic rats	Week 3: FBG (mg/100 mL blood) level at 50 and 100 mg/kg = 90.8 ± 6.03 and 99.3 ± 4.15, respectively Week 10: FBG (mg/100 mL blood) level at 50 and 100 mg/kg = 151 ± 3.26 and 136 ± 5.11, respectively	Sur et al. (2016)
		Antioxidant-DPPH	IC50 (μg/mg) = 5.25 ± 0.039	
L	MeOH	Antibacterial-disk diffusion	Zone of inhibition (mm) against BS, SA, STF, STP, EC, and PA = 9.97 ± 0.17, 19.56 ± 0.19, 15.74 ± 0.06, 11.31 ± 0.25, 5.63 ± 0.06, and 16.57 ± 0.22, respectively	Gurudeeban et al. (2015)
		Antioxidant-DPPH	%radical scavenging at 4, 8, 16, 32, and 64 μg/mL = 15.1 ± 0.2, 19.82 ± 0.61, 25.98 ± 0.46, 36.98 ± 0.04, and 42.98 ± 0.28, respectively	
L	C	Analgesic	Basal reaction time (s) after 15 min of administration = 7.40 ± 0.30, after 30 min = 11.34 ± 0.05, after 45 min = 13.13 ± 0.03, after 90 min = 9.01 ± 0.28	Ramanathan (2011)
B, F, Fr, L, R	MeOH	Antibacterial-disk diffusion	Zone of inhibition (mm) against SA for the respective plant parts extracts = 8.8, 7.5, 7.1, 6.1, and 7.6	Nurdiani et al. (2012)
L	NI	Anti-HIV-MTT assay	CC50 (μg/mL) = 798.39 ± 72.02, EC50 (μg/mL) = 492.29 ± 48.99, SI = 1.62	Premanathan et al. (1996)
L	MeOH	Antioxidant-DPPH, NO, SO	IC50 (μg/mg) = 5.25 ± 0.039, 3.44 ± 0.038, 6.04 ± 0.012, respectively	Sur et al. (2016)
St	E	Antimicrobial	MIC (mg/mL): EC = 17, SA = 16, ST = 19, CA = 15 at 10 mg/mL of extract	Jadhav and Jadhav (2012)
L	H, EA, MeOH	Anticholinesterase	IC50 (μg/mL): H = NR, EA = NR, Me = 222.48, Physostigmine (control) = 0.06	Wahyuni et al. (2015)

(Continued)

Table 24.2 Pharmacological activities of *Rhizophora mucronata. Continued*

Plant part (s)	Extract	Study	Results	References
AP	EA	Antimicrobial-agar disk diffusion	Overall activity (%) against SA, SM, KP, SF, ML, VM = 66.6	Manilal et al. (2015)
L	E	Hypoglycemic effect-Streptozotocin-induced diabetic rats	Dosage 100 and 200 mg/kg were administered for 6 h. Positive control (glibenclamide) = 0.5 mg/kg. Higher percentage decrease observed with control (27.2%) compared to 100 mg/kg extract (19.7%), 200 mg/kg extract (21.0%)	Pandey et al. (2014)
Tw	MeOH	Antioxidant-CUPRAC, FRAP	1336.88 ± 15.70 and 710.18 ± 21.04 mg TE/g, respectively	Sadeer et al. (2019)
L	MeOH	Antimicrobial	MIC (mg/mL) against MRSA = 0.19	

AAE, Ascorbic acid equivalent; *AFM, Aspergillus fumigatus*; *AN, Aspergillus niger*; *AP*, aerial part; *BS, Bacillus subtilis*; *C*, chloroform; *CA, Candida albicans*; *E*, ethanol; *EA*, ethyl acetate; *EC, Escherichia coli*; *H*, hexane; *KP, Klebsiella pneumonia*; *L*, leaf; *ML, Micrococcus luteus*; *MeOH*, methanol; *PA, Pseudomonas aeruginosa*; *PV, Proteus vulgaris*; *R*, root; *SA, Staphylococcus aureus*; *Sb*, stem bark; *SM, Serratia marcescens*; *ST, Salmonella typhi*; *St*, stem; *Tw*, twig.

24.7 Associated fungal endophytes

Compounds pestalotiopyrones A-H, pestalotiopisorin A, pestalotiollides A-B, pestalo-tiopin A, pestalotiopamides A-D, nigrosporapyrone D, p-hydroxy benzaldehyde, cytosporones J-L, tetradecanoic acid, nonanoic acid, pentadecanoic acid, suberic acid monomethyl ester, and tetrahydroedulan were produced by the fungus *Pestalotiopsis* sp. JCM2A4 (Li et al., 2013; Xu et al., 2011; Xu et al., 2009). Phomoxanthone A, 12-O-deacetyl-phomoxanthone A were identified in *Phomopsis* sp. IM 41−1 (Shiono et al., 2013). Seventeen genera belonging to 8 taxonomic orders of Ascomycota were discovered, specifically, *Botryosphaeriales, Capnodiales, Diaporthales, Eurotiales, Glomerellales, Hypocreales, Pleosporales*, and *Xylariales* (Zhou et al., 2018).

References

Alikunhi, N.M., Kandasamy, K., Manoharan, C., Subramanian, M., 2012. Insulin-like anti-gen of mangrove leaves and its anti-diabetic activity in alloxan-induced diabetic rats. Natural Product Research 26, 1161−1166.

Anjaneyulu, A.S.R., Lakshmana, R.V., 2003. Ceriopsins F and G, diterpenoids from *Ceriops decandra*. Phytochemistry 62, 1207−1211.

Balasubramanian, V., Rajesh, P., Rajaram, R., Kannan, V.R., 2015. A review on rhizophora genus: therapeutically important perspective phytochemical constituents. In: Gupta, V. K. (Ed.), Bioactive Phytochemicals: Perspectives for Modern Medicine. Daya Publishing House, New Delhi, India.

Banerjee, D., Chakrabarti, S., Hazra, A.K., Banerjee, S., Ray, J., Mukherjee, B., 2008. Antioxidant activity and total phenolics of some mangroves in Sundarbans. African Journal of Biotechnology 7.

Chakraborty, K., Raola, V.K., 2017. Two rare antioxidant and anti-inflammatory oleanenes from loop root Asiatic mangrove *Rhizophora mucronata*. Phytochemistry 135, 160−168.

GBIF, 2021. GBIF secretariat: GBIF backbone taxonomy. <https://www.gbif.org/> (accessed 27.02.21).

Gurudeeban, S., Ramanathan, T., Satyavani, K., 2015. Antimicrobial and radical scavenging effects of alkaloid extracts from *Rhizophora mucronata*. Pharmaceutical Chemistry Journal 49, 34−37.

Hardoko, H., Suprayitno, E., Puspitasari, Y., 2015. Study of ripe *Rhizophora mucronata* fruit flour as functional food for antidiabetic. International Food Research Journal 22, 953−959.

Jadhav, R., Jadhav, B., 2012. Evaluation of antimicrobial principles of *Rhizophora* species along Mumbai Coast. Journal of Advanced Scientific Research 3.

Joel, E.L., Bhimba, V., 2010. Isolation and characterization of secondary metabolites from the mangrove plant *Rhizophora mucronata*. Asian pacific journal of tropical Medicine 3, 602−604.

Kusuma, S., Kumar, P.A., Boopalan, K., 2012. Potent antimicrobial activity of *Rhizophora mucronata*. Journal of Ecobiotechnology 3 (11), 40−41.

Li, D., Yan, S., Proksch, P., Liang, Z., Li, Q., Xu, J., 2013. Volatile metabolites profiling of a Chinese mangrove endophytic *Pestalotiopsis* sp. strain. African Journal of Biotechnology 12.

Liebezeit, G., Rau, M.T., 2006. New Guinean mangroves—traditional usage and chemistry of natural products. Senckenbergiana maritima 36, 1−10.

Manilal, A., Merdekios, B., Idhayadhulla, A., Muthukumar, C., Melkie, M., 2015. An in vitro antagonistic efficacy validation of *Rhizophora mucronata*. Asian Pacific Journal of Tropical Disease 5, 28−32.

Miles, D., Kokpol, U., Chittawong, V., Tip-Pyang, S., Kwanjai, Nguyen, C., et al., 1999. Mangrove forests the importance of conservation as a bioresource for ecosystem diversity and utilization as a source of chemical constituents with potential medicinal and agricultural value. IUPAC, North Carolina, United States 1−9.

Nurdiani, R., Firdaus, M., Prihanto, A., 2012. Phytochemical screening and antibacterial activity of methanol extract of mangrove plant (*Rhyzophora mucronata*) from Porong River Estuary. Journal of Basic Science and Technology 1, 27−29.

Pandey, A.K., Gupta, P.P., Lal, V.K., 2014. Hypoglycemic effect of *Rhizophora mucronata* in streptozotocin induced diabetic rats. Journal of Complementary and Integrative Medicine 11, 179−183.

Pimpliskar, M.R., Jadhav, R.N., Jadhav, B.L., 2012. Evaluation of antimicrobial principles of Rhizophora species along Mumbai Coast. Journal of Advanced Scientific Research 3, 30−33.

Prabhu, V., Guruvayoorappan, C., 2014. Protective effect of marine mangrove *Rhizophora apiculata* on acetic acid induced experimental colitis by regulating anti-oxidant enzymes, inflammatory mediators and nuclear factor-kappa B subunits. International Immunopharmacology 18, 124−134.

Premanathan, M., Nokashima, H., Kathiresan, K., Rajendran, N., Yamamoto, N., 1996. In vitro anti human immunodeficiency virus activity of mangrove plants. Indian Journal of Medical Research 103, 278−281.

Ramanathan, T.A.H., 2011. Studies on analgesic activity of a mangrove species— *Rhizophora mucronata* Poir. In: Proc. of the Annual International Conference on Advances in Biotechnology, Bozen, Italy.

Ravindran, K., Venkatesan, K., Balakrishnan, V., Balasubramanian, K.P., 2005. Ethnomedicinal studies of Pichavaram mangroves of East coast, Tamil Nadu. Indian Journal of Traditional Knowledge 4, 409−411.

Revathi, P., Senthinath, T., Thirumalaikolundusubramanian, P., Nagarajan, P., 2014. An overview of antidiabetic profile of mangrove plants. International Journal of Pharmacy and Pharmaceutical Sciences 6, 1−5.

Rohini, R., Das, A., 2010. Antidiarrheal and anti inflammatory activities of lupeol, quercetin, β-sitosterol, adene-5-en-3-ol and caffeic acid isolated from *Rhizophora mucronata* bark. Der Pharmacia Lettre 2, 95−101.

Rollet, B., 1981. Bibliography on Mangrove Research 1600−1975. UNESCO, Paris, France.

Sadeer, N.B., Fawzi, M.M., Gokhan, Z., Rajesh, J., Nadeem, N., Kannan, R.R.R., et al., 2019. Ethnopharmacology, phytochemistry, and global distribution of mangroves-a comprehensive review. Marine Drugs 17.

Shiono, Y., Sasaki, T., Shibuya, F., Yasuda, Y., Koseki, T., Supratman, U., 2013. Isolation of a phomoxanthone A derivative, a new metabolite of tetrahydroxanthone, from a *Phomopsis* sp. isolated from the mangrove, *Rhizhopora mucronata*. Natural Product Communications 8, 1934578X1300801220.

Suganthy, N., Devi, K.P., 2016. In vitro antioxidant and anti-cholinesterase activities of *Rhizophora mucronata*. Pharmaceutical Biology 54, 118−129.

Sur, T.K., Hazra, A., Hazra, A.K., Bhattacharyya, D., 2016. Antioxidant and hepatoprotective properties of Indian Sunderban mangrove *Bruguiera gymnorrhiza* L. leave. Journal of Basic and Clinical Pharmacy 7, 75.

Wahyuni, W.T., Darusman, L.K., Surya, N.K., 2015. Potency of *Rhizopora* Spp. extracts as antioxidant and inhibitor of acetylcholinesterase. Procedia Chemistry 16, 681−686.

Xu, J., Aly, A.H., Wray, V., Proksch, P., 2011. Polyketide derivatives of endophytic fungus *Pestalotiopsis* sp. isolated from the Chinese mangrove plant *Rhizophora mucronata*. Tetrahedron Letters 52, 21−25.

Xu, J., Kjer, J., Sendker, J., Wray, V., Guan, H., Edrada, R., et al., 2009. Cytosporones, coumarins, and an alkaloid from the endophytic fungus *Pestalotiopsis* sp. isolated from the Chinese mangrove plant *Rhizophora mucronata*. Bioorganic and Medicinal Chemistry 17, 7362−7367.

Zhou, J., Diao, X., Wang, T., Chen, G., Lin, Q., Yang, X., et al., 2018. Phylogenetic diversity and antioxidant activities of culturable fungal endophytes associated with the mangrove species *Rhizophora stylosa* and *R. mucronata* in the South China Sea. PLoS One 13, e0197359.

Rhizophora mangle L.

25.1 General description

25.1.1 Botanical nomenclature

- *Rhizophora mangle* L. (Fig. 25.1)

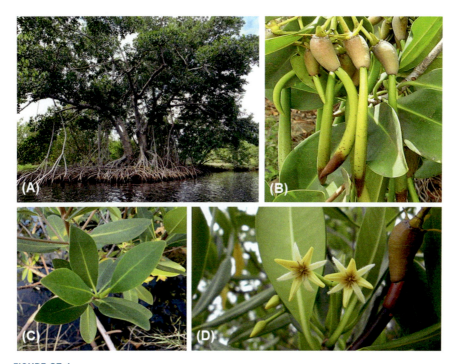

FIGURE 25.1

(A) Whole plant, (B) fruits, (C) leaves, and (D) flowers of *Rhizophora mangle* (GBIF, 2021).

25.1.2 Botanical family

- Rhizophoraceae

Mangroves with Therapeutic Potential for Human Health. DOI: https://doi.org/10.1016/B978-0-323-99332-6.00002-3

25.1.3 Vernacular names

- American mangrove, mangle, mangle colorado, mangrove, red mangrove (English)
- Aili kinnut (Panama language)

25.2 Geographical distribution

Rhizophora mangle is mostly distributed in Brazil, Colombia, Mexico, Central America, United States, West Africa as illustrated in Fig. 25.2. It is under human observation in the United States, Brazil, Martinique, Nicaragua, Dominican Republic, Mexico, Ecuador, Costa Rica.

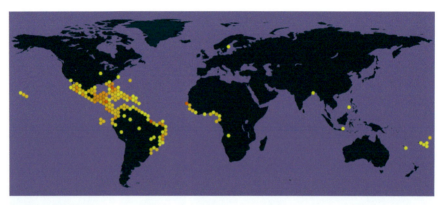

FIGURE 25.2

Distribution of *Rhizophora mangle* across the globe (GBIF, 2021).

25.3 Morphological characteristics

Rhizophora mangle attains a height of 24 m, has stilt roots, gray or gray-brown, smooth, thin bark, opposite, elliptical, acute apex, thick, shiny green on upper surface, yellow-green, black dots on bottom surface, 6−12 cm long, 2.5−6 cm wide leaves, yellowish-white petals, flowers usually in group of 3, individual flowers finally pendulous, seedling is the unit of dispersal (quatrocchi, sadeer).

25.4 Ethnobotanical uses

In India, the barks and leaves are used to treat diabetes (Revathi et al., 2014, Arora et al., 2014). The bark is used for sores and swellings. Dry fruit made into tea is taken on the onset of dysentery. Seeds infusion is used for bedwetting children (Quattrochi, 2012).

25.5 Phytochemicals

Revathi et al., (2014) and Kandil et al., (2004) reported the presence of tannins, triterpenes, flavonoids, glycosides, quercetin, myricetin, and kaempferol diglycosides in the bark and leaf extract. Cinchonain Ia, Ib, catechin-3-O-rhamnopyranoside, iyoniside, nudiposide, manool, jhanol, steviol and p-oxy-2-ethylhexyl benzaldehyde were identified (Andrade-Cetto et al., 2017, Martins et al., 2017)

25.6 Pharmacological activities

Rhizophora mangle possessed antioxidant and antiulcer activities. At dosage 50, 125, 250, 500, and 750 mg/kg of the aqueous bark extract, the lesion indices were 5.2 ± 0.84, 4.5 ± 0.58, 3.25 ± 1.71, 1.6 ± 1.95, and 4.6 ± 0.55, respectively. Lesion index (control-distilled water) $= 4.8 \pm 0.45$ (SÁnchez Perera et al., 2004). From antioxidant assay (SO), the IC50 values of leaf extract and polyphenolic fraction were 6.7 and 7.6 μg/mL, respectively (Sánchez et al., 2010) while from DPPH assay, the IC50 value of leaf extract was 89.83 μg/mL (Zhang et al., 2010).

25.7 Associated fungal endophytes

Not available

References

Andrade-Cetto, A., Escandón-Rivera, S.M., Torres-Valle, G.M., Quijano, L., 2017. Phytochemical composition and chronic hypoglycemic effect of *Rhizophora mangle* cortex on STZ-NA-induced diabetic rats. Revista Brasileira de Farmacognosia. 27, 744−750.

Arora, K., Nagpal, M., Jain, U., Jat, R., Jain, S., 2014. Mangroves: a novel gregarious phyto medicine for diabetes. International Journal of Research and Development in Pharmacy & Life Sciences 3, 1244−1257.

GBIF, 2021. GBIF Secretariat: GBIF Backbone Taxonomy. Available on: https://www.gbif.org/ (Accessed on: 24 February 2021).

Kandil, F.E., Grace, M.H., Seigler, D.S., Cheeseman, J.M., 2004. Polyphenolics in *Rhizophora mangle* L. leaves and their changes during leaf development and senescence. Trees 18, 518−528.

Martins, J.N., Figueiredo, F.S., Martins, G.R., Leitão, G.G., Costa, F.N., 2017. Diterpenes and a new benzaldehyde from the mangrove plant *Rhizophora mangle*. Revista Brasileira de Farmacognosia. 27, 175−178.

Quattrochi, U., 2012. CRC world of dictionary of medicinal and poisonous plants. CRC Press, Boca Raton, Florida.

Revathi, P., Senthinath, T.J., Thirumalaikolundusubramanian, P., Prabhu, N., 2014. An overview of antidiabetic profile of mangrove plants. International Journal of Pharmacy and Pharmaceutical Sciences 6, 1−5.

SÁnchez Perera, L.M., Batista, N.Y., Rodríguez, A., Farrada, F., Bulnes, C., 2004. Gastric and duodenal antiulcer effects of *Rhizophora mangle*. Le Pharmacien Biologiste 42, 225−229.

Sánchez, J.C., García, R.F., Cors, M.T.M., 2010. 1, 1-diphenyl-2-picrylhydrazyl radical and superoxide anion scavenging activity of *Rhizophora mangle* (L.) bark. Pharmacognosy Research 2, 279.

Zhang, L.-L., Lin, Y.-M., Zhou, H.-C., Wei, S.-D., Chen, J.-H., 2010. Condensed tannins from mangrove species Kandelia candel and *Rhizophora mangle* and their antioxidant activity. Molecules (Basel, Switzerland) 15, 420−431.

Rhizophora racemosa G. Mey.

26

26.1 General description

26.1.1 Botanical nomenclature

- *Rhizophora racemosa* G. Mey. (Fig. 26.1)

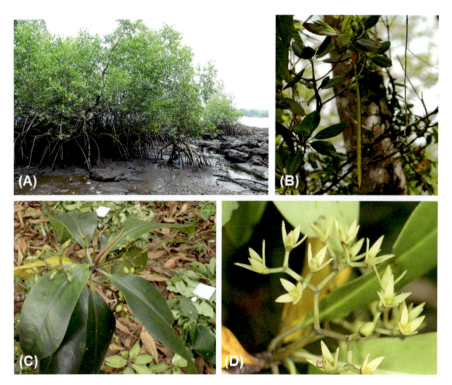

FIGURE 26.1

(A) Whole plant, (B) fruits, (C) leaves, and (D) flowers of *Rhizophora racemosa* (GBIF, 2021).

Mangroves with Therapeutic Potential for Human Health. DOI: https://doi.org/10.1016/B978-0-323-99332-6.00024-2

26.1.2 Botanical family

- Rhizophoraceae

26.1.3 Vernacular names

- Paletuvier (French)
- Ntan, ntana, tanda (Central African language)
- Tanda (Cameroon language)
- Ntan (Gabon language)
- Agala, egba, igba-dudu, litanda, ngala, odo nowe, odonowe, tanda, urher-nwere; egba (Yoruba); odo nowe (Edo); odo (Itsekiri); urheruwerim (Urhobo); agala (Ijaw); ngala (Igbo); nunung (Efik); nunung (Ibibio) (Nigerian language)
- Egba, igba dudu (Yoruba)

26.2 Geographical distribution

Rhizophora racemosa is distributed along the West coast of Africa, Brazil, and Central America (Fig. 26.2). It is under human observation in Panama and Benin.

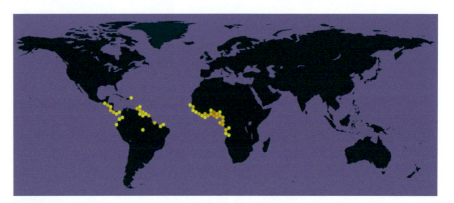

FIGURE 26.2

Distribution of *Rhizophora racemosa* across the globe (GBIF, 2021).

26.3 Morphological characteristics

Rhizophora racemosa is a tree reaching a height of up to 30 m developing stilt roots and elliptical leaves. This species has the potential to bloom 128 flowers on one axillary branch. Sepals of flowers are 8−10 mm long (Tomlinson, 2016).

26.4 Ethnobotanical uses

In Nigeria, the leaves are used to alleviate toothache and dysmenorrhea (Angalabiri-Owei and Isirima, 2014).

26.5 Phytochemicals

Revathi et al. (2014) reported the presence of inositols and steroids in the leaves, roots, and seeds extract. The methanolic leave and bark extracts were abounded with phenolics, flavonoids, phenolic acids and flavonols (Chiavaroli et al., 2020).

26.6 Pharmacological activities

Methanolic leaf and bark extracts (prepared by homogenizer-assisted extraction) exhibited the highest radical scavenging, reducing potential and total antioxidant capacity. Furthermore, findings showed that the highest enzymatic inhibitory activity recorded was with the tyrosinase enzyme (Chiavaroli et al., 2020).

26.7 Associated fungal endophytes

Hypoxylide was identified from the fungus *Annulohypoxylon* (Liu et al., 2018).

References

Angalabiri-Owei, B., Isirima, J., 2014. Evaluation of the lethal dose of the methanol extract of Rhizophora racemosa leaf using karbers method. African Journal of Cellular Pathology 2, 65−68.

Chiavaroli, A., Sinan, K.I., Zengin, G., Mahomoodally, M.F., Sadeer, N.B., Etienne, O.K., et al., 2020. Identification of chemical profiles and biological properties of *Rhizophora racemosa* G. Mey. extracts obtained by different methods and solvents. Antioxidants 9, 533.

GBIF, 2021. GBIF secretariat: GBIF backbone taxonomy. <https://www.gbif.org/> (accessed 03.03.21).

Liu, Z., Qiu, P., Li, J., Chen, G., Chen, Y., Liu, H., et al., 2018. Anti-inflammatory polyketides from the mangrove-derived fungus *Ascomycota* sp. SK2YWS-L. Tetrahedron 74, 746−751.

Revathi, P., Senthinath, T.J., Thirumalaikolundusubramanian, P., Prabhu, N., 2014. An overview of antidiabetic profile of mangrove plants. International Journal of Pharmacy and Pharmaceutical Sciences 6, 1−5.

Tomlinson, P.B., 2016. The Botany of Mangroves. Cambridge University Press, Cambridge.

Sonneratia apetala Buch.-Ham.

27

27.1 General description

27.1.1 Botanical nomenclature

- *Sonneratia apetala* Buch.-Ham. (Fig. 27.1)

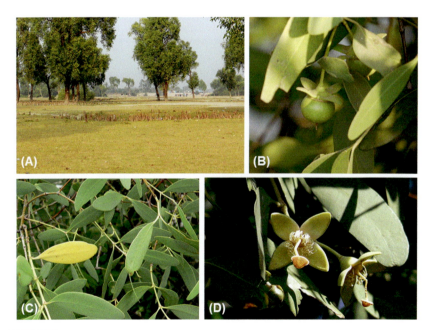

FIGURE 27.1

(A) Whole plant, (B) fruits, (C) leaves, and (D) flowers of *Sonneratia apetala* (GBIF, 2021).

Mangroves with Therapeutic Potential for Human Health. DOI: https://doi.org/10.1016/B978-0-323-99332-6.00015-1

27.1.2 Botanical family

- Lythraceae

27.1.3 Vernacular names

- Mangrove apple (English)
- Keora (Bengali)
- Wu ban hai sang (Chinese)
- Kerua, keruan (Hindi)

27.2 Geographical distribution

Sonneratia apetala is scarcely distributed across the globe as illustrated in Fig. 27.2. It is a preserved specimen in India, Hong Kong, China, Myanmar, Bangladesh, and Thailand and is under human observation in India and China.

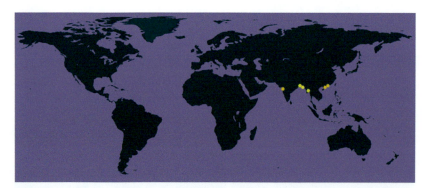

FIGURE 27.2

Distribution of *Sonneratia apetala* across the globe (GBIF, 2021).

27.3 Morphological characteristics

Sonneratia apetala is a fast-growing evergreen tree with a columnar crown (up to 15 to 20 m tall). The tree produces pneumatophores (vertical roots arising above the ground from shallow, horizontal roots) up to 1.5 m tall (Zhou et al., 2015).

27.4 Ethnobotanical uses

People in coastal Bangladesh, India, and Myanmar extensively consume the fruit by cooking and through other preparations. The ripe fruits are consumed by people from Africa to the Malayas and Javanese, and are said to taste like cheese. In many regions, the fruits are also processed to produce sour sauce which is marketed. Fermented juice of this fruit is useful in arresting hemorrhage. Fruits and barks of the plants belonging to genus *Sonneratia* have remedial activities against asthma, febrifuge, ulcers, swellings, sprains, bleeding, hemorrhages, and piles. The fruit can also be used in the treatment of gastrointestinal disorders, intestinal parasites, cough, dysentery, sprain, bruises, cataract, and sores in the ear. Different parts of the plant are also used in the treatment of hepatitis and cardiac diseases (Bandaranayake, 1998).

27.5 Phytochemicals

The fruit contains polyphenols, flavonoids, anthocyanins, ascorbic acid (vitamin C) (Hossain et al., 2013), alkaloids, reducing sugar, tannins, steroids, glycosides, and acidic compounds (Shefa et al., 2014). Ganguly et al. (1970) isolated a gibberellin from the leaves of the plant. The plant contains symgaresinol, betulinic acid, lupeol, lupeone, stigmast-5-ene3beta, 5β-cholestane-3α,7α-diol, β-amyrin hexadecaneate, and physcoion (Ji et al., 2005). Aerial parts of the plant contain terpenoid, steroid, alkaloid, flavonoid, tannins, saponins and polysaccharide (Panda et al., 2015). Leaf and bark contain alkaloids, glycosides (e.g., cardiac and anthraquinone), tannins, steroids, saponins, flavonoids, gums and steroids, carbohydrates, proteins and amino acids, terpenoids, vitamins (e.g., thiamin, riboflavin) and some minerals (Panda et al., 2015). The seeds also possess ethyl propanoate, n-propyl acetate, n-hexanal, 2,4-decadienal, oleic acid, 2-methyldecahydronaphthalene, methyl palmitate, β-sitosterol acetate (ascorbylpalmitate, palmitic acid, cyclodeca-cyclotetradecene, 14,15-didehydro-1,4,5,8,9,10,11,12,13,16,17,18,19,20-tetradecahydro-, margaric acid, 8,11-octadecadienoic acid methyl ester, oleic acid methyl ester, stearic acid and its methyl ester, linoleic acid, linoleic acid methyl ester, arachidic acid, tetracosanoic acid, cholesteryl bromide, stigmasta-5,22-dien-3-ol acetate, stigmast-5-en-3-ol, and oleate (Hossain et al., 2017).

27.6 Pharmacological activities

Methanol fraction of seeds strongly inhibited *Escherichia coli*, *Salmonella paratyphi* A, *Salmonella typhi*, *Shigella dysenteriae*, and *Staphylococcus aureus* except *Vibrio cholerae* at 500 μg/disk. The n-hexane, diethyl ether, chloroform, ethyl acetate, and methanol fractions strongly inhibited castor oil induced diarrheal episodes and onset time in mice at 500 mg extract/kg body weight (Hossain et al., 2017). *S. apetala* has diverse biological effects, including antioxidant, antiinflammatory, antimicrobial, anthelmintic, anticancer/cytotoxic, antidiarrheal, antidiabetic, analgesic, and antihyperlipidemic activities (Islam, 2020).

27.7 Associated fungal endophytes

Talaperoxides A–D, as well as one known analog, steperoxide B (5, or merulin A), have been isolated from the fungus, *Talaromyces flavus*. Talaperoxide B and D showed cytotoxicity against the five human cancer cell lines with IC50 values between 0.70 and 2.78 µg/mL (Li et al., 2011). Nine polyketides, including two new benzophenone derivatives, peniphenone and methyl peniphenone, along with seven known xanthones identified as conioxanthone A, methyl 8-hydroxy-6-methyl-9-oxo-9H-xanthene-1-carboxylate, pinselin, sydowinin B, sydowinin A, remisporine B, and epiremisporine B, were obtained from mangrove endophytic fungus *Penicillium* sp. ZJ-SY$_2$ isolated from the leaves. Peniphenone, conioxanthone A, pinselin and sydowinin A showed potent immunosuppressive activity with IC50 values ranging from 5.9 to 9.3 µg/mL (Liu et al., 2016).

References

Bandaranayake, W., 1998. Traditional and medicinal uses of mangroves. Mangroves and Salt Marshes 2, 133–148.

Ganguly, S., Sanyal, T., Sircar, P., Sircar, S., 1970. A new gibberellin (A25) in the leaves of *Sonneratia apetala* ham. Chemistry and Industry 25, 832–833.

GBIF, 2021. GBIF secretariat: GBIF backbone taxonomy. <https://www.gbif.org/> (accessed 7.03.21).

Hossain, S., Basar, M., Rokeya, B., Arif, K., Sultana, M., Rahman, M., 2013. Evaluation of antioxidant, antidiabetic and antibacterial activities of the fruit of *Sonneratia apetala* (Buch.-Ham.). Oriental Pharmacy and Experimental Medicine 13, 95–102.

Hossain, S.J., Islam, M.R., Pervin, T., Iftekharuzzaman, M., Hamdi, O.A., Mubassara, S., et al., 2017. Antibacterial, anti-diarrhoeal, analgesic, cytotoxic activities, and GC-MS profiling of *Sonneratia apetala* (Buch.-Ham.) seed. Preventive Nutrition and Food Science 22, 157.

Islam, M.T., 2020. Chemical profile and biological activities of *Sonneratia apetala* (Buch.-Ham.). Advances in Traditional Medicine 20, 123–132.

Ji, Q., Lin, W., Li, J., Li, W., Kazuo, K., Tamotsu, N., et al., 2005. Chemical investingation of Chinese mangrove *Sonneratia apetala* II. Zhongguo Zhong yao za zhi = Zhongguo zhongyao zazhi = China Journal of Chinese Materia Medica 30, 1258–1260.

Li, H., Huang, H., Shao, C., Huang, H., Jiang, J., Zhu, X., et al., 2011. Cytotoxic norsesquiterpene peroxides from the endophytic fungus Talaromyces flavus isolated from the mangrove plant *Sonneratia apetala*. Journal of Natural Products 74, 1230–1235.

Liu, H., Chen, S., Liu, W., Liu, Y., Huang, X., She, Z., 2016. Polyketides with immunosuppressive activities from mangrove endophytic fungus Penicillium sp. ZJ-SY$_2$. Marine Drugs 14.

Panda, S.K., Pati, D., Mishra, S.K., Sahu, S., Tripathy, B., Nayak, L., 2015. Phytochemical investigation and antimicrobial activity of methanolic extract of *Sonneratia apetala* Buch-Ham. International Journal of Pharmaceutical and Biological Archive 21, 274—285.

Shefa, A.A., Baishakhi, F.S., Islam, S., Sadhu, S.K., 2014. Phytochemical and pharmacological evaluation of fruits of *Sonneratia apetala*. Global Journal of Medical Research: B 14, 1—6.

Zhou, T., Liu, S., Feng, Z., Liu, G., Gan, Q., Peng, S., 2015. Use of exotic plants to control Spartina alterniflora invasion and promote mangrove restoration. Scientific Reports 5, 1—13.

Xylocarpus granatum J. Koenig

28

28.1 General description

28.1.1 Botanical nomenclature

- *Xylocarpus granatum* J. Koenig (Fig. 28.1)

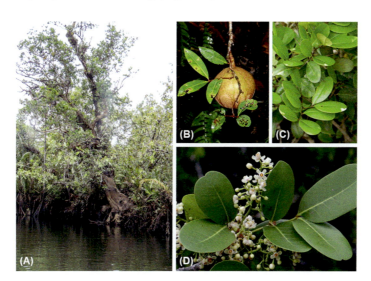

FIGURE 28.1

(A) Whole plant, (B) fruits, (C) leaves, and (D) flowers of *Xylocarpus granatum* (GBIF, 2021).

28.1.2 Botanical family

- Meliaceae

28.1.3 Vernacular names

- Cannonball mangrove, apple mangrove (English)
- Pinle on (Burma)
- Mu guo lian (Chinese)

Mangroves with Therapeutic Potential for Human Health. DOI: https://doi.org/10.1016/B978-0-323-99332-6.00026-6

- Adauipucha, adivipucca, comuntiri, conmuntiri, dhundol, dhundul, eel, kalikantai, kandalangay, karambola, parusha, pussur, shisumara, sisumbar (Hindi)
- Nireh, niri, nyireh, nyireh bunga, nyireh hudang, nyireh udang (Malayan)
- Nigi, nigue, tabigi (Philippines language)
- Dang dinh (Vietnamese)
- Fobo, foby, mkomafi, mtifi, mtonga, tavelo (East Africa language)
- Mkomabi (Tanzania language)
- Lekileki (Tonga language)

28.2 Geographical distribution

Xylocarpus granatum is distributed in Papua New Guinea, Indonesia, Malaysia, Vietnam, Thailand, Madagascar, and East Africa as illustrated in Fig. 28.2. It is a preserved specimen in Vanuatu, Madagascar, Solomon Islands, Cambodia, Micronesia, Malaysia, Tanzania, Indonesia, Papua New Guinea, Tonga, Fiji, Philippines, Palau, Brunei Darussalam, Mozambique, Singapore, New Caledonia, Kenya, Australia, and Seychelles.

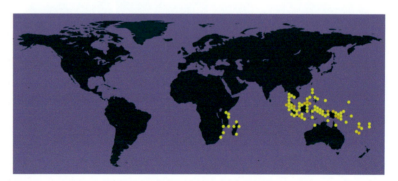

FIGURE 28.2

Distribution of *Xylocarpus granatum* across the globe (GBIF, 2021).

28.3 Morphological characteristics

This species is a small mangrove plant of height 3−8 m with a buttress root system. It has a light brown, yellowish, or greenish bark, and is smooth and flaky. The leaves are bright light green to dark green with a round apex (Peter and Sivasothi, 2001).

28.4 Ethnobotanical uses

In East Africa and South Asia, the local people use the bark and leaf as a natural remedy for cholera, diarrhea, fever, and malaria. The bark is used as an astringent and febrifuge; also, for diarrhea, dysentery, and abdominal problems. The fruit is used to treat elephantiasis and breast swelling; the seed kernel for a bitter tonic, and the seed (mixed with sulfur and coconut oil) in an ointment for itch. In Sidha, seeds are used for stomach ache and malaria; burned seeds against itch and rash; seed oil applied to cure breast tumor, also as mosquito repellent and to treat insect bites. Bark astringent, febrifuge, crushed and boiled in water, to treat diarrhea, dysentery. Fruit pulp applied to skin rashes; a decoction of the fruit and seeds used against diarrhea; crushed fruits decoction drunk as aphrodisiac; fruit to treat swellings of the breast (Das et al., 2014; Ravindran et al., 2005).

28.5 Phytochemicals

Wu et al. (2015) isolated three new limonoids, namely 2,3-dideacetylxyloccensin S, 30-deacetylxyloccensin W, and 7-hydroxy-21b-methoxy-3-oxo-24,25,26,27-tetranortirucalla-1,14-diene-23(21)-lactone from seeds. Xyloccensin O, xyloccensin P, gedunin, catechin, (-) epicatechin, procyanidin B1, procyanidin trimer, procyanidin pentamer were also identified from the plant (Simlai and Roy, 2013).

28.6 Pharmacological activities

Xylocarpus granatum has many pharmacological activities namely antioxidant, anticancer, antidiarrheal, and antimicrobial. Das et al. (2014) investigated the antimicrobial activity on the ethanolic stem extract against seven bacterial pathogens, namely *Escherichia coli, Enterobacter aerogenes, Pseudomonas aeruginosa, Salmonella typhi, Staphylococcus aureus, Klebsiella pneumoniae*, and *Vibrio cholerae*. The extract was active against all tested microorganisms. Methanolic bark extract at doses 250 and 500 mg/kg showed significant activity against castor oil and magnesium sulfate induced murine models (Simlai and Roy, 2013).

28.7 Associated fungal endophytes

Compounds namely (9R, 10R)-dihydro-harzianone and harzianelactone were identified in *Trichoderma* sp. Xy24 (Zhang et al., 2014; Zhang et al., 2016), merulinols A-G from endophytic fungus XG8D. Merulinol C and D selectively displayed cytotoxicity against KATO-3 cells with IC50 values of 35.0 and 25.3 μM, respectively (Choodej et al., 2016). Phomoxanthones F-K were identified from *Phomopsis* sp. xy21 (Hu et al., 2018). Merulin A displayed significant cytotoxicity against human breast (BT474) and colon (SW620) cancer cell lines (Chokpaiboon et al., 2010).

References

Chokpaiboon, S., Sommit, D., Teerawatananond, T., Muangsin, N., Bunyapaiboonsri, T., Pudhom, K., 2010. Cytotoxic nor-chamigrane and chamigrane endoperoxides from a basidiomycetous fungus. Journal of Natural Products 73, 1005−1007.

Choodej, S., Teerawatananond, T., Mitsunaga, T., Pudhom, K., 2016. Chamigrane sesquiterpenes from a basidiomycetous endophytic fungus XG8D associated with Thai mangrove *Xylocarpus granatum*. Marine Drugs 14, 132.

Das, S., Samantaray, D., Thatoi, H., 2014. Ethnomedicinal, antimicrobial and antidiarrhoeal studies on the mangrove plants of the genus Xylocarpus: a mini review. Journal of Bioanalysis and Biomedicine 12.

GBIF, 2021. GBIF secretariat: GBIF backbone taxonomy. <https://www.gbif.org/> (accessed 07.03.21.).

Hu, H.-B., Luo, Y.-F., Wang, P., Wang, W.-J., Wu, J., 2018. Xanthone-derived polyketides from the Thai mangrove endophytic fungus *Phomopsis* sp. xy21. Fitoterapia 131, 265−271.

Peter, K.L.N., Sivasothi, N., 2001. Guide to the mangroves of Singapore, Molluscs. Excerpt from A Guide to Mangroves of Singapore Volume 2: Animal Diversity., p.168.

Ravindran, K., Venkatesan, K., Balakrishnan, V., Chellappan, K., Balasubramanian, T., 2005. Ethnomedicinal studies of Pichavaram mangroves of East coast, Tamil Nadu. Indian Journal of Traditional Knowledge 4, 409−411.

Simlai, A., Roy, A., 2013. Biological activities and chemical constituents of some mangrove species from Sundarban estuary: an overview. Pharmacognosy Reviews 7, 170.

Wu, Y.B., Liu, D., Liu, P.Y., Yang, X.M., Liao, M., Lu, N.N., et al., 2015. New limonoids from the seeds of *Xylocarpus granatum*. Helvetica Chimica Acta 98, 691−698.

Zhang, M., Li, N., Chen, R., Zou, J., Wang, C., Dai, J., 2014. Two terpenoids and a polyketide from the endophytic fungus *Trichoderma* sp. Xy24 isolated from mangrove plant *Xylocarpus granatum*. Journal of Chinese Pharmaceutical Sciences 23, 421.

Zhang, M., Liu, J.-M., Zhao, J.-L., Li, N., Chen, R.-D., Xie, K.-B., et al., 2016. Two new diterpenoids from the endophytic fungus *Trichoderma* sp. Xy24 isolated from mangrove plant *Xylocarpus granatum*. Chinese Chemical Letters 27, 957−960.

Index

Printed in the United States
by Baker & Taylor Publisher Services